FASCIA

IN SPORT AND MOVEMENT

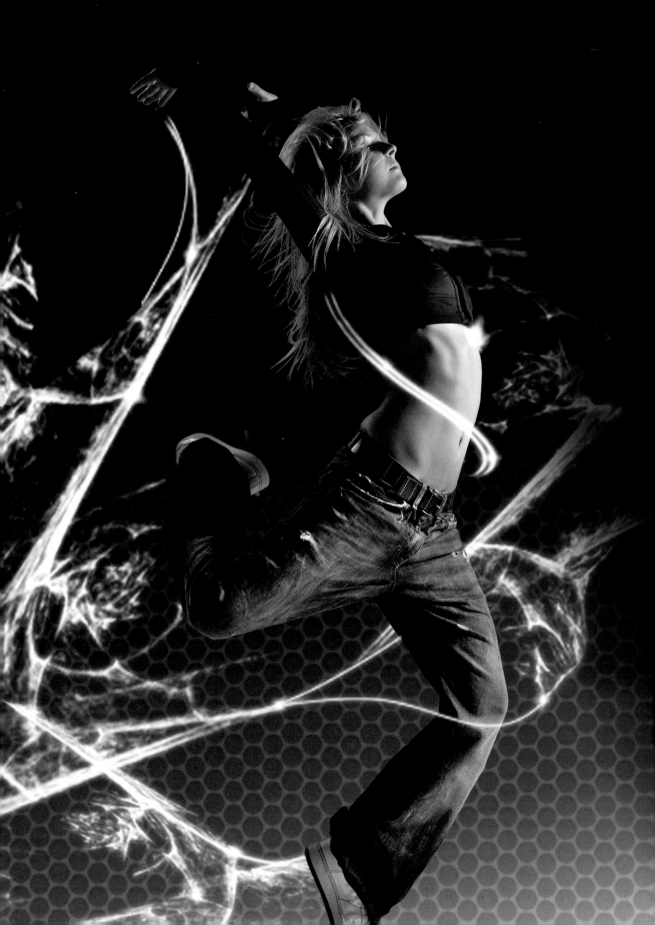

FASCIA
IN SPORT AND MOVEMENT

Editor
Robert Schleip PhD MA, Director Fascia Research Project, Division of Neurophysiology, Ulm University, Germany; Research Director European Rolfing Association; Vice President Ida P. Rolf Research Foundation; Certified Rolfing and Feldenkrais Teacher

Co-editor
Amanda Baker, MA, Experienced yoga teacher and Pilates instructor working in a clinical practice; Freelance journalist in the health and fitness industry; Qualified Fascial Fitness Trainer

With contributions by

Joanne Avison
Leon Chaitow
Stefan Dennenmoser
Donna Eddy
Klaus Eder
Raoul H.H. Engelbert
Piroska Frenzel
Fernando Galán del Río
Christopher Gordon
Robert Heiduk
Helmut Hoffmann
Birgit Juul-Kristensen
Wilbour E. Kelsick

Michael Kjaer
Werner Klingler
Elizabeth Jane Porter Larkam
Eyal Lederman
Divo Müller
Stephen Mutch
Thomas Myers
Sol Petersen
Lars Remvig
Philipp Richter
Raúl Martínez Rodríguez
Liane Simmel
Adjo Zorn

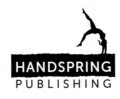

HANDSPRING
PUBLISHING

Edinburgh

HANDSPRING PUBLISHING LIMITED
The Old Manse, Fountainhall,
Pencaitland, East Lothian
EH34 5EY, Scotland
Tel: +44 1875 341 859
Website: www.handspringpublishing.com

First published 2015 in the United Kingdom by Handspring Publishing

Reprinted 2016, 2017

ISBN 978-1-909141-07-0

British Library Cataloguing in Publication Data
A catalogue record for this book is available from the British Library

Library of Congress Cataloguing in Publication Data
A catalog record for this book is available from the Library of Congress

Notice
Neither the Publisher nor the Author assumes any responsibility for any loss or injury and/or damage to persons or property arising out of or relating to any use of the material contained in this book. It is the responsibility of the treating practitioner, relying on independent expertise and knowledge of the patient, to determine the best treatment and method of application for the patient.

Commissioning Editor Sarena Wolfaard
Design direction Bruce Hogarth, kinesis-creative.com
Cover Design Gillian Richards
Index by Dr Laurence Errington
Typeset by DSM Soft
Printed in EU by Pulsio Print

The
Publisher's
policy is to use
paper manufactured
from sustainable forests

CONTENTS

FOREWORD

For many years both amateur and professional athletes have looked to exercise physiologists and trainers for ways to improve and maintain their performance, and avoid injury. Thirty years ago, there was research related to building muscle strength through concentric and eccentric exercise, with isometric, isokinetic and isotonic exercises as the building blocks, spaced over various repetitions and intervals. This was followed by research about muscle loss with inactivity and exercise to combat that loss, made particularly important by the space programme. Muscle biopsies showed slow twitch and fast twitch fibres, with little conversion of fibre types from one to the other. When changes in force generated by muscles were seen in a matter of days, long before there was any demonstrable change in muscle fibre size, this was attributed to changes in the innervations and activation of the muscle. However, all these studies led to the same conclusion: to improve performance in a specific activity, as opposed to strength in an isolated muscle, the best training is that activity itself which involves motion of the whole body.

At the same time, models of movement based on muscles and bones were challenged by the reality of motion that could not be explained. In the low back, lumbar fascia needed to be added to the model to account for movement capabilities. The running ability of the double amputee initially declared ineligible to compete in the regular 2008 Olympic games for fear that his bilateral below knee prostheses gave him an artificial advantage over athletes with normal calf muscles, shows that lower leg muscles are not sufficient or even necessary forces in propelling the human body. Studies of storage of energy in tendon and other connective tissues showed their importance in human gait. It turns out the normal myofascial locomotor system in humans is indeed slightly better than spring based prostheses

and in animals, such as the kangaroo, energy storage in tendons is critical to maintain the repetitive patterns of locomotion (Chapter 10).

More recently, studies have shown that energy storage in tissues around the shoulder allow humans to throw at speeds over 100 miles an hour, compared to a meager 20 miles per hour in our closely related primate species. Pre-contraction of the muscle stretches connective tissues, which then explosively releases to accomplish a movement for which muscle power alone would be insufficient. Whilst in the leg large tendons are found in obvious positions to store this energy, this is not the case in the shoulder. Instead, the storage is diffused across a network of as yet undefined tissues but the 'wind up' for the pitch indicates the whole body is involved.

The chapters in Part 1 provide a basis to understand principles of the body-wide tensional network of fascia. There is a continuity of fibrils from the extracellular matrix through the integrin receptor and the cell membrane to the nucleus. Manual massage after exercise can be seen to activate the force conducting pathways to the nucleus, followed within hours by changes in gene transcription. It is a useful concept to think of the body as a fascial network with connections to muscles and bones, rather than the more traditional view of a musculoskeletal system with fascia connections (Chapter 1). This suggests that the contraction of the trunk muscles prior to use of the superficial muscle slings, described in Chapter 7, may not be just stabilising the trunk. Rather, it may be taking the slack out of core fascial layers to allow 'prestretch' and energy storage for release later. Golfers and martial artists know the power in proper trunk rotation.

As described in Chapter 8, there are clear differences in mobility of tissues around the joints, with some people being more flexible than others. However, flexibility is not always a uniform function and the astute clinician will find patients with flexible elbows and tight hamstrings and vice versa. Indeed there are some rare muscle disorders characterised by certain tight and other loose joints. The theme of stretching to increase range in specific parts of the body is continued in Chapter 9 where, again, we find that practicing a task is the best way to prepare for that task performance. If we return to the notion that fascial tissues store energy for release during activities, we come to the logical conclusion that stretching these tissues to the point where their energy-absorbing properties are altered, will result in reduction in energy release and decreased subsequent performance. The mechanical interactions among muscle, tendon and fascia in humans have developed over many thousands of years to allow us to adapt to a wide range of activities. We are just beginning to understand these to be able to direct such adaptation by specific exercises and activities, which differ from the final desired task.

Skeletal muscle clearly responds to loading by hypertrophy and other adaptations, which increase its capacity for force generation. Chapter 5 takes this concept to connective tissue and explores loading in the context of adaptation or overloading pathology. For certain occupations, specific cycles of work/rest can be identified as tolerated or leading to functional loss. Again, task specificity is paramount. Adult tendons show little change or remodeling in the adult, unless there is wound healing to be repaired. However, to put this into perspective, connective tissue turnover every two days is found in the tiny fibres connecting a muscle to the nearby arteriole, which pull open the nitric oxide receptors and increase blood flow to the contracting muscle.

Additional aspects of fascial physiology and biochemistry are presented in Chapter 3, giving a wide range of factors to be taken into account to understand the basis for the broad spectrum of clinical applications presented in the next section. Some factors are specific to fascia. Others, such as work hardening, are general properties of hardening by plastic deformation, which have been used with copper, steel and other metals for thousands of years. To a greater or lesser extent, each of the chapters in Part 2 refers back to some of the basic physiology underlying these activities. By alternating study between Sections 1 and 2, the reader will develop a facility for analysing potentially beneficial therapies that will extend beyond the specific ones presented here. This is perhaps the most useful contribution of this book, to help the reader decide which of the many competing systems of therapy they will commit to studying further and which they will incorporate fully or partially into their own clinical approach to their patients and clients. Perhaps, most importantly, they will also to start to identify which particular approaches will work for particular patients.

Chapter 25 offers tools and techniques for assessment during the clinical examination to assist with gathering evidence to guide initiation of treatment and monitor progress. I expect this book will become a well-worn and dog-eared addition to the library of clinicians from many disciplines.

Thomas Findley
2014

Preface

Fascia certainly connects! It not only connects a large variety of collagenous tissues within the human body, ranging from tendons to joint capsules to muscular envelopes, but also the rapidly growing field of fascia-oriented explorations bringing together many different professional disciplines, personalities and perspectives. This includes scientists, dance professionals, stretch gurus and sports medicine celebrities. This book is nothing less than the first interdisciplinary publication to review scientific and practical approaches investigating the importance of fascia in sports and movement therapies.

We editors are proud of what has been accomplished in the following pages. In an extensive and intense collaboration, we have managed to include as contributing team members the top scientific experts in their fields as well as leading figures from different practical approaches such as athletic training, yoga, Pilates, sports rehabilitation, kettlebell training, martial arts, plyometrics, dance medicine and others.

Note that the range of professional perspectives varies about as much as the different fibrous tissues that are connected with each other as parts of the body-wide fascial net. Based on this, the scope of this textbook purposely embraces different opinions, such as the provocatively sceptical suggestions presented in the stretching chapter, which are subsequently complemented by different views on the same topic by other authors. Similarly the myofascial transmission lines of our colleague, Thomas Myers, are described with

their most recent and impressive advances together with detailed practical applications. However, other models of myofascial force transmission across the human body are presented as well. Yes, this book presents many exciting answers and a multitude of reliable and novel information. However, in addition, it also offers new inspiring questions, careful hypothetical speculations, as well as clinical observations that we editors consider well founded and clinically valuable.

A huge thank you has to be expressed to our 26 authors, all of whom have endeavoured to deliver an optimal contribution from their field for this first book in a new and promising territory. In addition, the team at Handspring Publishing has been wonderful in their enthusiastic support of our project. Their extensive publishing experience and personal familiarity with the field have been beyond anything that we could have imagined. The pioneering excitement, which was almost palpable at the first *'Connective Tissues in Sports Medicine'* congress (Ulm University, April 2013), and which has been shaping the different networking projects within this expanding field since then, has provided a strong motivational backdrop for all involved in this book. We trust that the reader will not only notice the exciting collaborative spirit of this new adventure but will also benefit from the resulting wealth of information and the quality of contributions from our whole international team.

Robert Schleip and Amanda Baker
Munich and Brighton, November 2014

Contributors

Joanne Avison, KMI, CTK, E-RYT500, CMED
Director, Art of Contemporary Yoga, Teacher
Training, London, UK
Co-chair Presentation Committee:
Biotensegrity Interest Group

Leon Chaitow, ND DO
Director, Ida P. Rolf Research Foundation
Honorary Fellow, University of Westminster,
London, UK

Stefan Dennenmoser, MA in Sports Science
PhD-student at the Fascia Research Project
Institute of Applied Physiology,
Ulm University, Ulm
Germany
Cert. Adv. Rolfer, Gyrotonic/
Gyrokinesis-Instructor
Fascial-Fitness-Master Trainer (FFA)

Donna Eddy, BHSc TCM,
Grad Dip Counselling, Dip RM,
Cert IV Pilates & Fitness
Physical Therapist & Movement Specialist
Owner & Creator Posture Plus
Co-owner & Creator Everything Movement &
The Swinging Weights Academy
Bondi, Sydney, Australia

Klaus Eder, PT
Lecturer at the Institute of Sport Science,
University of Regensburg,
Instructor for sports physiotherapy at the
German Olympic Sport Confederation,
Donaustauf, Germany

Raoul H.H. Engelbert, PhD, PT
Professor of Physiotherapy, University of
Amsterdam, Department of Rehabilitation,
AMC Amsterdam
Director, School of Physiotherapy, Amsterdam
School of Health Professions, University of
Applied Sciences, The Netherlands

Piroska Frenzel, MD
Master student of the Vienna School for
Osteopathy at the Danube University Krems,
Austria

Member of the Fascia Research Project
Division of Neurophysiology,
Ulm University, Ulm, Germany

Fernando Galán del Río, PhD, PT, DO
Spanish National Football Federation.
Physiotherapy Team
Professor at Department of Physical Therapy,
Occupational Therapy,
Rehabilitation and Physical Medicine, Rey
Juan Carlos University, Madrid, Spain

Christopher-Marc Gordon SRP, hcpc, HP
Physiotherapist, Naturopath,
Founder of the Center of Integrative Therapy
Stuttgart
Myofascial Pain Researcher
Lecturer Institute for Medical Psychology and
Behavioural Neurobiology
University Tübingen, Germany

Robert Heiduk, MSc,
Sports Science Director, German Strength
and Conditioning Conference Sports Coach,
Bochum, Germany

Helmut Hoffmann, MSS, MBA
Owner Eden Sport Private Institute for
Performance Diagnostics
Sportscientific Director Eden Reha Private
Clinic for Sport Rehabilitation
Donaustauf, Germany

Birgit Juul-Kristensen, PhD, PT
Associate professor,
Research Unit of Musculoskeletal Function,
and Head of Centre for Research in Adapted
Physical Activity and Participation, Institute
of Sports Science and Clinical Biomechanics
University of Southern Denmark, Odense,
Denmark
Professor, Bergen University College,
Institute of Occupational Therapy,
Physiotherapy and Radiography,
Department of Health Sciences,
Bergen, Norway

Wilbour E. Kelsick, BSC(kin), PhD, DC, FRCCSS(C), FCCRS(C)
Sports Chiropractic Lead
Athletics Olympic Team Canada
Clinical Director
MaxFit Movement Institute
Vancouver, Canada

Michael Kjaer, MD DMSci
Professor, Chief physician
Institute of Sports Medicine, Bispebjerg
Hospital and Centre for Healthy Aging
Faculty of Health and Medical Sciences
University of Copenhagen, Copenhagen, Denmark

Werner Klingler, MD, PhD
Director, Neurophysiological Laboratory,
Neuroanaesthesiology, Ulm University
Fascia Research Group, Division of Neurophysiology,
Ulm University, Ulm, Germany
Department of Neuroanaesthesiology, Ulm University, Guenzburg, Germany

Elizabeth Larkam
Pilates Method Alliance-Gold CPT
Balanced Body Faculty/Mentor
PMA Heroes in Motion® Pioneer
Distinguished Instructor, Pilates Anytime
GYROTONIC®/GYROKINESIS® Teacher
GCFP®
San Francisco, California, USA

Eyal Lederman, DO, PhD
Director, CPDO Ltd, Self Care Education Ltd.
Senior Honorary Lecturer and Research Supervisor
Institute of Orthopaedics & Musculoskeletal Health, University College London (UCL), UK

Divo G. Müller
FF Mastertrainer
CEO Fascial Fitness Association
Director Somatic Academy
Munich, Germany

Stephen Mutch, MSc (Sports Physiotherapy)
BSc (Physiotherapy) MCSP
Clinical Director Spaceclinics.com,
Physiotherapist, Scotland Rugby Team

Vice President Association of Chartered Physiotherapists in Sports & Exercise Medicine, Edinburgh, UK

Thomas W. Myers, LMT, NCTMB
Director: Kinesis LLC,
Walpole, Maine, USA

Sol Petersen, B Phys Ed
Rehabilitation Specialist and Psychotherapist,
Tai Ji & Qi Gong Instructor
Founder, Mana Retreat Centre, Coromandel, New Zealand

Lars Remvig, MD, DMSc
Senior Consultant,
Department of Infectious Medicine and Rheumatology
Rigshospitalet, University of Copenhagen, Copenhagen, Denmark

Philipp Richter, DO
Osteopath, Belgium; Head of the IFAO (Institut für angewandte Osteopathie), Germany

Raúl Martínez Rodríguez, PT, DO
Spanish National Football Federation, Physiotherapy Team
Director of Tensegrity Clinic Physiotherapy & Osteopathy
Health Area, European University of Madrid, Madrid, Spain

Liane Simmel PhD**,** MD, DO
Director, Institute for Dance Medicine 'Fit for Dance', Munich
Medical Consultant, University for Theatre and Performing Arts, Dance Department, Munich
Lecturer for Dance Medicine, Palucca University for Dance, Dresden
Senior Consultant, Dance Medicine Germany eV, Munich, Germany

Adjo Zorn, PhD
Fascia Research Project
Institute of Applied Physiology
Ulm University, Ulm;
European Rolfing Association
Munich, Germany

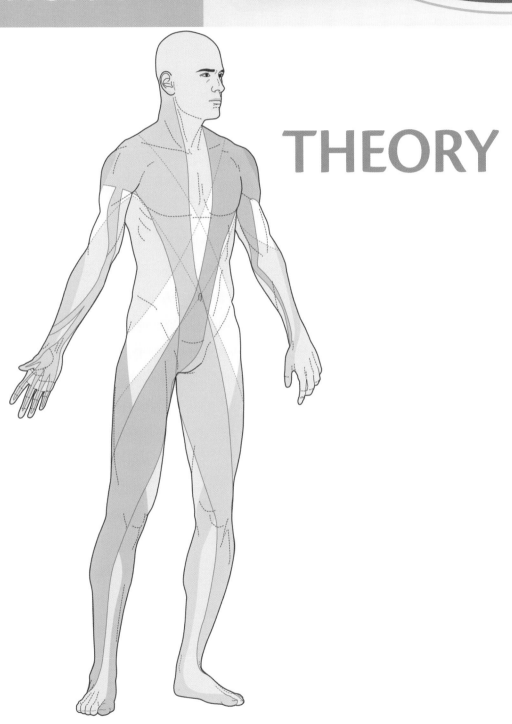

THEORY

CHAPTER 1

Fascia as a body-wide tensional network: Anatomy, biomechanics and physiology

Werner Klinger and Robert Schleip

Fascia the forgotten organ

After several decades of a Cinderella-like neglect, fascia has suddenly entered the limelight within the field of human life sciences. While literally thrown away in most anatomical dissections, this colourless fibrous tissue had mostly been treated like a dull and inert packaging organ. There were several reasons for this neglect. One of which is the lack of clear distinctions based on the ubiquitous and seemingly disordered nature of this tissue, compared with the shiny muscles and organs underneath. Another and more important reason for the severe neglect of scientific attention was the lack of adequate measurement tools. While x-ray imaging allowed detailed study of bones and electromyography of muscles, for many decades, changes in fascia were hard to measure. For example, the fascia lata or lumbar fascia is typically less than 2 mm thick and a local increase in thickness of 20% was too small to be seen on ultrasound (or other affordable imaging technology in clinical practice) although it may be easily palpable to the hand of the therapist and may also be felt by the client during movement.

This unfortunate situation has changed significantly in recent years. Advances in ultrasound measurement, as well as in histology, have resulted in a dramatic increase of fascia-related studies (Chaitow et al., 2012). Clinical fields whose practitioners have an avid interest and participation in this process include manual therapies, physiotherapy, scar treatment, oncology (based on the matrix-dependent behaviour of cancer cells), surgery and rehabilitative medicine, amongst others. Similarly, sports science is embracing these developments. The first congress on 'Connective tissues in sports medicine', hosted at Ulm University in 2013, served as important impetus for the development of this field. Today, fascia has become a favoured new subject in conferences for sports sciences as well as among movement teachers.

What is fascia?

Based on the inter-connected nature of fascial tissues, the new terminology proposed at the first Fascia Research Congress defines fascia as all collagenous fibrous connective tissues that can be seen as elements of a body-wide tensional force transmission network. In contrast to bones or cartilage, the specific morphology of these fibrous tissues is shaped by a dominance of tensional – rather than compressional – loading. The specific shape of a fascial tissue depends on the local history of these tensional forces. If the local tensional demands are mostly unidirectional and have involved high loads, then the fascial net will express these in the shape of a tendon or ligament. In other circumstances it may express them as a lattice-like membrane or as a loose fibrous arealor safron (see Figure 1.1). The term 'fascia' is, then, fairly synonymous with the layperson's understanding of the term 'connective tissue' (although in medical science the term 'connective tissue' includes bones, cartilage and even blood, all of which derive from the embryonic mesenchym layer).

A body-wide interconnected tensional network

An advantage of this new and more encompassing terminology is that it recognises the widespread continuities of this fibrous network, while still allowing for a detailed description of the local architecture. Note that in contrast to

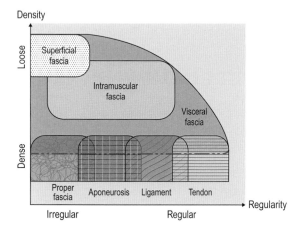

Density

Loose

Superficial fascia

Intramuscular fascia

Visceral fascia

Dense

Proper fascia   Aponeurosis   Ligament   Tendon

Irregular   Regular

Regularity

Figure 1.1

Different connective tissues as specialisations of the global fascial net

In the new terminology, proposed at the first Fascia Research Congress, all collagenous fibrous connective tissues are considered as 'fascia'. These tissues differ in terms of their density and directional alignment of collagen fibres. For example, superficial fascia is characterised by a relatively low density and mostly multidirectional or irregular fibre alignment, whereas in the denser tendons or ligaments the fibres are mostly unidirectional. Note that the intramuscular fasciae – septi, perimysium and endomysium – may express varying degrees of directionality and density. The same is true for the visceral fasciae, like the very soft greater omentum in the belly or the much tougher pericardium. Depending on local loading history, fascia proper can express a uni-directional, lattice-like, or multi-directional arrangement. (Illustration courtesy of fascialnet.com.).

the simplified anatomical textbook illustrations, the collagenous tissues around major joints in the human body express large areas of gradual transition, where a clear distinction between ligament, capsule, tendon, septum or muscular envelope is virtually impossible.

Force transmission from the muscle to the skeleton also involves more extramuscular myofascial delineations than was classically assumed. The work of Huijing et al., 2007 has shown impressively how muscles transmit up to 40% of their contraction force not into their respective tendon but rather via fascial connections into other muscles that are positioned next to them. Interestingly, this often involves force transmission to antagonistic muscles, which are then co-stiffened and tend to increase resistance to this primary movement. An increase of this particular force transmission to antagonistic muscles has been shown to be an important complication in many spastic contractures (Huijing et al., 2007).

Important muscular force transmissions, via their fascial connections, have been shown between:

• latissimus dorsi and contralateral gluteus maximus via the lumbodorsal fascia (Barker et al., 2004)

• biceps femoris to the erector spinae fascia via the sacrotuberous ligament (Vleeming et al., 1995)

• biceps brachii and the flexor muscles of the lower arm via the lacertus fibrosis (Brasseur, 2012)

• gluteus maximus and lower leg muscles via the fascial lata (Stecco et al., 2013).

Don Ingber showed that the architecture of cells can be understood to behave like a tensegrity structure. In a tensegrity structure the compressional elements (struts) are suspended without any compressional contact towards each other, whereas the tensional elements (elastic bands or membranes) are all connected with one another in a global tension-transmitting network (Ingber, 1998). This model served as a basic inspiration for the field of fascia research. Driven by the observation that healthy human bodies express a higher degree of tensegrity-like qualities in their movements, many clinicians as well as scientists have started to see the fascial web as the elastic elements of a tensegrity structure, in which bones and cartilage are suspended as spacers, rather than as classical weight bearing structures (Levin, 2003). While this is based on the assumption that the human body is a pure tensegrity structure, since it also contains hydraulic elements that behave in a sponge-like manner, the above examples of myofascial force transmission across several joints show that a tensegrity-inspired perspective offers an improved understanding of the fascial net and its role in musculoskeletal dynamics.

Components of fascial tissues

Fascial connective tissues basically consist of two components: cells plus the extracellular matrix (Figure 1.2). Unlike most other tissues, the cells take up a very minor part of the total volume (usually less than 5%). Most of the cells are fibroblasts, which function as construction and maintenance workers for the surrounding matrix. The matrix consists again of two parts: ground substance and fibres. The ground substance consists mostly of water, which is bound by proteoglycans. Most of the fibres are collagen fibres, except for few elastin fibres.

A common misconception is that sometimes ground substance and the matrix are taken as synonyms. However, the net of collagen fibre is an important matrix element. The overall architecture of the matrix can be compared to a composite structure in engineering, in which a mesh of sturdy cables is combined with a more amorphic material to provide optimum mechanical strength in multidirectional loading.

Except for water (which is extruded by the small arterioles in fascia) most of the constituents are produced, remodeled and maintained by the resident fibroblasts. These cells are responsive to mechanical stimulation as well as to biochemical stimulation. Biochemical stimulation includes the effect of inflammatory cytokines, several other cytokines, hormones, as well as changes in pH level (acidity of the ground substance). For example, human growth hormone (HGH) – most of which is produced during sleep – is an important requirement for collagen production. As many body builders who have experimented with HGH have discovered, muscle growth is not affected by this important hormone. However, there is a clear effect on collagen production and proper collagen synthesis as renewal is dependent on a sufficient supply of HGH which effectively acts as an important fertiliser (Kjaer et al., 2009).

Biomechanical stimulation is at least as important for tissue health as the biochemical environment. In fact, without proper mechanical stimulation fascial fibroblasts will not create an adequate fibrous matrix, no matter how good or bad their biochemical environment is. While nutritional care can improve the biochemical milieu, sports and movement therapies are potent tools for fostering optimal biomechanical stimulation for the matrix remodelling behaviour of the fibroblasts. Fibroblasts are equipped with numerous devices to 'sense' tensional and mechanical shear stimulation exerted upon them. In response to this, they constantly change their metabolic function.

Adaptability to mechanical loading

For a connective tissue oriented training approach, it is as important to understand that the local architecture of this network adapts to the specific history of previous strain-loading demands (Blechschmidt, 1978) (Chaitow, 1988). Collagen shows an enormous adaptability to the

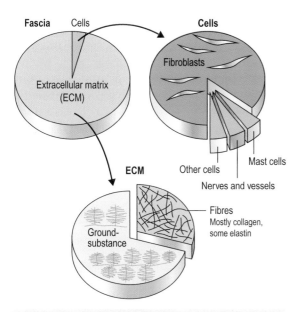

Figure 1.2

Components of fascia

The basic constituents are cells (mostly fibroblasts) and extracellular matrix (ECM), the latter of which consists of fibres plus the watery ground substance. (Illustration courtesy of fascialnet.com)

demands in the gravitational field. For example, the human biped has developed a unique structure: the dense fascia lata on the outside of the thigh, which enables us to stabilise the hips in walking, running and hopping. No other animal, not even our genetically closest relative the chimpanzee, shows this kind of fascial feature. These fascial sheets on the lateral side of the thigh will develop a more palpable firmness than on the medial side in those who walk or run regularly. In a couch potato, who prefers a sedentary lifestyle or a wheelchair patient with almost no leg movement, this difference in tissue stiffness is scarcely found. In contrast, for regular horse riders the opposite would be the case. After a few months, the fascia on the inner leg would become dense and strong (El-Labban et al., 1993).

Good news for tissue renewal: if the connective structures are loaded properly, the inherent networking cells, called fibroblasts, adapt their matrix remodelling activity so that the tissue architecture responds even better to daily demands. Not only does the density of bone change, as happens with astronauts who spend time in zero gravity wherein the bones become more porous (Ingber, 2008), fascial tissues also react to their dominant loading patterns. With the help of the fibroblasts, they slowly but constantly react to everyday strain as well as to specific training (Kjaer et al., 2009). Their remodelling activity is particularly responsive to repeated challenges from the mechanical integrity of their surrounding matrix. Challenges to the tissue's strength, extensibility and ability to shear will stimulate the fibroblasts to respond in a process of constant reconstructing and re-arrangement of the fascial web.

Fascia in sports science

In sports science, and in recent sports education, the prevailing emphasis has been on the classical triad of muscular training, cardiovascular conditioning and neuromuscular coordination (Jenkins, 2005). Comparatively little attention had been given to a specifically targeted training of the connective tissues involved. This widespread practice has not taken into consideration the huge role that the collagenous connective tissues play in sports associated with overuse injuries. Whether in running, soccer, baseball,

swimming or gymnastics, the vast majority of associated repetitive strain injuries occur in the muscular collagenous connective tissues, such as tendons, ligaments or joint capsules. Even in so-called 'muscle tears', the specific ruptures rarely occur within the red myofibres but rather within the white collagenous portions of the overall muscle structure. It seems that in these instances, the respective collagenous tissues have been less adequately prepared – and less well adapted to their loading challenge – than their muscular or skeletal counterparts (Renström & Johnson, 1985) (Hyman & Rodeo, 2000) (Counsel & Breidahl, 2010).

Of course, any muscular training also 'trains' the connective tissues involved, although in a non-specific and usually non-optimal manner. This is comparable to the suboptimal effect of cardiovascular endurance training on muscular strength and vice versa. Similarly, all sports training will stimulate collagen remodelling 'somehow'. Recent fascia-oriented training suggestions, therefore, propose that a specifically tailored connective tissue training may yield the same training enhancements as a tailored strength training, coordination training or cardiovascular fitness programme does for their specific target functions.

Getting the spring back in your step

One of the most inspiring aspects for movement and sports practitioners, within this rapidly advancing field of new scientific revelations about fascia is the ability of tendons and aponeuroses to store and release kinetic energy. This will be addressed in detail in Chapter 10. Given the right architecture of the loaded collagenous structures, and given sufficient sensorimotor refinement for sensing the appropriate resonance frequency, seemingly effortless elastic recoil motions can then be performed.

The usually higher elastic storage quality in young people is reflected in their fascial tissues showing a typical two-directional lattice arrangement, like the regular arrangement of fibres in a woman's stocking (Staubesand et al., 1997). Ageing is usually associated with a loss of elasticity, bounce and springiness in our gait and this is also reflected in the fascial architecture (Figure 1.3). Here, the fibres proliferate and take on an irregular arrangement. Animal experiments have shown that immobilisation quickly leads to a dysregulation in fibre arrangement and to a multidirectional growth of additional cross-links between dense collagen fibres. As a result, the fibres lose their elasticity as well as the smooth gliding motion against one another. They then stick together forming tissue adhesions over time and, at worst, they become matted together (Jarvinen et al., 2002).

Taking a closer look into the microstructure of the collagen fibres, it shows undulations, called crimp, which is reminiscent of elastic springs. In older people, or those whose fascial fibres suffer immobilisation, the structure of the fibre appears rather flattened, losing both crimp and springiness (Staubesand et al., 1997). Research has confirmed the previously optimistic assumption that proper exercise loading of the fibres, if applied regularly, can induce a more youthful collagen architecture. This regains a more wavy fibre

arrangement (Wood et al., 1988) (Jarniven et al., 2002), and expresses a significantly increased elastic storage capacity (Figure 1.4) (Reeves et al., 2006) (Witvrouw et al., 2007).

Given a proper elastic resilience in the fascial tissues of feet and legs, less cushioning may be required as external shock absorption in one's shoes. Habitual barefoot running, as well as running with minimalistic shoes, tends to involve an earlier forefoot contact with the ground compared to conventionally shod running. This seems to involve a higher storage capacity within the fasciae of foot and lower leg when compared to shod running (Tam et al., 2014). Interestingly, this increase in elastic storage quality is more strong-

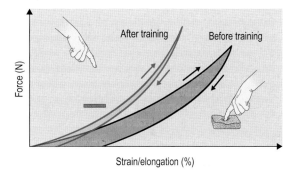

Figure 1.4

Decreased hysteresis in trained tendons

In the tendinous tissues of rats, which had to practice rapid treadmill running on a regular schedule, there were increases in elastic storage capacity, compared with their non-running peers. See the double curve on the left. The area between the respective loading versus unloading curves represents the amount of 'hysteresis', which is a measure for the loss of kinetic energy. The smaller hysteresis of the trained animals (left double curve) reveals their more 'elastic' tissue storage capacity. The larger hysteresis of their peers, in contrast, signifies their more 'visco-elastic' tissue properties, also referred to as inertia. Note that compared with the original data the relative differences between the two double curves have been exaggerated for better understanding. (Illustration courtesy of fascialnet. com, modified after Reeves et al., 2006)

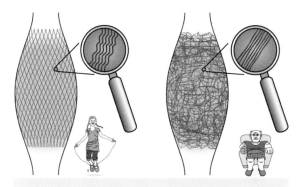

Figure 1.3

Collagen fibres respond to loading

Healthy fasciae (left image) express a clear two-directional (lattice) orientation of their collagen fibre network. In addition, the individual collagen fibres show a stronger crimp formation. Lack of exercise on the other hand, has been shown to induce a multidirectional fibre network and a reduction in crimp formation leading to a loss of springiness and elastic recoil (right image). (Illustration courtesy of fascialnet.com)

ly expressed in barefoot running than in running with minimalistic shoes, (Bonacci et al., 2013) possibly due to the role of proprioceptive stimulation involvement by barefoot contact with the ground. However, due to the slow speed of fascial adaption (see page 9), transition to more 'natural' footwear should be performed even more gradually than is recommended by conservative instructions, due to the high likelihood of overuse injuries such as bone marrow oedema during the change-over time (Ridge et al., 2013).

Hydration and renewal

It is helpful to note that approximately two thirds of the volume of fascial tissues is made up of water. During application of mechanical load, whether by stretching or via local compression, a significant amount of water is pushed out of the more stressed zones, similar to squeezing a sponge (Schleip et al., 2012). During the subsequent release time this area is again filled with new fluid, which comes from surrounding tissue as well as the local arterioles. The sponge-like connective tissue can lack adequate hydration at places that are not reached during everyday movements. Application of external loading to fascial tissues can result in a refreshed hydration in such places in the body (Chaitow, 2009).

It also seems to matter what kind of water is stored in the tissue. In healthy fascia, a large percentage of the extracellular water is in a state of bound water (as opposed to bulk water) where its behaviour can be characterised as that of a liquid crystal (Pollack, 2013). Many pathologies, such as inflammatory conditions, oedema, or the increased accumulation of free radicals and other waste products, tend to go along with a shift towards a higher percentage of bulk water within the ground substance. Recent reports by Sommer and Zhu (2008) suggest that when local connective tissue gets squeezed like a sponge and subsequently rehydrated, some of the previous bulk water zones (in which the water had been 'polluted' with inflammatory cytokines as well as with free radicals as a by-product of stress or ageing) may then be replaced by 'fresh' water from blood plasma which instantly forms bound water zones, which could lead to a more healthy water constitution within the ground substance. As shown by the work of Pollack, bound water has higher elastic storage ability and behaves like a liquid crystal (Pollack, 2013). It is likely that some of the tissue effects of stretching, yoga as well as foam roller self-treatments may be related to such water renewal dynamics. It is possible that a relatively dehydrated tissue area can be rehydrated again through such treatments (Schleip et al., 2012). It is additionally possible that not only can the total water content be improved but also the water quality in the direction of a higher percentage of bound water, with subsequent improvements in the viscoelastic tissue properties.

How fast does it change?

How rapid is the described adaptation process? This seems to depend on which elements are looked at. Some of the denser collagen cables in the Achilles tendon – which are composed of particularly thick collagen type 1 fibre bundles – are not replaced until the end of the skeletal growth period and show zero turnover after that age. At the other end of the spectrum, many of the proteoglycans in the water-binding ground substance are constantly remodeled in only a matter of days . For the particular collagen fibres in cartilage, the half-life has been calculated as 100 years while in skin this was estimated as 15 years. More recent labelling techniques examining collagen proteins from Achilles and patellar tendons suggested a fractional of 1% per day for the collagen of intramuscular fasciae. The same study estimated the turnover rate of collagen tissues to be approximately two to three times slower than the respective rate for skeletal muscle fibres (Miller et al., 2005). In summary, the renewal speed of the body-wide fascial network is quite slow, with a half-life between months and years, rather than days or weeks.

Fascia science put into daily practice

It is suggested that in order to build up an injury resistant and elastic fascial body network it is essential to translate current insights from the field of fascia research into practical training programmes. Adequately tailored training can improve the elastic storage capacity of the stimulated fascial tissues (Figure 1.4). For the respective tissue remodelling, it apparently makes a difference which kind of exercise movements are applied: a controlled exercise study with a group of senior women using slow-velocity and low-load contractions only demonstrated an increase in muscular strength and volume. However, it failed to yield any change in the elastic storage capacity of the collagenous structures (Kubo et al., 2003). While the latter response could possibly be also related to age differences, more recent studies by Arampatzis et al. (2010) have confirmed that, in order to yield adaptation effects in human tendons, the strain magnitude applied should exceed the value that occurs during habitual activities.

These studies provide evidence of the existence of a threshold in the magnitude of the applied strain at which transduction of the mechanical stimulus influences tendon homeostasis (Arampatzis et al., 2007). For tendinous tissue, the required loading magnitude seems to be fairly high and is usually not reached with loads comparable to normal everyday activities. Whereas for intramuscular fasciae, much lower forces are sufficient (Kjaer, personal communication).

Recent studies have shown that during the first three hours after appropriate exercise loading, collagen synthesis is increased. However, collagen degradation is also increased and, interestingly, during the first 1½ days the degradation outweighs the synthesis (Figure 1.5). Only afterwards, the resulting net synthesis of collagen production becomes positive. It is, therefore, assumed that daily strong exercise loading could lead towards a weaker collagen structure. Based on this it is recommended that fascial tissues should be properly exercised two to three times per week only, in order to allow for adequate collagen renewal (Magnusson et al., 2010).

Several training recommendations for fostering an optimal remodelling of fascial tissues have been proposed and will be explored in the second portion of this book. They attempt to translate an understanding of fascial properties into specific movement instructions or treatment

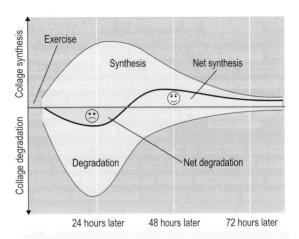

Figure 1.5

Collagen turnover after exercise

The upper curve demonstrates how collagen synthesis is increased after exercise. After 24 hours the synthesis is increased two fold compared with the previous condition at rest. However, as an additional effect of exercise, the stimulated fibroblasts also increase their rate of collagen degradation. Interestingly during the first 1–2 days, collagen degradation outweighs the collagen synthesis, whereas afterwards this situation is reversed. Based on this, training recommendations aimed at improving connective tissue strength suggest exercising 2–3 times per week only. Data based on Miller et al. 2009. (Illustration courtesy of fascialnet.com, modified after Magnusson et al., 2010)

recommendations. Based on their particular emphasis, they promise to foster a stronger, faster, younger, more elastic, refined, resilient, flexible, and, above all, more injury-resistant mobility of our body. As this general field is fairly new within sports science, very few of these promises have, so far, been clinically proven (these are mentioned in the respective chapters). For the vast majority of these claims, only anecdotal evidence exists, which of course may be prone to multiple biases based on evangelic expectations. Future critical research, possibly based on the measurement tools described in the last sections of this book, will reveal to what degree these promising beneficial effects are achieved.

References

Arampatzis, A., Karamanidis, K. & Albracht, K. (2007) Adaptational responses of the human Achilles tendon by modulation of the applied cyclic strain magnitude. *J Exp Biol*. 210: 2743–2753.

Arampatzis, A., Peper, A., Bierbaum, S. & Albracht, K. (2010) Plasticity of human Achilles tendon mechanical and morphological properties in response to cyclic strain. *J Biomech*. 43: 3073–3079.

Barker, P.J., Briggs, C.A. & Bogeski, G. (2004) Tensile transmission across the lumbar fasciae in unembalmed cadavers: effects of tension to various muscular attachments. *Spine* 29(2): 129–138.

Blechschmidt, E. (1978). In: Charles, C. (Ed.), *Biokinetics and Biodynamics of Human Differentiation: Principles and Applications*. Thomas Pub Ltd, Springfield, Illinois.

Bonacci, J., Saunders, P.U., Hicks, A.,Rantalainen, T.,Vicenzino, B.G. & Spratford, W. (2013) Running in a minimalist and lightweight shoe is not the same as running barefoot: a biomechanical study. *Br J Sports Med*. 47(6): 387–392.

Brasseur, J.L. (2012) The biceps tendons: From the top and from the bottom. *J Ultrasound*. 15(1): 29–38.

Chaitow, L. (1988) *Soft-tissue Manipulation: A Practitioner's Guide to the Diagnosis and Treatment of Soft-tissue Dysfunction and Reflex Activity*. Healing Arts Press, Rochester, Vermont.

Chaitow, L. (2009) Research in water and fascia. Micro-tornadoes, hydrogenated diamonds & nanocrystals. *Massage Today* 09(6): 1–3.

Chaitow, L., Findley, T.W. & Schleip, R. (Eds.) (2012) *Fascia research III – Basic science and implications for conventional and complementary health care*. Kiener Press, Munich.

Counsel, P. & Breidahl, W. (2010) Muscle injuries of the lower leg. *Seminars in Musculoskelet Radiol* 14: 162–175.

El-Labban, N.G., Hopper, C. & Barber, P. (1993) Ultrastructural finding of vascular degeneration in myositis ossificans circum-scripta (fibrodysplasia ossificans). *J Oral Pathol Med*. 22: 428–431.

Huijing, P.A. (2007) Epimuscular myofascial force transmission between antagonistic and synergistic muscles can explain movement limitation in spastic paresis. *J Electromyogr Kinesiol*. 17(6): 708–724.

Hyman, J. & Rodeo, S.A. (2000) Injury and repair of tendons and ligaments. *Phys Med Rehabil Clin N Am*. 11: 267–288.

Ingber, D.E. (1998) The architecture of life. *Scientific American*. January, 48–57.

Ingber, D.E. (2008) Tensegrity and mechanotransduction. *J Bodyw Mov Ther*. 12: 198–200.

Jarvinen, T.A., Jozsa, L., Kannus, P., Jarvinen, T.L., & Jarvinen, M. (2002) Organization and distribution of intramuscular connective tissue in normal and immobilized skeletal muscles. An immunohistochemical, polarization and scanning electron microscopic study. *J Musc Res Cell Mot*. 23: 245–254.

Jenkins, S. (2005) Sports Science Handbook. In: *The Essential Guide to Kinesiology, Sport & Exercise Science*, vol. 1. Multi-science Publishing Co. Ltd., Essex, UK.

Kjaer, M., Langberg, H., Heinemeier, K., Bayer, M.L., Hanse, M., Holm, L., Doessing, S., Kongsgaard, M., Krogsgaard, M.R. & Magnusson, S.P. (2009) From mechanical loading to collagen synthesis, structural changes and function in human tendon. *Scand J Med Sci Sports* 19(4): 500–510.

Kubo, K., Kanehisa, H., Miyatani, M., Tachi, M., Fukunaga, T. (2003). Effect of low-load resistance training on the tendon properties in middle-aged and elderly women. *Acta Physiol Scand*. 178: 25–32.

Levin, S.L. & Martin, D. (2012) Biotensegrity: The mechanics of fascia. In: Schleip, R. et al. *Fascia – the tensional network of the human body*. Edinburgh: Elsevier, 137–142.

Magnusson, S.P., Langberg, H. & Kjaer, M. (2010). The pathogenesis of tendinopathy: balancing the response to loading. *Nature Rev Rheumat*. 6: 262–268.

Miller, B.F., Olesen, J.L., Hansen M., Døssing, S., Crameri, R.M., Welling, R.J., Langberg, H., Flyvbjerg, A., Kjaer, M., Babraj, J.A., Smith, K. & Rennie, M.J. (2005) Coordinated collagen and muscle protein synthesis in human patella tendon and quadriceps muscle after exercise. *J Physiol*. 567(Pt 3): 1021–1033.

Pollack, G.H. (2013) *The fourth phase of water. Beyond solid, liquid and vapor*. Ebner and Sons Publishers, Seattle, Washington.

Reeves, N.D., Narici, M.V. & Maganaris, C.N. (2006). Myo-tendinous plasticity to aging and resistance exercise in humans. *Exp Physiol*. 91: 483–498.

Renström, P. & Johnson, R.J. (1985) Overuse injuries in sports. A review. *Sports Med*. 2: 316–333.

Ridge, S.T., Johnson, A.W., Mitchell, U.H., Hunter, I., Robinson, E., Rich, B.S. & Brown, S.D. (2013) Foot bone marrow edema after a 10-wk transition to minimalist running shoes. *Med Sci Sports Exerc*. 45(7): 1363–1368.

Schleip, R., Duerselen, L., Vleeming, A., Naylor, I.L., Lehmann-Horn, F., Zorn, A., Jaeger, H. & Klingler, W. (2012) Strain hardening of fascia: static stretching of dense fibrous connective tissues can induce a temporary stiffness increase accompanied by enhanced matrix hydration. *J Bodyw Mov Ther*. 16(1): 94–100.

Staubesand, J. & Baumbach KUK, Li Y (1997) La structure find de l'aponeurose jambiere. *Phlebologie*. 50: 105–113.

Stecco, A., Gilliar, W., Hill, R., Fullerton, B., & Stecco, C. (2013) The anatomical and functional relation between gluteus maximus and fascia lata. *J Bodyw Mov Ther*. 17(4): 512–517.

Tam, N., Astephen Wilson, J.L., Noakes, T.D. & Tucker, R. (2014) Barefoot running: an evaluation of current hypothesis, future research and clinical applications. *Br J Sports Med*. 48(5): 349–355.

Vleeming, A., Pool-Goudzwaard, A.L., Stoeckart, R., van Wingerden, J.P. & Snijders C.J (1995) The posterior layer of the thoracolumbar fascia. Its function in load transfer from spine to legs. *Spine* 20(7): 753–758.

Witvrouw, E., Mahieu, N., Roosen, P. & McNair, P. (2007) The role of stretching in tendon injuries. *Br J Sports Med.* 41: 224–226.

Wood, T.O., Cooke, P.H. & Goodship, A.E. (1988) The effect of exercise and anabolic steroids on the mechanical properties and crimp morphology of the rat tendon. *Am J Sports Med.* 16: 153–158.

CHAPTER 2

Myofascial force transmission

Stephen Mutch

'Connectivity' and the effect of exercise

Fascia, defined as the 'soft tissue component of the connective tissue system that permeates the human body' is effectively a network recognised as part of a body-wide tensional force transmission system (Schleip et al., 2012). Fascia has a key role to play in musculoskeletal dynamics: its ability to spontaneously adapt and adjust to strain or stretch, establishes it as an active contributor to stability and mobility (Chapter 1). The adaptation process is essentially one of stimulus-response.

This process of conversion from the stimulus of mechanical loading to cellular response is called mechanotransduction. Actual structural change occurs as a result of this conversion process and practically takes place with the application of manual compression load or through movement or stretch (Chaitow, 2013) (Khan & Scott, 2009). The potential impact of this process for practitioners is enormous. Their ability to elicit specific biological changes and manipulate a physiological process, by their treatment and exercise methods, is only just beginning to be understood and recognised.

In addition to local dense regular connective tissue formations, broadly known as ligaments and tendons, planar tissue sheets such as septa, muscle envelopes, joint or visceral capsules and retinacula are included in this inter-connected fascial net. Also included are the softer collagenous areolar connective tissue of the superficial fascia and the intra-muscular layer of epimysium, perimysium and endomysium. These have the greatest diversity of cell types, all with their own distinct individual composition and structure, but fundamentally they are all made up of collagen fibres in an amorphous matrix of hydrated proteoglycans. This is fundamental for the mechanical linkage of this connective tissue network (Purslow, 2010). Areolar fibroblasts are integral to mechanotransduction, communicating with each other via gap junctions, responding to tissue stretch by shape changes mediated via the cytoskelton (Langevin et al., 2005).

It is apparent that a muscle cannot exist as an isolated entity. It is connected mechanically to adjacent neighbouring structures that collectively have a substantial myofascial force transmission effect on muscle force-length characteristics (Yucesoy et al., 2003b) (Yucesoy, 2010). Intramuscular, intermuscular and extramuscular force transmissions all have the capability to alter the distribution of lengths of sarcomeres within muscle fibres.

For controlled movement of the human skeleton, forces must be exerted onto the bony frame in order to create a biomechanical moment, with respect to articular joints. Additional force is exerted on the tissues of the joints to establish mechanically stable conditions, and thus contribute towards muscle mechanics and function (Yucesoy et al., 2003a).

Experimental evidence, from early this century, has demonstrated that there are significant additional extramuscular myofascial force transmissions that supplement muscle function. Tension, initially generated in actomyosin filaments of sarcomeres, is transmitted across the muscle fibre surface to the surrounding connective tissues via complex mechanomolecular pathways (Masi et al., 2010). Myofibrils were seen to transmit force both longitudinally and to adjacent myofibrils, as well as the sarcolemma. Muscle fibres then transmit force along tendons, which are arranged partly in series and partly parallel with muscle fibres (Yucesoy et al., 2003a). This continuous connecting matrix of connective tissue, and adjacent muscle fibres, coordinates force transmission between fibres in a fascicle and keep fibres uniform (Purslow, 2010).

Force transmission through epi-, peri- and endomysium

Each muscle is enveloped by epimysium, a connective tissue layer continuous with tendons. Epimysium can be two parallel sets of wavy collagen embedded in a proteocollagen matrix crossed-ply arrangement in some long strap-like muscles or, in pennate muscles, the collagen is arranged parallel to the long axis of the muscle forming a dense surface layer that functions as a surface tendon (Purslow, 2010).

At the muscle surface, perimysium merges seamlessly into epimysium and they are connected mechanically. The perimysium is a continuous connective tissue network that divides the muscle up into fascicles, or muscle fibre bundles that run the muscle length from tendon to tendon. The folded interdigitating ends of these muscle fibres form the myotendinous junctions.

Within each fascicle or muscle fibre bundle, the endomysium is a continuous network of connective tissue that uniquely separates but links individual muscle fibres. As the endomysium is compliant in tension, force transmission may be by shear linkage through its thickness, which offers a highly efficient force transduction pathway from one muscle cell to its neighbours. In this way, uniform sarcomere lengths are maintained by the coordination of non-contracting fibres with adjacently lying contracting fibres. Due to its low tensile stiffness, the endomysium can deform easily in the plane of the network and, therefore, does not restrict changes in muscle fibre length and diameter as muscles contract and relax (Purslow, 2010).

This form of lateral load sharing through the endomysium offers an explanation as to how muscles can grow, add and repair damaged sarcomeres without any loss of contractile function. Endomysial connections between adjacent fibres can ensure the maintenance of this highly desirable uniform strain throughout tissue. Even when damaged, myofibrils are being remodelled after injury demonstrating an inbuilt protection from overexertion and further tearing at the site of traumatic injury (Maas & Sandercock, 2010).

The shear strains within working muscle are both substantial and diverse and perimysium exists in different thicknesses. Thus perimysium is able to adapt and accommodate these large and shear strains (Purslow, 2010). There is, generally,

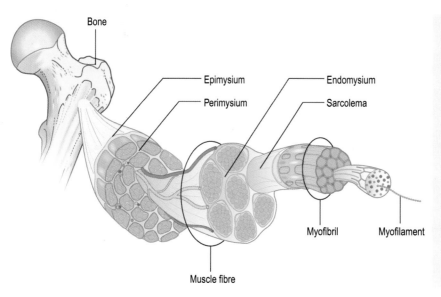

Bone
Epimysium
Perimysium
Endomysium
Sarcolema
Myofibril
Myofilament
Muscle fibre

Figure 2.1
Interrelating anatomical structures contributing to force transmission

a consistency to composition, amount and resulting thickness of endomysium but there are significant differences in the size and shape of muscle fascicles of the perimysium, which is, as a result, up to 50 times thicker than the endomysium (Purslow, 2010).

There are two sizes of fascicles, with small primary fascicles delineated by what is termed primary perimysium, and larger, thicker secondary fascicles that are made up of groups of primary fascicles, organised by secondary perimysium. The perimysial layer is primarily composed of crossed-plies of wavy collagen fibre bundles in a proteoglycan matrix and functions in separating and sharing two adjacent fascicles. This layered and fenestrated network extends across the cross sectional area of the entire muscle. The diameter of collagen fibre bundles are larger in perimysium than endomysium and lie parallel to each other, between 20° to 80° to the muscle fibre axis, at the resting length of any muscle (Purslow, 2010).

In effect, the tensile properties of perimysium and endomysium are similar, with changes in length and diameter causing initial deformation following the contraction or lengthening of antagonistic muscles affecting muscle fibres and fascicles. Very little shear displacement occurs within a fascicle, with most shear deformation occurring at boundaries between fascicles (Purslow, 2010).

It has been postulated that muscle is divided into fascicles to facilitate shear deformations, which allow muscles to change their shape on contraction (Purslow, 2010). This may explain why the perimysium diameter and shape demonstrates such variation across muscles, with thinner perimysium in long strap-like muscles associated with small shear displacements and large perimysial sheets and primary fascicles involved in larger shear displacements. The connective tissue network thus allows for accommodation of a variety in shear strains, whilst maintaining the advantages of the tight shear linkage of endomysium. Whilst the epimysium and perimysium are recognised as complex mechanomolecular pathways for myofascial force transmission, the latter also allows for large slip plane displacements between muscle fascicles to occur during muscular contraction (Purslow, 2010).

When the muscles are at shorter lengths, endomysial collagen fibres are arranged circumferentially, whilst at longer muscle lengths they are more likely to be oriented longitudinally. Irrespective of sarcomere length, a large proportion of collagen fibres are wavy. Accordingly, the soft tissue network is compliant in tension at any appropriate physiological length but can easily deform to track changing muscle lengths in vivo. This is advantageous as provision of protection from overload at high deformations when muscle lengths exceed those of normal function. Once rodent studies had demonstrated that there were myofascial force transmission effects between sarcomeres and the extra-cellular matrix of muscle, in addition to extra-muscular effects on muscle length-force characteristics, any individual muscle could not be considered as a fully independent unit of force generation and movement (Huijing & Baan, 2003) (Masi et al., 2010) (Yucesoy, 2010).

Different levels of organisation are required, from the cellular to the compartmental level, and the extra-cellular matrix structures assist the synergistic skeletal muscles in force transmission throughout the profoundly complex connective tissue linkages described (Maas & Sandercock, 2010) (Masi et al., 2010). In conclusion, muscle should not be seen as being either mechanically independent, or solely responsible for the generation of force and, for 'contraction' to occur, a cascade of multi-cellular events is triggered that ultimately leads to simultaneous forces being exerted upon the skeleton (Huijing et al., 2011).

The evidence for adaptation

Wound healing and 'myofibroblasts'

Connective tissue fibroblasts are dynamically responsive to tissue stretch and mechanical stimuli. Collagen assembly and turnover is the responsibility of the predominant cell type of the tendon, the tenocyte, and its mechanobiology (Benjamin et al., 2008). These specialised fibroblasts are typically arranged in longitudinal rows, and in close proximity to collagen fibrils, surrounded by matrix proteoglycans such as biglycan and fibromodulin. These are involved in the expression of scleraxis, a transcription factor for collagen synthesis and tendon differentiation

(Magnusson et al., 2010). Tenocytes are responsible for secretion of the extracellular matrix and, it has been suggested, that the extent of the collagen synthesis is probably regulated by the strain experienced by these fibroblasts.

Myofibroblasts are specific connective tissue cells that regulate connective tissue remodelling. Their role is reparative for injured tissue, achieved by the combination of the secretion of new extra-cellular matrix-synthesising features of fibroblasts, with cytoskeletal characteristics of contractile smooth muscle cells influencing the exertion of contractile force (Wipff & Hinz, 2009) (Hinz et al., 2012). This is correlated to the degree of a-smooth muscle actin expression (Hinz et al., 2001a). Fibroblasts, chondroblasts and osteoblasts have an innate capacity to express the gene for a-smooth muscle actin and to display contractile behaviour (Spector, 2002). Expression is triggered pathologically, such as in wound healing or through injury, as well as mechanically (Hinz et al., 2007).

There exists a mechanism whereby cell forces and mechanical forces from the extracellular matrix may be translated into biochemical signals by the actions of transmembranous proteins called integrins (Zollner et al., 2012). Mechanical stress causes activation of the pro-fibrotic cytokine transforming growth factor beta (TGF β1) by myofibroblasts as an aspect of their contractile function (Wipff et al., 2007). TGF β1 is synthesised as a protein compound and is secreted by the majority of cell types as part of the large latent complex. Integrins are used by myofibroblasts to transmit stress fibre contraction to the extracellular matrix. They are also used for detection of mechanical change in the microenvironment (Wipff & Hinz, 2009).

Activity of the myofibroblasts should occur to promote adaptation appropriate to the level of stress in their surrounding tissue but excessive activity and extracellular matrix secretion contributes to maladaptation and the retractile phenomenon that characterises the majority of fibrocontractive diseases, such as in heart, liver, kidney, scleredoma, Dupuytren's contractures and hypertrophic scars (Wipff & Hinz, 2009) (Hinz et al., 2007).

Fascia appears to have the ability to actively contract when challenged in periods of mechanical and/or emotional stress. This is mediated by mechanical strain and specific stress related cytokines. Does this just occur in unhealthy or injured tissue? The presence of contractile fibroblasts in normal healthy fascia suggests that the regular expression of the cellular phenotype probably serves a functional purpose, i.e. these cells are, at times, used for smooth muscle-like contractions in addition to the aiding of fascial stiffness (Schleip et al., 2005).

Therefore active cellular contraction of fibroblasts and myofibroblasts contribute, in part, to the strain hardening effect, in addition to changes in the water content of the local fascial tissues (Schleip et al., 2012). A temporary alteration in the tissue matrix may contribute to the fascial tissue stiffness in dense connective tissue areas, such as tendons, joint capsules, ligaments, retinaculae, and aponeuroses.

Influences and effects of the central nervous system

Interaction with connective tissue and the pelvic girdle

The central nervous system is consistently sampling the internal and external environments, interpreting the contemporary and immediate status of stability and movement, as well as planning for predictable tasks. It needs to be able to manage and cope with unpredictable loads and challenges (Hodges & Mosley, 2003). An examination of the fascial characteristics to local and stability challenges affecting lumbo-pelvic 'stability' and pelvic girdle or low back pain is instructive and beneficial in how the central nervous system interacts for optimum motor control. The key role that the pelvis plays, as the link between the trunk and lower limbs, needs to be acknowledged (Cusi, 2010), as does the fact that pelvic girdle or sacro-iliac incompetence can have a correlation with low back pain, injury, incontinence and breathing issues.

The neuromotor control of the fascial tension depends on the passive and active tensioning of muscles with direct attachments (transversus abdominis) and those that are enclosed in fascia such as erector spinae and multifidus. Central nervous system independent, thereby passive, resting tension present in the myofascial system provides postural stability (Masi et al., 2010). Lumbar multifidus has been described as having passive stiffness properties and fascial interrelationships that contribute to its functionality in lumbar and postural stability.

Intersegmental control is augmented by LaPlace's Law of Hoop Tension comprising the radius of the abdomen and increased intra-abdominal pressure. However it also increases bladder pressure and presents a challenge to continence as striated urethral activity increases proportionally with intra-abdominal pressure (Stafford et al., 2012).

For a satisfactory contribution to stability, intra-abdominal pressure depends on the floor of the pelvic canister being competent so it is easy to see the relationship between respiration and continence to the static maintenance of posture in addition to the dynamic control of movement. Transversus abdominis never switches off and, critically, is involved with the fascial system in anticipation and pre-activation, such as peripheral unilateral movements of arm raising or leg movement.

Sacro-iliac joint stabilisation is enhanced by the specific extensive myofascial contributions to force closure and ligamentous tensioning, for example, the sacrotuberous (van Wingerden et al., 2004). Force closure has been defined as 'the effect of changing joint reaction forces generated by tension in ligaments, fasciae and muscles and ground reaction forces' in order to overcome the forces of gravity by the provision of strong compression (Cusi, 2010).

Evidence of beneficial force transmission exists in the extensive connections of the gluteus maximus, biceps femoris, latissimus dorsi, paraspinal muscles, transversus abdominis/internal oblique aponeurosis and the thoracolumbar fascia (Carvalhais et al., 2013). The thoracolumbar fascia is critical to the integrity of the inferior lumbar spine and sacro-iliac joint. This is particularly due to its three-dimensional structure, which is built out of 'aponeurotic and fascial planes uniting together to surround the paraspinal muscles and stabilise the lumbosacral spine' (Willard et al., 2012).

This has been experimentally demonstrated in vivo by a study showing definitive myofascial transmission from the latissimus dorsi to

contralateral gluteus maximus on the opposite side of the body through the thoracolumbar fascia (Chapter 1). The dynamics of myofascial activity, along with the structural quality and integrity, unquestionably influence the pelvic girdle as well as lumbar stability and stiffness. This appears critical to movement function, as the sacro-iliac joints are essential for effective load transfer between the spine and limbs via these functional interactions and slings (Cusi, 2010) (Vleeming et al., 2012).

The antero-lateral abdominal muscles, attached to the thoracolumbar fascia, have been implicated in spinal stabilisation (Hodges et al., 1996, 2003) (Hodges & Richardson, 1997) (Hides et al., 2011) with alterations in activation patterns present in lumbopelvic pain (Hodges & Richardson, 1996) (Hungerford et al., 2003). The tension across the lateral raphe and thoracolumbar fascia is part of the complex interactive mechanism of load transfer in the lumbopelvic region, with muscles transmitting forces longitudinally and adjacently via endomysial connections (Huijing, 2007). Thus the increased regional fascial density, receiving direct and indirect muscular force transmission, allied to active fascial contraction, across the extracellular matrix significantly enhances local and global stability.

Brown & McGill (2009) report rodent studies showing that even when the transversus abdominis aponeurosis was cut, meaning that an anticipated route of force transmission was severed, effective force percentages of original 'muscle' output could still be generated: the connective tissues were demonstrated to transfer the vast majority (73%) of force and stiffness! This astonishing degree of efficient transmission is credited to the three sheet-like muscles of the obliques and transversus abdominis being so tightly bound together through their attachments of complex connective tissue. This must be considered as contributory to the effective stabilisation of the spinal column, enhancing local musculature to work synergistically.

The structure of the tissue not only implies there is significant linkage between muscle and fascia but also that there is optimisation of fascia due to local composition. A fat-filled lumbar interfascial triangle is described along the lateral border of the paraspinal muscles, from the 12th rib to the iliac crest, as a result of the unification of fascial sheaths along the lateral border of the thoraco-lumbar fascia. This ridged-union of dense connective tissue has been previously portrayed as the lateral raphe, initially coined by Bogduk & Mackintosh in 1984. The function of the lumbar interfascial triangle may be to minimise fascial friction between adjacent fasciae under tension, to accommodate lateral expansion of paraspinal muscles when contracting or, as has recently been suggested, to act as a fulcrum to distribute laterally mediated tension to 'balance different viscoelastic moduli along either the middle or posterior layers of the thoracolumbar fascia' (Schuenke et al., 2012).

Hoffman & Gabel (2013) propose an updated model to the classic Punjabi model of stability from 1992, with fascia contributing to the six proposed subsytems presented. It is suggested that a breakdown in any of the individual subsytems will inevitably result in movement impairment, regardless of the cause and irrespective of stability or mobility, whether passive, active or neutral. This is a progression of original ideas derived from experimentally induced pain leading to altered activation timings, which affected stability and mobility muscles (Hodges & Moseley, 2003).

A controlled study showed that there is a significant loss of local proprioception in low back pain subjects (Taimela et al., 1999). Without the sensory feedback from mechanoreceptors situated in broad fascial sheets as well as arthrogenic and ligamentous mechanoreceptors, neuromuscular coordination can be impaired.

Multi-segmental innervation patterns might exist offering potential therapeutic solutions to back pain, the fitness of myofascial regions and rehabilitative exercise (Schuenke et al., 2012). The linkage of connective tissues with the muscular, respiratory and urinary-continent systems can promote a more synergistic and unified mechanical stabilising system for the promotion of trunk control. The challenges of sport, disease, or habitual improper functioning of these interrelated systems can injuriously affect the multifaceted movement patterns and postural control mechanisms.

Clinical summary

- Muscular force is transmitted by complex pathways via endo-, peri- and epimysial fasciae.
- Resident connective tissue cells are responsive to mechanical stress and are readily adaptive. Exercise stimulation can therefore influence the metabolic and contractile behavior of these cells.
- Intersegmental stability – such as in dynamic trunk/core stability – involves adequate fascial architecture and adequate fascial force transmission.

References

Benjamin, M., Kaiser, E. & Milz, S. (2008) Structure-function relationships in tendons: a review. *J Anat.* 212: 211–228.

Brown, S.H. & McGill, S.M. (2009) Transmission of muscularly generated force and stiffness between layers of the rat abdominal wall. *Spine* 15; 34(2): 70–75.

Carvalhais, V.O.D., Ocarino, Jde, M., Araujo, V.L., Souza, T.R., Silva, P.L. & Fonseca, S.T. (2013) Myofascial force transmission between the latissimus dorsi and gluteus maximus muscles: An in vivo experiment. *J Biomech.* 46: 1003–1007.

Chaitow, L. (2013) Understanding mechanotransduction and biotensegrity from an adaptation perspective. *J Bodyw Mov Ther.* 17: 141–142.

Corey, S.M., Vizzard, M.A., Bouffard, N.A., Badger, G.J. & Langevin, H.M. (2012) Stretching of the Back Improves Gait, Mechanical Sensitivity and Connective Tissue Inflammation in a Rodent Model. *PLoS ONE* 7(1): 1–8.

Cusi, M.F. (2010) Paradigm for assessment and treatment of SIJ mechanical dysfunction. *J Bodyw Mov Ther.* 14: 152–161.

Hides, J., Stanton, W., Mendis, M.D. & Sexton, M. (2011) The relationship of transversus abdominis and lumbar multifidus clinical muscle tests in patients with chronic low back pain. *Man Ther.* 16: 573–577.

Hinz, B., Celetta, G., Tomasek, J.J., Gabbiani, G. & Chaponnier, C. (2001a) Smooth muscle actin expression upregulates fibroblast contractile activity. *Mol Biol Cell.* 12: 2730–2734.

Hinz, B. Phan, S.H., Thannickal, V.J., Galli, A., Bochaton-Piallat, M.L., Gabbiani, G. (2007) Biological Perspectives. The Myofibroblast. One Function, Multiple Origins. *Am J Pathol.* 170(6): 1807–1819.

Hinz, B., Phan, S.H., Thannickal, V.J., Prunotto, M., Desmoulière, A., Varga, J., De Wever, O., Mareel, M. & Gabbiani, G. (2012) Recent Developments in Myofibroblast

Biology: Paradigms for Connective Tissue Remodeling. *Am J Pathol.* 180(4): 1340–1355.

Hodges, P.W. & Moseley, G.L. (2003) Pain and motor control of the lumbopelvic region: effect and possible mechanisms. *J Electromyogr Kinesiol.* 13(4): 361–370.

Hodges, P.W. & Richardson, C.A. (1996) Inefficient muscular stabilization of the lumbar spine associated with low back pain. A motor control evaluation of transversus abdominis. *Spine* 21: 2640–2650.

Hodges, P.W. & Richardson, C.A. (1997) Contraction of the abdominal muscles associated with movement of the lower limb. *Phys Ther.* 77: 132–142.

Hodges, P.W., Richardson, C.A. & Jull, G. (1996) Evaluation of the relationship between laboratory and clinical tests of transversus abdominis function. *Physiother Res Int.* 1: 30–40.

Hodges, P.W., Holm, A.K., Holm, S., Ekstrom, L., Cresswell, A., Hansson, T. & Thorstensson, A. (2003) Intervertebral stiffness of the spine is increased by evoked contraction of transversus abdominis and the diaphragm: in vivo porcine studies. *Spine.* 28: 2594–2601.

Hoffman, J. & Gabel, P. (2013) Expanding Panjabi's stability model to express movement: A theoretical model. *Med Hypotheses* Apr. 1–5.

Huijing, P.A. & Baan, G.C. (2003) Myofascial force transmission: muscle relative position and length determine agonist and synergist muscle force. *J Appl Physiol.* 94: 1092–1107.

Huijing, P.A., Yaman, A., Ozturk, C. & Yucesoy, C.A. (2011) Effects of knee angle on global and local strains within human triceps surae muscle: MRI analysis indicating in vivo myofascial force transmission between synergistic muscles. *Surg Radiol Anat.* 33(10): 869–879.

Hungerford, B., Gilleard, W. & Hodges, P. (2003) Evidence of altered lumbopelvic muscle recruitment in the presence of sacroiliac joint pain. *Spine* 28: 1593–1600.

Khan, K.M. & Scott, A. (2009) Mechanotherapy: how physical therapists' prescription of exercise promotes tissue repair. *Br J Sports Med.* 43: 247–252.

Kim, A.C. & Spector, M. (2000) Distribution of chondrocytes containing α-smooth muscle actin in human articular cartilage. *J. Orthop. Res.* 18(5): 749–755.

Langevin, H.M., Bouffard, N.A., Badger, G.J., Iatridis, J.C. & Howe, A.K. (2005) Dynamic fibroblast cytoskeletal response to subcutaneous tissue stretch ex vivo and in vivo. *Am J Physiol Cell Physiol.* 288: C747–C756.

Maas, H. & Sandercock, T.G. (2010) Force Transmission between Synergistic Skeletal Muscles through Connective Tissue Linkages. *J Biom Biotechnol.* 1–9.

Magnusson, S.P., Langberg, H. & Kjaer, M. (2010) The pathogenesis of tendinopathy: balancing the response to loading. *Nat Rev Rheumatol.* 6: 262–268.

Masi, A.T., Nair, K., Evans, T. & Ghandour, Y. (2010) Clinical, biomechanical, and physiological translational interpretations of human resting myofascial tone or tension. *Int J Ther Massage Bodywork* 3(4): 16–28.

Purslow, P. (2010) Muscle fascia and force transmission. *J Bodyw Mov Ther.* 14: 411–417.

Schleip, R., Klingler, W. & Lehmann-Horn, F. (2005) Active fascial contractility: Fascia may be able to contract in a smooth muscle-like manner and thereby influence musculoskeletal dynamics. *Med Hypotheses* 65: 273–277.

Schleip, R., Duerselen L., Vleeming A., Naylor, I.L., Lehmann–Horn, F., Zorn, A., Jaeger, H. & Klingler, W. (2012) Strain hardening of fascia: static stretching of dense fibrous connective tissues can induce a temporary stiffness increase accompanied by enhanced matrix hydration. *J Bodyw Mov Ther.* 16: 94–100.

Schuenke, M.D., Vleeming, A., Van Hoof, T. & Willard, F.H. (2012) A description of the lumbar interfascial triangle and its relation with the lateral raphe: anatomical constituents of load transfer through the lateral margin of the thoracolumbar fascia. *J Anat.* 221(6): 568–576.

Spector, M. (2002) Musculoskeletal connective tissue cells with muscle: expression of muscle actin in and contraction of fibroblasts, chondrocytes, and osteoblasts. *Wound Repair Regen.* 9(1): 11–8.

Stafford, R.E., Ashton-Miller, J.A., Sapsford, R. & Hodges, P.W. (2012) Activation of the striated urethral sphincter to maintain continence during dynamic tasks in healthy men. *Neurourol Urodyn.* 31(1): 36–3.

Stecco, C. & Day, J.A. (2010) The Fascial Manipulation Technique and Its Biomechanical Model: A Guide to the Human Fascial System. *Int J Ther Massage Bodywork* 3(1): 38–40.

Taimela, S., Kankaanpaa, M. & Luoto, S. (1999) The effect of lumbar fatigue on the ability to sense a change in lumbar position. A controlled study. *Spine.* 24: 1322–1327.

Tesarz, J., Hoheisel, U., Wiedenhofer, B. & Mense, S. (2011) Sensory innervation of the thoracolumbar fascia in rats and humans. *Neuroscience* 194: 302–308.

Van der Waal, J. (2009) The Architecture of the Connective Tissue in the Musculoskeletal System—An Often Overlooked Functional Parameter as to Proprioception in the Locomotor Apparatus. *Int J Ther Massage Bodywork* 2(4): 9–23.

Van Wingerden, J.P., Vleeming, A., Buyruk, H.M. & Raissadat, K. (2004) Stabilization of the sacroiliac joint in vivo: verification of muscular contribution to force closure of the pelvis. *Eur Spine J.* 13: 199–205.

Willard, F.H., Vleeming, A., Schuenke, M.D., Danneels, L. & Schleip, R. (2012) The thoracolumbar fascia: anatomy, function and clinical considerations. *J Anat.* 221(6): 507–536.

Wipff, P-J. & Hinz, B. (2009) Myofibroblasts work best under stress. *J Bodyw Mov Ther.* 13(2): 121–127.

Wipff, P.J., Rifkin, D.B., Meister J.J. & Hinz B. (2007). Myofibroblast contraction activates latent TGF- 1 from the extracellular matrix. *J Cell Biol.* 179: 1311 – 1323.

Yucesoy, C.A. (2010) Epimuscular myofascial force transmission implies novel principles for muscular mechanics. *Exerc Sport Sci Rev.* 38(3): 128–134.

Yucesoy, C.A., Koopman, B.H.F.J.M., Baan, G.C., Grootenboer, H.J. & Huijing, P.A. (2003a) Extramuscular myofascial force transmission: experiments and finite element modeling. *Arch Physiol Biochem.*111(4): 377–388.

Yucesoy, C.A., Koopman, B.H.F.J.M., Baan, G.C., Grootenboer, H.J. & Huijing, P.A. (2003b) Effects of inter- and extramuscular myofascial force transmission on adjacent synergistic muscles: assessment by experiments and finite-element modeling. *J Biomech.* 36(12): 1797–1811.

Zollner, A.M., Tepole, A.B. & Kuhl, E. (2012) On the biomechanics and mechanobiology on growing skin. *J Theor Biol.* 297: 166–175.

Further reading

Arampatzis, A. (2010) Plasticity of human Achilles tendon mechanical and morphological properties in response to cyclic strain. *J Biomech.* 43: 3073–3079.

Barker, P., Briggs, C.A. & Bogeski, G. (2004) Tensile transmission across the lumbar fasciae in unembalmed cadavers: effects of tension to various muscular attachments. *Spine.* 29(2): 129–138.

Benjamin, M. (2009) The fascia of the limbs and back – a review. *J Anat.* 214: 1–18.

Bogduk, N. & MacIntosh, J.E. (1984) The applied anatomy of the thoracolumbar fascia. *Spine* 9: 164–170.

Chaudhry, H., Schleip, R., Ji, Z., Bukiet, B., Maney, M. & Findley, T. (2008) Three-dimensional mathematical model for deformation of human fasciae in manual therapy. *J Am Osteopath Assoc.* 108(8): 379–390

DellaGrotte, J., Ridi, R., Landi, M. & Stephens, J. (2008) Postural improvement using core integration to lengthen myofascia. *J Bodyw Mov Ther.* 12: 231–245.

Fukashiro, S., Hay, D.C. & Nagano, A. (2006) Biomechanical behavior of muscle-tendon complex during dynamic human movements. *J Appl Biomech.* 22(2): 131–147.

Fukunaga, T., Kawakami, Y., Kubo, K., Kanehisa, H. (2002) Muscle and tendon interaction during human movements. *Exercise Sport Sci R.* 30(3): 106–110.

Hashemirad, F., Talebian, S., Olyaei, G. & Hatef, B. (2010) Compensatory behaviour of the postural control system to flexion-relaxation phenomena. *J Bodyw Mov Ther.* 14(2): 418–423.

Hinz, B. & Gabbiani, G. (2003) Mechanisms of force generation and transmission by myofibroblasts. *Curr Opin Biotechnol.* 14: 538–546.

Hinz, B. (2010) The myofibroblast: paradigm for a mechanically active cell. *J Biomech.* 43: 146–155.

Hinz, B., Phan, S.H., Thannickal, V.J., Prunotto, M., Desmoulière, A., Varga, J., De Wever, O., Mareel, M. & Gabbiani, G. (2012) Recent Developments in Myofibroblast Biology: Paradigms for Connective Tissue Remodeling. *Am J Pathol.* 180(4): 1340–1355.

Huijing, P.A. & Baan, G.C. (2003) Myofascial force transmission: muscle relative position and length determine agonist and synergist muscle force. *J Appl Physiol.* 94: 1092–1107.

Huijing, P.A. (2007) Epimuscular myofascial force transmission between antagonistic and synergistic muscles can explain movement limitation in spastic paresis. *J Electromyogr Kinesiol.* 17: 708–724.

Ianuzzi, A., Pickar, J.G. & Khalsa, P.S. (2011) Relationships between joint motion and facet joint capsule strain during cat and human lumbar spinal motions. *JPMT.* 34: 420–431.

Kawakami, Y. (2012) Morphological and functional characteristics of the muscle-tendon unit. *J Phys Fit Sports Med.* 1(2): 287–296.

Killian, M.L., Cavinatto, L., Galatz, L.M. & Thomopoulos, S. 2012. The role of mechanobiology in tendon healing. *J Shoulder Elbow Surg.* 21(2): 228–37.

Kjaer, M., Langberg, H., Heinemeier, K., Bayer, M.L., Hansen, M., Holm, L., Doessing, S., Konsgaard, M., Krogsgaard, M.R. & Magnusson, S.P. (2009) From mechanical loading to collagen synthesis, structural changes and function in human tendon. *Scand. J. Med. Sci. Sports.* 19(4): 500–510.

Moseley, G.L., Zalucki, N.M. & Wiech, K. (2008) Tactile discrimination, but not tactile stimulation alone, reduces chronic limb pain. *Pain*, 137: 600–608.

Myers, T. (2001) *The Anatomy Trains.* Churchill Livingstone.

Sawicki, G.S., Lewis, C.L. & Ferris, D.P. (2009) It pays to have a spring in your step. *Exerc Sport Sci Rev.* July, 37(3): 130.

Schleip, R. & Klingler, W. (2007) Fascial strain hardening correlates with matrix hydration changes. In: Findley, T.W., Schleip, R. (Eds.), *Fascia research – basic science and implications to conventional and complementary health care.* Munich: Elsevier GmbH, 51.

Schleip, R. & Müller, D.G. (2012) Training principles for fascial connective tissues: Scientific foundation and suggested practical applications. *J Bodyw Mov Ther.* 1–13.

Stecco, C., Porzionato, A., Lancerotto, L., Stecco, A., Macchi, V., Day, J.A. & De Caro, R. (2008) Histological study of the deep fasciae of the limbs. *J Bodyw Mov Ther.* 12: 225–230.

Vleeming, A., Schuenke, M.D., Masi, A.T., Carreiro, J.E. Danneels, L. & Willard, F.H. (2012) The sacroiliac joint: an overview of its anatomy, function and potential clinical implications. *J Anat.* 221(6): 537–567.

Vleeming, A., Snijders, C., Stoeckart, R. & Mens, J. (1997) The role of the sacroiliac joins in coupling between spine, pelvis, legs and arms. In: Vleeming et al. (Eds.), *Movement, Stability & Low Back Pain.* Churchill Livingstone, 53–71.

Wallden, M. (2010) Chains, trains and contractile fields. *J Bodyw Mov Ther.* 14: 403–410.

CHAPTER 3

Physiology and biochemistry

Werner Klingler

Myofascial tissue is composed of cellular and non-cellular elements. Both components are sensitive to physical strain, temperature, pH and humoral factors. This chapter describes the physiological and biochemical properties of fascial tissue, as well as the interaction with connected tissue, most notably skeletal muscle. Knowledge of underlying neurophysiological pathways is indispensable because 'you can't depend on your eyes when your imagination is out of focus' (Mark Twain, 1889).

Neurophysiological fundamentals

Movement, first and foremost in sport, involves a sophisticated interaction of the central and peripheral central nervous system, force-generating muscle and connective tissues, such as fascia, which is intrinsically tied to skeletal muscle.

Upper and lower motor neuron

The protocol of a movement (engram) is generated in the motor cortex of the brain. The electrical impulses originating from pyramidal neurons propagate along their axons, crossing over to the contralateral side at the brain stem level. This is the reason why the left hemisphere of the brain controls the right side of the body. In most cases, the left hemisphere is dominant. This fact is proven not only in right-handed people but, surprisingly, also in the vast majority of left-handed individuals. Aside from the brain, left predominance is also found in other matched organs like kidneys or testicles, which are slightly bigger on the left side. The heart is also localised on the left. Why the body is asymmetrically in favour of the left side is unknown.

The pyramidal tract carries information from the brain to the spinal cord and includes the systematic denomination corticospinal tract or upper motor neurons. The signal from the upper motor neuron is then transmitted in the anterior horn of the spinal cord to the lower motor neuron, which finally carries the information to the skeletal muscle (Figure 3.1). By definition, an injury of the upper motoneuron leads to a spastic palsy due to disinhibition of motor reflexes. In contrast, loss of peripheral nerve function, lower motoneuron lesion, results in flaccid paralysis. Connective tissue reacts to such disturbances of the reflex circuit in due course. For example, after injury to upper motor neurons, such as in a stroke or spinal chord injury, there is significant fascial stiffening which in some cases may require surgical relief. In a nutshell, exactly two nerve cells, including their long axons, carry the motor information from the brain to the muscle. On the sensory side, three nerve cells are assembled. The peripheral sensory neuron is switched to the central part in the dorsal horn of the spinal cord. The central part of the sensory system is composed of two neurons that are interconnected at a nut-like part of the brain, the thalamus. The thalamus is located at the centre of the brain and is also known as 'the door to consciousness'.

Extrapyramidal movement coordination

This directly addressable and mechanistic system of motor control is subject to a variety of influences and modifications, which collectively are known as the extrapyramidal motor system. Important anatomical components of the extrapyramidal motor system are the basal ganglia, the cerebellum and numerous interneurons, which interconnect pyramidal axons recursively, side by side and with brain nuclei. The extrapyramidal system is designed to enhance or hamper signal

Interestingly, other inputs converging in the thalamic nuclei also influence the extrapyramidal movement coordination. Here, important factors are emotion and pain. Emotion is thought to be generated by a circular flow of electrical impulses along a set of anatomical brain structures known as the limbic system. Furthermore, the limbic system is a key element for memory, olfaction and evolutionary survival. It includes several anatomical brain structures, notably interfering with the thalamic nuclei and thereby giving one explanation as to why emotional state can influence movements and vice versa. In this context, it is interesting that regular sport activity improves learning, reduces the probability for dementia and significantly prolongs life expectancy.

Another pathway can be found in cerebral hormones, which mostly have multiple functions. Dopamine and serotonin are key promoters for movement but also for happiness. This coherence can be observed, for example, in patients with psychiatric mania, who are restlessly in motion until they are treated with neuroleptic drugs, i.e. dopamin-antagonists. Then, rather robotic movements may be observed. On the positive side, good mood is often associated with physical activity, such as dancing. Another example is the need for movement in children, especially as an expression of happiness. Direct effects of these hormones on fascial tissue have only been shown indirectly so far. For example, long-term medication with potent dopamine-agonists leads to fibrosis in the lungs and around the kidneys as well as thickening and stiffening of cardiac valves (Antonini & Poewe, 2007).

Pain is a complex topic involving humoral factors, peripheral nervous structures and higher brain centres, e.g. thalamic nuclei. Briefly, fascia contains numerous nociceptors, such as free nerve endings. In contrast to the aforementioned somatosensory neurons that have conduction speeds in the order of 10-100 m/s, the 'so-called' C-fibres are not surrounded by a myelin sheat and, therefore, conduct impulses more slowly, at roughly 0.5 to 2 m/s. The resulting pain sensation is dull and less localised. Nerve endings whose stimulation triggers pain sensations are called nociceptors. These nerve endings are linked to the autonomic nervous system. Irritation and

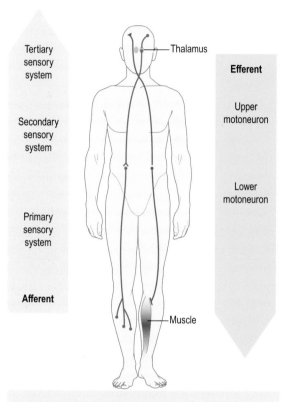

Figure 3.1

Basic neuronal elements of movement control

Exactly two efferent nerve cells, upper and lower motor neuron, conduct specific movement information encoded as action potential frequency to the target organ, i.e. skeletal muscle. On the sensory side, there are three neurons interconnected. The extrapyramidal system integrates information such as optic, acoustic and sensory input and modulates the efferent coricospinal tract, i.e. the upper motoneuron. A major component of the extrapyramidal motor system is the thalamic nuclei. Formation of the peripheral nerve plexus is not shown in this sketch.

transduction. It assesses afferent signals, such as the aforementioned somatosensory input, and computes the necessary amplification factor. In this way, the extrapyramidal system coordinates and fine-tunes movements (Chaitow & DeLany 2000). A loss of function of this system, e.g. in Parkinson's disease, leads to a very specific akinetic and rigid movement disorder.

coupling of sympathetic fibres is one mechanism for the development of chronic pain, such as in the so-called Complex Regional Pain Syndrome (also called Sudeck's disease). Moreover, neurons containing substance P or calcitonin-gene related peptide have been found in fascia. Both humoral mediators are associated with chronic and self-sustaining pain (Tesarz et al., 2011) (Chapter 4).

Muscle and fascia – a dream team

Skeletal muscle is composed of myofibres, which develop as a merger of several single muscle cells via multiple cell fusions. Microscopically, myofibres are readily identifiable by regular arrangement of the contractile proteins. The subcellular contractile units are called sarcomeres, in which effective force generation requires optimum interdigitation of actin and myosin filaments. Experiments have shown that, after surgical excision of a muscle bundle, the elastic fibres shrink by roughly one third of their length in vivo. Therefore, force registration measurements in a laboratory cell-dish environment require an experimental pre-stretching of the bundle.

For efficient contraction development, this pre-stretch may be dynamically regulated in the body by fascial tissue. Depending on the cross-link tension, hydration, elastic content and even active fascial contraction, the strain on myofibres can be regulated in order to intensify or weaken muscular force generation. In other words, fascia acts as an energy-saving and intelligent servo-mechanism.

Myofascial tone

Muscle tone is a feature that is regularly assessed by a broad variety of medical professionals. However, diagnosis is based on the experience of the examiner, as reference standards are lacking for symptoms like body aches or subjective stiffness. Manually assessed elevations in muscle tone is also often attributed to postural pain syndromes. Semantically it is more precise to use the term 'myofascial tone' because the tensional properties originate not only from the muscle tissue itself but also from the fascial tissue, such as the epi-, peri- and endomysium.

Interestingly, the amount of connective tissue found in a specific muscle is dependent on its function. Tonic muscle contains significantly more and firmer fascial components than phasic muscle. Differences are also found between species. Meat from mountain goats has a much higher percentage of collagenous connective tissue compared to domestic pigs, for example. In hereditary muscle diseases, fibrosis is one of the most prominent features and may even be the first symptom of the disease. Therapeutic efforts aim to reduce the fibrosis in muscle disease, such as Duchenne myopathy. Here, corticosteroids are effective inhibitors of fibroblast proliferation and collagen synthesis. Corticosteroid treatment then significantly postpones the onset of disability, in relation to walking. Due to the adverse effects of high corticosteroid doses, alternative treatment options are currently being explored with management of such pathologies (Klingler et al., 2012). In summary, the contribution of fascia and myofibres to muscle tone is highly variable and adaptive to external and internal factors.

Resting tone

What is **resting** myofascial tone? This question is not trivial and will be addressed in the following paragraph. By definition, resting muscle tone is electrically silent. This means that the voluntary innervation is zero and the reflex circuit is quiescent. In theory, this is a clear condition and should be easy to assess by examining a resting muscle in terms of resistance to passive movement and firmness of the tissue (Masi & Hannon, 2008). However, from a practical point of view, it can be observed that in awake and even sleeping subjects resting muscle is far from being electrically silent. In most patients who undergo electromyography (EMG), a neural activity in the muscle tissue can be seen, even if the muscle is voluntarily slack. Indeed, the creaky sound of the EMG-device can be used as a biofeedback method in order to calm and relax the subject. Another problem during clinical examination is that many people tend to innervate ('unconscious helping') the muscle/limb under investigation or suffer from disinhibition of monosynaptic reflexes, for example, in encephalomyelitis disseminata, stroke or other pathologies of the central nervous system. A long-term neuronal overstimulation leads to a fascial remodeling, increase of collagen fibres and more rigid and less hydrated connective fascial tissue. From a purpose or function oriented point of view, fascial hypertrophy is not only a compensation for muscle overstimulation but also a reaction to inflammatory processes. This fits with altered tissue microperfusion, hydration and nutrition.

A complete inhibition of innervation can be observed during general anaesthesia in the hospital. Here, neuromuscular blocking agents are used for induction and tracheal intubation. For training purposes, it is helpful for any movement professional to visit an operating theatre and get an impression of the effect of a complete neuromuscular block on myofascial tissue.

Physical strain

Experiments on isolated fascia specimens show that repetitive stretch leads to changes in peak force and stiffness. This feature of fascial tissue has been described as strain hardening. This effect also occurs after pre-treatment with deep freezing and rapid thawing. In this way, cellular components were reliably devitalised. This is a strong indication that strain hardening is not caused by active cellular contraction of fibroblasts/myofibroblasts. Additional investigations reveal that the same protocol leads to an enhanced tissue hydration accompanying the increase in tissue stiffness. Hence, strain hardening is probably caused, at least partially, by temporarily enhanced matrix hydration. The clinical implications are considered as enhanced load transfer promoting a more direct muscle, tendon interaction (Schleip et al., 2012).

Stretching is a controversial debate in sports science. For fascial tissue it can be stated that stretching immediately before exercise increases the range of motion possibly by influencing tissue hydration and fibre alignment. This might be helpful in sports such as swimming, for example in front crawl. Here, optimum propulsion significantly depends on the leverage produced by elongation of the shoulder and arm. Other sports, such as hurdling may benefit from firm fascial structures because of more direct force transmission and reduction of ground contact time.

Cellular components also react to physical strain. Fibroblasts are involved in remodelling fascial tissue. Fibroblasts can express contractile proteins under special conditions such as mechanical or chemical stimuli (Figure 3.3). Several growth factors are expressed in response to mechanical loading. Examples are transforming growth factor-β1 (TGF-β1), insulin-like growth factor-I (IGF-I) and connective tissue growth factor (CTGF). These factors induce proliferation of fibroblasts, myofibroblasts and synthesis of collagenous fibres (Table 3.1). These processes are similar to those found in skin wound healing (Klingler et al., 2012).

Factors influencing the fascial system	Example	Clinical impact
upper motor neuron	injury in stroke	spastic palsy
lower motor neuron	injury in herniated lumbar disc	flaccid palsy
extrapyramidal system	Parkinson syndrome	rigid, hypokinetic movement disorder
cerebral hormones	serotonine, dopamine	mood, need for movement
microenvironmental conditions	pH, temperature, hydration	effects on extracellular matrix and (myo)fibroblasts
humoral factors	Transforming growth factor-β1 (TGF-β1), connective tissue growth factor (CTGF), relaxin, interleukins, cortisol	effects on extracellular matrix and (myo)fibroblasts
physical strain	sporting activity, stretching	effects on all discussed levels

Table 3.1

Factors influencing the fascial system

Temperature

Temperature is highly variable in myofascial tissue and unevenly distributed throughout the body. Biological reactions obey the logarithmic Arrhenius law. In other words, temperature is a main determinant for allocation of myofascial tonus. The core temperature is regulated between 36.5 and 38.5°C. Outside the core body, temperature greatly depends on environmental conditions and muscle activity. At rest, a limb can cool down to roughly 30°C whereas during sports 40°C can be reached. Higher temperatures, in fever or sustained exercise for example, increase metabolism roughly 10–20% per degree Celsius. Contraction in skeletal muscle is solely dependent on calcium release from internal stores, the so-called sarcoplasmic reticulum. Calcium unmasks the binding site of the contractile enzyme myosin, which is a temperature dependent ATPase. ATP is replenished by cellular respiration and glycolysis. In turn, these biochemical reactions lead to accumulation of the metabolite lactate, which promotes the synthesis of growth factors and collagen (see below).

Higher temperatures lead to enhanced excitability and calcium turnover of muscle cells. On excised myofibres an increased basal tension as well as increased twitch force can be observed. Interestingly, the fascial components show a different reaction to temperature changes. Fascia shows a higher peak force and stiffness in cold conditions. In other words, an important fascial feature is heat relaxation (Mason & Rigby, 1963), (Muraoka et al., 2008).

At first glance the different temperature characteristics of muscle fibres and fascial tissue seems conflicting. However, the opposite is true. Under resting, i.e. cool conditions, the viscoelastic properties of fascial tissue are adapted to serve stabilisation and load bearing function (Figure 3.2). When myofascial tissue is warmed up, i.e. during sports, fascia shows heat relaxation allowing an expansion of range of movement. Lower temperature induced fascial relaxation can promote injuries in some instances, which is attributed to more rigid tissue response. On the other hand, this strongly depends on the degree and type of tissue stress.

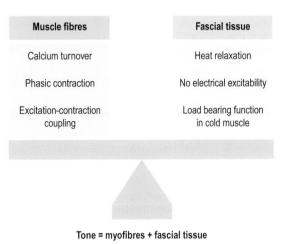

Figure 3.2
Temperature balance

During physical activity the temperature in myofascial structures outside the body core can increase by up to 10°C. Warmth leads to enhanced skeletal muscle excitability, faster contraction and relaxation parameters, as well as increased force generation. This effect is mainly caused by an increased calcium turnover and temperature-induced facilitation of enzymatic processes promoting contractile activity. In fascial tissue, however, higher temperature leads to heat relaxation and reduced myofascial stiffness in vitro. Given, that there is no voluntary innervation, this effect can also be observed in vivo. The lesson we learn from the differential temperature effects on fasciae and myofibrils also helps us to understand passive muscle tone. At rest, i.e. in cold conditions, there is an augmentation of the load bearing function of fascial tissue whereas in sports, temperatures of more than 41°C are reached, allowing fascial release and increase of range of motion.

Tissue pH and lactic acid

Tissue pH

pH (*potentia Hydrogenii*) is an indicator for acidic or alkaline conditions. It is tightly regulated in all biological systems because it is a key element of all organic processes in the body, such as oxygen uptake, coagulation and immune response. A pH-optimum is necessary for effective enzymatic function. pH values below 7.35 indicate a high concentration of protons (H$^+$ ions), i.e. acidic conditions. Vice versa, blood pH values above 7.45 are defined as alkalosis. Potassium is an ion, which can penetrate the lipid bilayer of cell membranes and, therefore, serves as a counterion to protons. In other words potassium concentration increases with dropping pH.

Physical exercise leads to a drop in myofascial tissue pH caused by a production of lactate and carbon dioxide, due to glycolysis and the cellular respiratory chain. Acidic metabolites accumulate and are exhaled by the lungs as carbonic acid and more slowly excreted by the kidneys. To a lesser extent, acids are egested by the skin, liver and bowels. Deeper breathing after exercise is not only necessary for replenishment of oxygen but also for elimination of carbonic acid. Abnormal chronic breathing patterns, which influence pH-regulation may also have an impact on myofascial tissue (Chaitow, 2007). Muscle activation can lead to tissue acidosis, as can inflammations of various causes, be it traumatic, infectious or autoimmune.

Lactate

Lactate plays a major role in tissue regeneration not only because it promotes blood perfusion and exchange of nutrients but also because of its effects on collagen synthesis and angiogenesis.

In vitro data show that acidic conditions enhance contractility of myofibroblasts (Pipelzadeh & Naylor IL, 1998). This feature is important in tissue repair. The opposite effects can be observed in skeletal muscle fibres. Here, increasing concentrations of protons, potassium and lactate reduce contractility and mediate fatigue by inhibition of membrane excitability and the enzymatic activity of the myosin ATPase, as well as reduction of the glycolytic rate and calcium turnover (Gladden, 2004).

Lactate concentration is increased nearly 2-fold in healing of Achilles tendon rupture, indicating a key factor of the metabolic response after tissue damage (Greve et al., 2012). Lactate has been shown to stimulate vascular endothelial growth factor (VEGF) production. Furthermore, it induces myofibroblast differentiation via pH-dependent activation of transforming growth factor-β(TGF-β), which has been shown in lung fibrosis. The authors, therefore, speculate that acidotic microenvironment and the metabolite lactic acid play an important role, respectively, in connective fascial tissue remodelling (Trabold et al., 2003) (Kottmann et al., 2012)

Extracellular matrix and humoral factors

Extracellular matrix

The extracellular matrix (ECM) is a dynamic complex that constantly modifies its viscoelastic properties. It adapts to changes in physiological as well as mechanical demands. It is composed of a gelatinous ground substance made up of glycoproteins and proteoglycans, which is interwoven by stiffer fibrous proteins. It serves a mechanical buffer system similar to a water bed. Hydration can influence the mechanic properties of the ECM (Figure 3.3). Transforming growth factor-β1 (TGF-β1) promotes the build-up of ground substance as well as regulating expression of catabolic enzymes and other mediators.

From a mechanical perspective, it can be observed, that shortly after strain in the Achilles and patella tendon, the tendon's cross-sectional area decreases significantly. In transverse strain, recovery was prolonged. The authors speculate that decrease of tendon diameter resembles a squeeze of water. The resulting rehydration in recovery may be an important contributor to a slow-acting exchange of nutrients, electrolytes and other humoral factors, such as cytokines (Wearing et al., 2013).

Notably, the excretion of humoral factors depends on the direction of strain on (myo)fibroblasts. Irregular strain, such as in injury, leads to significantly higher release of interleukin-6, a substance involved in regenerative processes and an increased production of nitric oxide (NO), which is a gaseous neurotransmitter and vasodilator (Murrell, 2007).

Growth factors

In fascial tissue, several growth factors are produced in response to mechanostimulation, for example, in sports, but also after tissue damage. The interaction of multiple humoral factors is a complex orchestra of biochemical processes, which does not allow simple cause-and-effect conclusions. The most prominent growth hormones in fascial tissue are TGF-β, insulin-like growth factor-I (IGF-I), platelet-derived growth factor (PDGF) and connective tissue growth factor (CTGF). Growth factors regulate in collaboration with several cytokines, (for example, interleukin 1, 6 and 8) proliferation and differentiation of fibroblasts and myofibroblasts and production of collagen and extracellular matrix proteins. These humoral factors also influence blood perfusion, tissue hydration, pain generation and nutrition, as well as cell migration due to chemotactic properties (Kjaer et al., 2009) D'Ambrosia et al., 2010 (Kjaer et al., 2013).

Hormones

Hormonal influences, as well as growth factors, are important to fascial tissue. Insulin has anabolic effects and enhances (myo)fibroblast proliferation in vitro. Oestrogen and thyroid hormone receptors have also been found in fibroblasts. Preliminary experiments suggest that thyroid hormones promote fibroblast expansion and counteract apoptosis in connective tissue. Oestrogen challenge leads to a more than 40% reduction in collagen synthesis, a reduction in fibroblast proliferation in vitro and a reduction of bioavailability of growth factors. Female subjects on oral contraceptives had a reduced

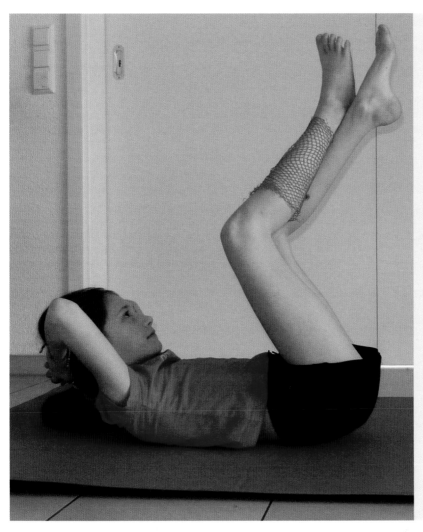

Figure 3.3

Physiology and biochemistry of myofascial tissue

Fascial tissue forms an interconnected three-dimensional network throughout the whole body. Physiological and biochemical processes determine tissue characteristics, such as collagen turnover, extracellular matrix hydration and stiffness of fascial components. The photograph shows a fictitious illustration of fascia on the lower leg. Here, a loose 'fascial stocking' might contribute to the development of varicosis. On the other hand, tight fascial tissue can lead to exercise-induced pain, mismatch of blood perfusion and muscle metabolism in the calf. Indeed, compartment syndrome is a feared post-exercise complication in running athletes.

collagen synthesis in response to sporting activity. The authors speculate that this finding might explain the greater risk to female athletes of certain kinds of injury in, for example, cruciate ligament rupture and pelvic joint instability (Hansen et al., 2009).

Endogenous cortisol is the main opponent of insulin and a regulator of tissue metabolism and inflammation. Several studies show that high doses of corticosteroid hormones and derivatives lead to a reduction in the proliferation and activity of fibroblasts and collagen synthesis, leading to delayed and hampered healing response, i.e. after tissue damage. Conversely, cortisol at physiological levels is indispensable for cellular energy metabolism. Hence, the dose-dependent interaction with cells and other factors is decisive for the anabolic or catabolic effects of corticosteroid hormones. Corticosteroids can be an effective treatment for the prevention of pulmonary fibrosis, for example, in asthma. However, because of the catabolic effects at high concentrations, injections of corticosteroids in injuries or chronic pain in fascial structures should be avoided whenever possible.

Relaxin is a peptide hormone that is structurally related to the insulin family of petides and up-regulated during pregnancy, for example. The most consistent biological effect of relaxin is a regulatory effect on collagen synthesis and its ability to stimulate the breakdown of collagen.

Interestingly, relaxin gene knock out (RLX-/-) mice are characterised by a significant increase in type I and III collagen, resulting in severe scleroderma and interstitial fibrosis leading to multi-organ failure. This effect could be inhibited by administration of recombinant relaxin (Samuel et al., 2005).

Clinical summary

- Sensory input from myofascial tissue is indispensable for nervous movement control.
- Myofascial tone depends on nervous excitation, activation level of intracellular calcium turnover, mechanic properties of myofibres and, to a great extent, on the amount and nature of interwoven, adjacent and attached fascial components.
- Sporting activity leads to significant micro-environmental changes, such as temperature increase, accumulation of metabolites, hydration shift in the extracellular matrix and alteration of protein expression including growth factors and cytokines. Adaptation processes in fascial tissue can explain parts of post-exercise phenomena.
- Knowledge about fascial tissue may help to improve movement and should be integrated in sport and exercise science and practical application. Depending on the type of sports, the fascial characteristics may be decisive for optimum performance.

References

Antonini, A. & Poewe, W. (2007) Fibrotic heart-valve reactions to dopamine-agonist treatment in Parkinson's disease. *Lancet Neurol* 6(9): 826–829.

Chaitow, L. & DeLany, J.W. (2000) *Clinical Application of Neuromuscular Techniques.* Vol. 1 The Upper Body. Churchill Livingstone, Edinburgh, 131–134.

Chaitow, L. (2007) Chronic pelvic pain: Pelvic floor problems, sacro-iliac dysfunction and the trigger point connection. *J Bodyw Mov Ther* 11(4): 327–339.

D'Ambrosia, P., King, K., Davidson, B., Zhou, B.H., Lu, Y. & Solomonow, M. (2010) Pro-inflammatory cytokines expression increases following low- and high-magnitude cyclic loading of lumbar ligaments. *Eur Spine J* 19(8): 1330–1339.

Gladden, L.B. (2004) Lactate metabolism: a new paradigm for the third millennium. *J Physiol* 558(1): 5–30.

Greve, K., Domeij-Arverud, E., Labruto, F., Edman, G., Bring, D., Nilsson, G. & Ackermann, P.W. (2012) Metabolic activity in early tendon repair can be enhanced by intermittent pneumatic compression. *Scand J Med Sci Sports* 22(4): 55–63.

Hansen, M., Miller, B.F., Holm, L., Doessing, S., Petersen, S.G., Skovgaard, D., Frystyk, J., Flyvbjerg, A., Koskinen, S., Pingel, J., Kjaer, M. & Langberg, H. (2009) Effect of administration of oral contraceptives in vivo on collagen synthesis in tendon and muscle connective tissue in young women. *J Appl Physiol* 106(4): 1435–1443.

Kjaer, M., Langberg, H., Heinemeier, K., Bayer, M.L., Hansen, M., Holm, L., Doessing, S., Kongsgaard, M., Krogsgaard, M.R. & Magnusson, S.P. (2009) From mechanical loading to collagen synthesis, structural changes and function in human tendon. *Scand J Med Sci Sports* 19(4): 500–510.

Kjaer, M., Bayer, M.L., Eliasson, P. & Heinemeier, K.M. (2013). What is the impact of inflammation on the critical interplay between mechanical signaling and biochemical changes in tendon matrix? *J Appl Physiol* [Epub April 2013]

Klingler, W., Jurkat-Rott, K., Lehmann-Horn, F. & Schleip, R. (2012) The role of fibrosis in Duchenne muscular dystrophy. *Acta myologica* 31: 184–195.

Kottmann, R.M., Kulkarni, A.A., Smolnycki, K.A., Lyda, E., Dahanayake, T., Salibi, R., Honnons, S., Jones, C., Isern, N.G., Hu, J.Z., Nathan, S.D., Grant, G., Phipps, R.P. & Sime, P.J. (2012) Lactic acid is elevated in idiopathic pulmonary fibrosis and induces myofibroblast differentiation via pH-dependent activation of transforming growth factor-β. *Am J Respir Crit Care Med* 186(8): 740–751.

Masi, A.T. & Hannon, J.C. (2008) Human resting muscle tone (HRMT): Narrative introduction and modern concepts. *J Bodyw Mov Ther* 12(4): 320–332.

Mason, T. & Rigby, B.J. (1963). Thermal transition in collagen. *Biochemica et Biophysica Acta*, 79: 448–450.

Muraoka, T., Omuro, K., Wakahara, T., Muramatsu, T., Kanehisa, H., Fukunaga, T. & Kanosue, K. (2008). Effects of Muscle Cooling on the Stiffness of the Human Gastrocnemius Muscle in vivo. *Cells Tissues Organs* 187(2): 152–160.

Murrell, G.A. (2007) Oxygen free radicals and tendon healing. *J Shoulder Elbow Surg* 16(5): 208–214.

Pipelzadeh, M.H. & Naylor, I.L. (1998) The in vitro enhancement of rat myofibroblast contractility by alterations to the pH of the physiological solution. *Eur J Pharmacol* 357(2): 257–259.

Samuel, C.S., Zhao, C., Bathgate, R.A., DU X.J., Summers R.J., Amento, E.P., Walker, L.L., McBurnie, M., Zhao, L. & Tregear G.W. (2005) The relaxin gene-knockout mouse: a model of progressive fibrosis. *Ann N Y Acad Sci* 1041: 173–181.

Schleip, R., Duerselen, L., Vleeming, A., Naylor, I.L., Lehmann-Horn, F., Zorn, A., Jaeger, H. & Klingler, W. (2012) Strain hardening of fascia: Static stretching of dense fibrous connective tissues can induce a temporary stiffness increase accompanied by enhanced matrix hydration. *J Bodyw Mov Ther* 16: 94–100.

Tesarz, J., Hoheisel, U., Wiedenhöfer, B. & Mense, S. (2011) Sensory innervation of the thoracolumbar fascia in rats and humans. *Neuroscience* 194: 302–308.

Trabold, O., Wagner, S., Wicke, C., Scheuenstuhl, H., Hussain, M.Z., Rosen, N., Seremetiev A., Becker, H.D. & Hunt, T.K. (2003) Lactate and oxygen constitute a fundamental regulatory mechanism in wound healing. *Wound Repair Regen* 11(6): 504–509.

Wearing, S.C., Smeathers, J.E., Hooper, S.L., Locke, S., Purdam, C. & Cook, J.L. (2013) The time course of in vivo recovery of transverse strain in high-stress tendons following exercise. *Br J Sports Med* [Epub ahead of print April 2013]

Bibliography

Chaitow, L., Gilbert, C. & Morrison, D. (2013). *Recognizing and Treating Breathing Disorders: A Multidisciplinary Approach*, 2e. Edinburgh, Churchill Livingstone The International Fascia Research Society: www.fasciaresearchsociety.org

Schleip, R., Findley, T., Chaitow, L. & Huijing, P. (eds.), (2012). *Fascia- The Tensional Network of the Human Body* Edinburgh, Elsevier.

CHAPTER 4

Fascia as sensory organ

Robert Schleip

The surprising miracle gift wrap

For most anatomical researchers, fascia was mainly considered an inert wrapping organ, giving mechanical support to our muscles and most other organs. Yes, there were some early histological reports about the presence of sensory nerves in fascia (Stilwell, 1957) (Sakada, 1974) but these were largely disregarded and did not affect the common understanding of musculoskeletal dynamics. While Moshe Feldenkrais as well as Ida Rolf, the founders of the related somatic therapies, were apparently not aware of the importance of fascia as a sensory organ, Andrew Taylor Still, the founder of osteopathy, proclaimed that, 'No doubt nerves exist in the fascia ...' and suggested that all fascial tissues should be treated with the same degree of respect as if dealing with 'the branch offices of the brain' (Still, 1902).

Van der Wal reported, with painstaking detail, the substantial presence of sensory nerve endings in the fascia of rats, yet this finding was ignored for several decades (van der Wal, 1988). As far as ligaments were concerned, their proprioceptive innervation was recognised during the 1990s, which subsequently influenced the guidelines for joint injury surgeries (Johansson et al., 1991). Similarly, the plantar fascia was found to contribute to the sensorimotor regulation of postural control in standing (Erdemir & Piazza, 2004). However, what really changed the 'view' in a more powerful manner was the first international Fascia Research Congress, held at Harvard Medical School in Boston in 2007. During the Congress, three teams from different countries reported, independently, their findings of a rich presence of sensory nerves in fascial tissues (Findley & Schleip, 2007).

Figure 4.1 gives an example of the density of sensory nerves in a piece of lumbar fascia, gained by using immunohistochemistry. When the intricate system of intramuscular sacs and septi of collagenous connective tissues is included as contributing elements of this body-wide tensional network, then the fascial web can be seen as our largest sensory organ in terms of overall surface area. Additionally, with regards to the sheer quantity and richness of nerve endings, this network can 'match' our sense of sight, not to mention hearing or any of our other normally considered sensory organs (Mitchell & Schmidt, 1977).

The following analogy may well serve to express the magnitude of the general perceptual shift

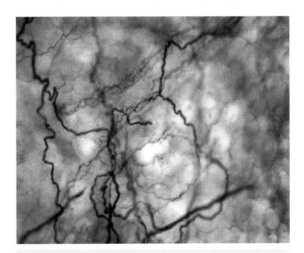

Figure 4.1

Demonstration of the rich presence of nerves in a piece of fascia

Immunostaining of a piece of rodent lumbar with a pan-neuronal marker reveals the rich network of visible nerves. Image length: approx. 0.5 mm. (Photo from Tesarz et al., 2011, with permission of Elsevier.)

elicited by the first fascia congress: Imagine receiving a Christmas present from a dear friend, who hands it to you with a very meaningful expression. At first glance it looks like a bottle of wine wrapped in ordinary newspaper. After unwrapping the newspaper you find only a bottle of apple juice from a nearby grocery shop … and you may be overplaying your disappointment by thanking your friend for 'this very nice bottle'. However, after a minute you notice that the discarded wrapping paper on the floor starts to change its colour in response to your facial expressions. It even starts to slowly contract and move in relation to your personal movements. You then realise that it is not the bottle that is special but its packaging, which clearly is more alive and fascinating than you had expected.

Different types of sensory receptors in the fascial net

From a morphological and embryological perspective, the fascial net has been described to consist of those connective tissues that have adapted their architecture in response to a local dominance of tensional, rather than compressive, loading (Schleip et al., 2012). It is, therefore, not surprising that the majority of intrafascial sensory nerve endings, also called nerve receptors, are particularly responsive to either stretch or shear loading.

Figure 4.2 illustrates the typical composition of a musculoskeletal nerve bundle, such as the sciatic nerve in the legs or the radial nerve in the arms.

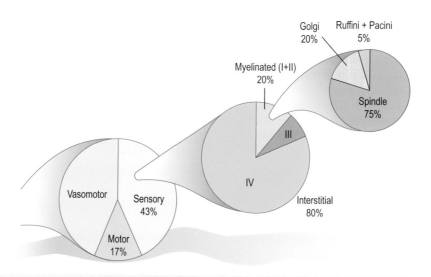

Figure 4.2

Composition of neurons in musculoskeletal connective tissues

The quantities of respective axons shown were derived from detailed analysis of the combined nerve supplying the lateral gastrocnemius and soleus muscle of a cat. While a small portion of the interstitial neurons may terminate inside bone, the remaining neurons can all be considered to terminate in fascial tissues. Even the sensory devices called muscle spindles are nestled within fibrous collagenous intramuscular tissues. Interstitial neurons terminate in free nerve endings. Some of these clearly have a proprioceptive, interoceptive or nociceptive function. Recent investigations however suggest that the majoriy of the interstitial neurons in fascia serve a polymodal function, meaning that they are open for stimulation from more than one of these mentioned sensorial categories. (Illustration courtesy of fascialnet.com)

One of the many interesting aspects about this composition is that a vast number of nerves are devoted to the fine-tuning of nutrient delivery via the vascular supply, which is regulated by the sympathetic nervous system. The remaining portion, dealing with sensorimotor regulation, is then not at all equally devoted to motor and sensory pathways. In contrast, the body architecture devotes more than twice as many neurons for the 'listening' or feeling aspect of communication as it does to 'talking' and giving instructions towards the periphery. Could this wise architectural principle be one of the explanations why sometimes the body's innate intelligence achieves much smarter results than an old-fashioned CEO, who directs the company, would?

A quarter of the sensory nerves contain relatively fast conducting myelinated axons. These include the Pacini, Golgi and Ruffini corpuscles. All of these clearly serve a proprioceptive function. They usually terminate in fascial tissues, whether it is in the epimysial or tendinous portions or in the intramuscular connective tissues. Note that the muscle spindles, which are a fairly recent invention in evolutionary terms for fine tuning the movement of land animals, can be considered to be sensory devices that are also located within perimysial or endomysial collagenous tissues of the intramuscular fascial network. It is plausible that if the surrounding collagenous tissues suffer from a loss of elasticity, then the functioning of these spindles may be corrupted. Possibly this could be a contributing factor in conditions such as fibromyalgia or in chronic muscle stiffness, as an increased thickness of the endomysium has been shown to characterise fibromyalgia patients (Liptan, 2010). Furthermore, an increased thickness of the perimysium seems to provide the main architectural difference between tough meat muscles versus tender meat muscles within the same animal (Schleip et al., 2006).

While much is known about the functioning of these different mechanosensitive neurons, the majority of sensory nerves in fascial tissue belong to the interstitial neurons, which are much less understood and are still considered as intriguingly mysterious by those who investigate. Their axons terminate in so-called free nerve endings. Classical neurology divides these further into the type III neurons, whose axons contain a very thin myelin sheet, and type IV neurons, with unmyelinated axons. For our purpose however, they can largely be considered to behave in a similar manner, although the speed of the type IV neurons (also called C-fibres in another classification category) is even a little slower than the type III axons (also called A-delta fibres).

Functional properties of these neurons

What are the respective functions of the different sensory neurons in fascia? For the regularly myelinated neurons, it is clear that they mainly serve as proprioceptive devices. Some of them, like the Ruffini endings, are highly sensitive to shear loading (i.e. a directional difference in tensional loading between one tissue layer and an adjacent one). Others like the Pacini endings, respond to rapid changes only as their endings filter out any non-changing stimulations. While the Golgi receptors were previously considered to exist in tendinous tissues only, their presence in other fascial tissues has been securely confirmed by several independent studies (Yahia et al., 1992) (Stecco et al., 2007). Stimulation of Golgi receptors tends to trigger a relaxation response in skeletal muscle fibres that are directly linked with the respectively tensioned collagen fibres. However, if tendinous extramuscular tissues are stretched in a condition in which they are arranged in series with relaxed muscle fibres, then most of the respective elongation will be 'swallowed' by the more compliant myofibres. In this way, the respective stretching impulse may not provide sufficient stimulation for eliciting any muscular tonus change (Jami, 1992). A practical conclusion of this may be that a stretching impulse, aimed at reaching the tendinous tissues, may profit from including some moments in which the lengthened muscle fibres are actively contracting or are temporarily resisting their overall elongation.

Neurons terminating in free nerve endings are frequently understood to be nociceptive, i.e. signalling stimulations that are associated with potential tissue damage, which is usually associated with a perception of pain. Such nociceptive neurons have recently been clearly identified in fascial tissues. Provocation tests, with intrafascial injection of hypertonic saline, have also confirmed that fascia can be the origin of pain perception.

Most clearly this has been shown from the human lumbar fascia (Schilder et al., 2014) in which the related interstitial neurons seem to be particularly responsive, in terms of a subsequently long lasting hyper-sensitivity, to repeated mechanical or biochemical irritation. Similar provocation tests, with hypertonic saline, revealed that much of the sensation known as delayed onset muscle soreness (DOMS) after strenuous eccentric exercise seems to originate from nociceptive interstitial neurons in the fascial layer of the muscular epimysium (Gibson et al., 2009).

Polymodal receptors in fascia

For health-oriented practitioners, it is important to realise that not all interstitial neurons can be classified as nociceptive. Some of them are sensory devices for thermoception. Others monitor muscular activity to the sympathetic nervous system in order to allow for a locally specific fine-tuning of the blood flow to respective muscle portions, which is then called ergoreception. Interestingly, in fascial tissues the majority of the interstitial neurons are so called polymodal receptors, meaning that they are responsive to more than one kind of stimulation. While their respective synapses in the posterior horn of the spinal cord are hungry and eager for 'any' kind of stimulation, they seem to be easily satisfied if sufficient proprioceptive information is supplied to them via these polymodal receptors. However, in cases of insufficient supply with proprioceptive stimulation (because of alterations in the connective tissue matrix surrounding the respective nerve endings, for example) these neurons tend to actively lower their threshold for nociceptive stimulation. In addition, they may actively extrude cytokines that sensitise polymodal neurons in their neighbourhood and predispose them towards a nociceptive function. A seemingly miniscule mechanical stimulation, such as a leg length difference of 1 mm only, can then lead to a nociceptive response within the intricate network of these intrafascial polymodal receptors.

Based on the mutually inhibiting dynamics between proprioceptive and nociceptive intrafascial stimulation, many therapeutic approaches are exploring the use of movement and/or touch in order to supply the respective polymodal receptors with refined proprioceptive input. This can be done with many different methods, whether it be the guided exploration of new movement patterns (as in the Feldenkrais method), the use of active micro-movements of the client at an amplitude of few millimetres only (as in Continuum Movement) or use of a calliper to improve two point discrimination when touched at decreasing two-point distances on the skin, amongst many others. Since fascia constitutes the most important organ for proprioception, it also makes sense to focus particularly on the stimulation of fascial mechanoreceptors when following this general therapeutic strategy.

Within the fields of complementary therapies, different opinions exist as to whether mental attention of the patient is a necessary requirement for the described 'proprioception against potential nociception' strategy. While some schools teach that it is completely fine if the cortical attention of the client shifts away from their specific somatic sensations, others are constantly engaging mindful attention of their clients as a pre-requisite to gain therapeutic effects. While this meaningful debate has been hard to advance by philosophical argumentation or by random clinical observation only, an elegant study by Lorimer Moseley has provided strong support for those advocates who insist on fostering mindful attention of their clients. When applying a newly developed tactile therapy, which involved stimulation of mechanoreceptors in the skin and superficial fascia of the hand with patients suffering from complex regional pain syndrome, the examiners treated half the patients in a setup that required full mental attention to the respective touch. The other group of patients were treated with exactly the same stimulations but their mental attention was distracted away from the specific bodily stimulation by allowing them to read a book during the treatment. The outcome showed that only the mental attention group achieved a significant improvement, whereas no significant improvement could be witnessed in the mentally distracted group (Moseley et al., 2007). It is unclear whether the impressive findings of this study can be used to generalise for other similar or non-similar musculoskeletal conditions, as well as therapeutic approaches. It can be concluded however, that the mental attention, or state of mindfulness, of the patient seems to provide an augmenting effect, if not a necessary requirement, in at least some therapeutic approaches that aim to follow the above described 'proprioception against potential nociception' avenue.

Not all fasciae are equal

Does it make a difference which locations of the body-wide fascial network are stimulated in order to supply the spinal cord with new proprioceptive input? Two new insights regarding the density of sensory receptors in fascia provide valuable insight into this question. First, the recent studies from the group around Mense at the University of Heidelberg have shown that in human, as well as rat, lumbar fascia, the density of sensory neurons is significantly higher in the superficial tissue layers between the dermis and fascia profunda when compared to the respective density within the deeper tissue layer, called lumbodorsal fascia, just underneath these superficial layers (Tesarz et al., 2011). In our own experimental examinations at Ulm University, we also observed an increased density of visible nerves in the transitional shearing zone between fascia profunda and fascia superficialis. In healthy body regions, this zone is where a lateral 'skin sliding' movement, in relation to the underlying tissues, can easily be induced. It is also the zone whose architecture determines whether a skin fold can be pulled away from the body or not. It makes sense to assume that the lateral gliding movements provided by everyday movements provide an important source of fascial proprioception. It is also an intriguing thought that the often profound reported therapeutic effects of various skin taping techniques in sports medicine may partially be explained by their local amplification of respective skin movements in normal joint functioning.

The second recent insight regarding areas of increased density of sensory nerves in the fascial net comes from the Stecco group at Padua University in Italy (Stecco et al., 2007). Their histological examinations of upper and lower limb fasciae in human cadavers revealed huge differences in the density of proprioceptive nerve endings, such as Golgi, Pacini and Ruffini corpuscles. This recent data indicated that fascial tissues, which clearly serve an important force-transmitting function (such as the lacertus fibrosus on the upper forearm as an extension of the biceps femoris), hardly contain any proprioceptive endings. On the other hand, they observed that some fascial structures seem to have very little role in force transmission, as witnessed when cutting them away, as is the case of the retinacula around ankle and wrist region. Interestingly, these more obliquely running fascial bands seem to be located at specific approximations to major joints and they contain a very high density of proprioceptive nerve endings. Some researchers even suggest that the prime function of these fascial bands may not be their biomechanical but their sensorial function in providing detailed proprioception to the central nervous system. If verified, this could suggest that proprioception enhancing approaches, whether in skin taping, yoga, stretching, foam roller self-treatment, or Continuum Movement-like micro movements, could possibly be augmented in their respective therapeutic effectiveness by stimulating fascial tissue movements in regions with an increased proprioceptive innervation.

Interoception and the insular cortex

An often overlooked aspect of fascial stimulation is the presence of interstitial nerves in fascia that serve an interoceptive, rather than proprioceptive or nociceptive, function. Stimulation of those free nerve endings provides the brain with information about the condition of the body in its constant search for homeostasis in relation to its physiological needs. Many of the respective free nerve endings are located in visceral connective tissues and constitute an important part of what is frequently referred to as the enteric brain. However, other interoceptive interstitial neurons are located within endomysial and perimysial intramuscular connective tissues. Interoceptive signalling is associated with feelings like warmth, nausea, hunger, soreness, effort, heaviness or lightness, as well as a sense of belonging or alienation regarding specific body regions, etc. (Craig, 2002).

The neural stimulation from the respective nerve endings does not follow the usual afferent pathways towards the somatomotor cortex of the brain, rather these neurons project to the so-called insular cortex, an internally folded area of cortical gray matter located inside the forebrain. In this walnut-sized cortical area, perceptions about internal somatic sensations are associated with emotional preferences and feelings. People with disturbed functioning of the insula may still have full biomechanical functioning and achieve high IQ levels in respective tests, however they are usually socially dysfunctional and are unable to make reasonable decisions in complex situations (Damasio, 1999).

Whereas some health related conditions, such as low back pain, scoliosis or complex regional pain syndrome, are associated with a diminished proprioceptive acuity, other conditions seem to be more clearly related to dysfunctional interoceptive processing. These latter conditions include anorexia, anxiety, depression, irritable bowel syndrome, alexithymia (inability in recognising and expressing one's own emotional states) and possibly fibromyalgia. It therefore makes sense that movement instructors, whether in yoga, Pilates, or martial arts, carefully examine their habitual preferences in fostering the direction of the suggested somatic curiosity of their clients. A rigid reliance on proprioceptive perception, 'Where exactly is your lower back touching the ground?', may provide limited long-term effects if applied to clients for whom a more interoceptive perceptual refinement approach may be required. In these cases, a skilful fostering of visceral fascial sensations, via specific yoga postures for example, may sometimes provide more profound effects than the often habitual focus on musculoskeletal sensations (Table 4.1).

Table 4.1

Health conditions associated with dysfunctions in proprioceptive or interoceptive processing

Several pathologies have been shown to be associated with dysfunctions in proprioception. Other conditions are associated with an altered interoceptive processing. In the pathways of interoception the insular cortex plays a leading role, in which all sensory input is combined with affective associations. In prioprioception the somatomotor cortex and its representational mapping of the body ('body schema') are of central importance. Dependent on the involved pathway of dysfunction a different emphasis in fascia oriented therapies may be indicated. Receptive nerve endings for proprioception tend to be located in fascial shearing zones between superficial and deep fascia. Respective sensory nerve endings for interoception are found directly below non-glabrous skin as well as in visceral connective tissues. Note that in fibromyalgia an augmented temperature signalling from the superficial fascia has recently been documented. However the hypothesis of augmented interoception as a major player in fibromyalgia and chronic fatigue syndrome remains to be confirmed.

Proprioceptive impairment	Interoceptive dysregulation
Low back pain	Irritable bowel syndrome
Whiplash	Anxiety, depression
Complex regional pain syndrome (CRPS)	Alexythymia ('emotional blindness')
Attention deficit hyperactivity disorder (ADHS)	Schizophrenia
Scoliosis	Anorexia and other eating disorders
Other myofascial pain syndromes	Fibromyalgia/chronic fatigue syndrome?

A surprising new finding is the discovery of the so-called tactile C-fibres in the superficial fascia of humans and other primates. These interstitial neurons are present in body areas where our ancestors had furry skin (for example, not on the palms of the hands or the soles of the feet) and they are associated with grooming behaviour as a social health function in primates. When stimulated, these intrafascial neurons do not signal any proprioceptive information (and the brain cannot apparently locate the regional origin of the stimulation), however they trigger activation in the insular cortex, which is expressed as a sense of peaceful well-being and social belonging (McGlone et al., 2014).

Clinical summary

- Fascia constitutes a body-wide tensional network, which serves as our richest and most important sensory organ for feeling changes in our own body.
- Related sensory nerves include receptors that clearly signal proprioceptive information.
- Proprioceptive signalling tends to inhibit potential myofascial nociception, particularly if accompanied by a state of mindfulness.
- Other smaller receptor neurons in fascia are focused on interoceptive or nociceptive sensations.
- Therapeutic enhancement of proprioceptive stimulation can be beneficial in many myofascial pain conditions.
- A skilful facilitation of interoceptive perceptions, on the other hand, may work equally well in several complex somatic dysfunctions by fostering an improved insular processing.

References

Bednar, D.A.1., Orr, F.W. & Simon, G.T. (1995) Observations on the pathomorphology of the thoracolumbar fascia in chronic mechanical back pain. A microscopic study. *Spine*. 15;20(10): 1161–1164.

Craig, A.D. (2002) How do you feel? Interoception: the sense of the physiological condition of the body. *Nat Rev Neurosci*. 3(8): 655–666.

Damasio, A. (1999) *The feeling of what happens: body and emotion in the making of consciousness*. Harcourt-Brace, New York.

Erdemir, A. & Piazza, S.J. (2004) Changes in foot loading following plantar fasciotomy: a computer modeling study. *J Biomech Eng*. 126(2): 237–243.

Findley T., Schleip R. (eds.) (2007) *Fascia research - Basic science and implications for conventional and complementary health care*. Elsevier Urban & Fischer, Munich.

Gibson, W., Arendt-Nielsen, L., Taguchi, T., Mizumura, K. & Graven-Nielsen, T. (2009) Increased pain from muscle fascia following eccentric exercise: animal and human findings. *Exp Brain Res* 194(2): 299–308.

Jami, A. (1992) Golgi tendon organs in mammalian skeletal muscles: functional properties and central actions. *Physiol Rev*. 72(3): 623–666.

Johansson, H., Sjölander, P. & Sojka, P. (1991) A sensory role for the cruciate ligaments. *Clin Orthop Relat Res*. 268: 161–178.

Liptan, G.L. (2010) Fascia: A missing link in our understanding of the pathology of fibromyalgia. *J Bodyw Mov Ther*. 14(1): 3–12.

McGlone, F., Wessberg, J. & Olausson, H. (2014) Discriminative and affective touch: sensing and feeling. *Neuron* 82(4): 737–755.

Mitchell, J.H. & Schmidt, R.F. (1977) Cardiovascular reflex control by afferent fibers from skeletal muscle receptors. In: Shepherd JT et al. (eds.) *Handbook of physiology*, Section 2, Vol. III, Part 2: 623–658.

Moseley, G.L.1., Zalucki, N.M. & Wiech, K. (2007) Tactile discrimination, but not tactile stimulation alone, reduces chronic limb pain. *Pain*. 137(3): 600–608.

Sakada, S. (1974) Mechanoreceptors in fascia, periosteum and periodontal ligament. *Bull Tokyo Med Dent Univ*. 21 Suppl(0): 11–13.

Sandkühler, J. (2009) Models and mechanisms of hyperalgesia and allodynia. *Physiol Rev*. 89(2): 707–758.

Schilder, A., Hoheisel, U., Magerl, W., Benrath, J., Klein, T. & Treede, R.D. (2014) Sensory findings after stimulation of the thoracolumbar fascia with hypertonic saline suggest its contribution to low back pain. *Pain* 155(2): 222–231.

Schleip, R., Naylor, I.L., Ursu, D., Melzer, W., Zorn, A., Wilke, H.J., Lehmann-Horn, F. & Klingler, W. (2006) *Med Hypotheses* 66(1): 66–71.

Schleip, R., Jäger, H. & Klingler, W. (2012) What is 'fascia'? A review of different nomenclatures. *J Bodyw Mov Ther*. 16(4): 496–502.

Stecco, C., Gagey, O., Belloni, A., Pozzuoli, A., Porzionato, A., Macchi, V., Aldegheri, R., De Caro, R. & Delmas, V. (2007) Anatomy of the deep fascia of the upper limb. Second part: study of innervation. *Morphologie* 91(292): 38–43.

Still, A.T. (1902) *The philosophy and mechanical principles of osteopathy*. Hudson-Kimberly Publishing Company, Kansas City, 62.

Stillwell, D.L. (1957) Regional variations in the innervation of deep fasciae and aponeuroses. *Anat Rec* 127: 635–648.

Tesarz, J., Hoheisel, U., Wiedenhöfer, B. & Mense, S. (2011) Sensory innervation of the thoracolumbar fascia in rats and humans. *Neuroscience* 194: 302–308.

van der Wal, J.C. (1988) The organization of the substrate of proprioception in the elbow region of the rat. [PhD thesis]. Maastricht, Netherlands: Maastricht University, Faculty of Medicine.

Yahia, L., Rhalmi, S., Newman, N. & Isler, M. (1992) Sensory innervation of human thoracolumbar fascia. An immunohistochemical study. *Acta Orthop Scand*. 63(2): 195–197.

CHAPTER 5

Stress loading and matrix remodeling in tendon and skeletal muscle: Cellular mechano-stimulation and tissue remodeling

Michael Kjaer

Introduction – the concept of mechanical loading on tissue and cells

Loading of connective tissue is a dominant part of all body movement, from light recreational walking to high-level running and athletic activities, such as jumping or throwing. The connective tissue has to resist high levels of loading from muscular contractile activity and, clearly, very high loads will result in acute injuries of connective tissue structures like ligaments, tendons or bones. These present themselves as a tissue rupture or fracture due to a single mechanical load that surpasses the load tolerance.

With regards to repeated loading on the connective tissue there is a fine, yet undefined, line between tissue tolerance of loading and potential adaptation and the development of tissue pathology and associated clinical symptoms. It is, however, clear that very intense physical training, in elite level sports requiring repeated movements of specific body parts, does demonstrate a kind of upper limit of tolerance in the body. Table 5.1 illustrates how elite athletes within sports, including running, swimming and rowing, experience loading of the lower extremity, shoulder or upper body of up to 40,000–50,000 repetitions per week. Clearly, genetic differences will provide a varying degree of tolerance towards repetitive loading but, in general, it is accepted among athletes that if you extend the amount of training further, than that given in Table 5.1, most athletes will experience decreased performance within their sports. In general, this decrease in performance is unlikely to be as a result of the total number of training hours, since several sports that have a more varied loading of the body than the examples provided in Table 5.1, for example, triathletes, are able to train for up to 35–38 hours a week without any resulting decrease in performance or the accumulation of injuries. Thus, Table 5.1 seems to show that each specific regional connective tissue has an upper limit for repeated loading.

Connective tissue in the body is able to withstand substantial load, varying for clear tensile loading to more compressive loading. Data, primarily animal literature but also more recently from human experiments, shows that increased loading results in improved size and strength of tendons, ligaments, bone and cartilage (Table 5.2). It is, however, clear that the improvement is very moderate and that the adaptation requires considerable time. Compared to skeletal muscle adaptation, the response to training in matrix tissue is moderate. On the other hand, findings on the influence of inactivity, upon different connective tissues, normally indicate some kind of loss in tissue strength and mechanical characteristics (Table 5.2). These findings illustrate that connective

	Training-dose/wk	Tissue loading reps/wk
Dist. Running	120 km/wk (steps 1.5 m)	~40,000 steps/legs
Swimming	3–4 h/day (30–40 str/min)	~26,000 strokes/arm
Rowing	3–4 h/day (22–35 str/min)	~38,000 strokes

Table 5.1

Tissue tolerance in elite athhletes

Function	Capacity (acute)	Training (% increase)	Inactivity (% decrease 4–8 wks)	
Connective tissue		**Months-years**		
Tendon	100 MPa	10	30	(+ stiff./cross-links)
Ligament	60–100 MPa	10	30	(+ stiffness/elastin)
Bone	50–200 MPa	5–10	30	(+ mineraliz./Ca++)
Cartilage	5–40 MPa	5–10	30	(+ water/proteogl)
Skeletal muscle		**Months-years**		
Strength		100	60	
Muscle Mass		60	20–30	

Table 5.2

Examples of connective tissue adaptation to long-term physical training and inactivity

tissue is highly dependent upon normal daily loading and is very vulnerable when not being mechanically loaded. When subjected to inactivity, the connective tissue doesn't diminish quickly in size, but does demonstrate a quick (within 1–2 weeks) alteration in passive mechanical properties. The explanation for this is currently unknown but indicates that molecular structures, that are of importance for mechanical properties, can change quickly when unloaded. In artificial tendons it has been shown that just a few days of unloading in tendon-like structures results in a disorganisation of the fibrils. In humans, the quick changes in mechanical properties of the tendon is accompanied by a change in the expression of enzymes of importance for the formation of cross-link molecules.

Mechanotransduction – signaling and outcome

Mechanical loading of connective tissue is a complex process that involves several steps, from the initial conversion of mechanical stress upon the tissue into chemical signals. Initially, integrin receptors will be activated and this will result in adhesion and activation of mechanotransduction pathways (Kjaer, 2004) (Magnusson et al., 2010). An important pathway for mechanotransduction is the Rho-Rock pathway and, in several studies, the importance of this pathway for mechanotransduction has been documented. The resulting activation of protein synthesis,

from the cell nucleus, will lead to formation of matrix proteins, such as collagens, and subsequent tissue structure changes, whether this be more dense tissue, larger tissue volume or altered organisation of fibrillar and other structures. This will then ultimately contribute to the mechanical properties of the matrix tissue.

Mechanical loading will also lead to local upregulation (i.e. more pronounced gene expression and incresed synthesis of the protein) of growth factors, such as IGF-I and TGF-beta. These will probably be released from the fibroblasts of the connective tissue. Whether these growth factors will act in an autocrine or a paracrine fashion is yet to be explained, but the upregulation of these factors can be found to be associated with an exercise induced upregulation of collagen protein synthesis. This suggests a direct association between growth factor release and matrix protein formation (Table 5.3). There is also some indication that mechanical loading and growth factors can stimulate the matrix tissue in an additive or even synergistic way (Magnusson, 2010).

Mechanical loading increases both collagen expression and protein synthesis in animal studies (Heinemeier et al., 2007). In humans an upregulation of protein synthesis has been demonstrated both in the peri-tendinous tissue and, as determined from incorporation of labeled amino acids, into tendon tissue (Miller et al., 2005). Furthermore, a degradation of collagen tissue has also been demonstrated in humans. Despite these rather dynamic changes of collagen turnover in tendon tissue, this does not prove any major exchange of tendon structure with mechanical loading. Very recent data indicates that the exchange of tendon structures takes place in the first 17 years of life and that, thereafter, a more stable structure is maintained in an intact uninjured tendon (Heinemeier et al., 2013). The fact that well trained individuals have higher cross-sectional areas of Achilles and Patella tendons than untrained ones, and that within the same individual one stronger leg also shows a larger diameter tendon than on the contralateral side (Couppe et al., 2008), indicates that either the growth of tendon with training occurs in the early years, or that it represents an addition of tissue on the surface of the tendon not unlike the addition of layers on a tree from year to year.

Cellular responses to mechanical loading: In vitro to in vivo

During mechanical loading of connective tissue, tendons for example, the cell within the tendon responds, as mentioned above, with an increase in mRNA and protein synthesis in the central elements of the matrix (collagen type I). The studies show that interstitial concentrations of collagen propeptide fragments in the peritendinous space rose after exercise. Furthermore, when infusing amino acids, labeled with stable isotopes, and determining the incorporation of these into the relevant connective tissue, it has been shown that this incorporation into hydroxyl-proline, and thus into collagen, was almost doubled in both tendon and skeletal muscle after intense exercise (Miller et al., 2005). Conversely, with inactivity over 2–3 weeks it can be shown that such incorporation would be diminished. It therefore seems that the collagen production in tendon and skeletal muscle matrix is affected by the degree of mechanical loading. Interestingly, both in tendon and muscle it seems that the dose-response curve for the relation between intensity of loading and the responding protein synthesis outcome is leveling off relatively early. This means that, already at a relatively moderate loading of the tissue, a sufficient connective tissue response is observed. As adaptation of connective tissue in general

is relatively slow, it presents an advantage that also relatively moderate loading will result in an increase in protein synthesis. This means that during rehabilitation, after an injury, humans may stimulate their connective tissue with low levels of intensity, at a time where the tissue would otherwise be too weak to tolerate heavy muscle resistance training.

The question now is whether or not this reflects a true tissue renewal and replacement of existing fibrillar structures or rather represents a tool by which mechanical loading provides collagen for potential incorporation in the case of injury. It could be that only a minor fraction of adult tendon is turned over and that a large part of the tendon is more inert and, therefore, less dynamic. In order to determine this, an experiment can be performed in which the atmospheric content of the radioactive carbon isotope 14C can be used to mark the age of connective tissue. This is possible because the content of 14C peaked with atom bomb trials in the late 1950s and early 1960s, whereafter it was banned and the 14C content in the air dropped over the years. Using this methodology, it can be shown that, by taking into account the increased turnover of tissue in the first 17 years of life during height growth, it would appear that no major collagen turnover occurred in the adult tendon (Heinemeier et al., 2013). This implies that, in spite of loading, the tendon remains relatively inert during adult life and that only mechanical damage can cause changes. It is, therefore, suggested that the cells in the adult tendon are predominantly dormant and will only be activated in emergency situations.

When the adult tendon is prepared so that cells are isolated and grown in 3D culture systems where, due to attachment patterns, they will be subjected to tension, it can be observed that new and artificial tendon constructs are formed. These artificial tendons are cell rich, produce new fibrils, display an aligned fibril structure and have the same qualitative type of mechanical properties as natural cells. They express proteins important for tendon structure, like fibrillar collagens, as well as proteins that are phenotypical for tendons, like tenomodulin. Interestingly, when tension is released from these tendon constructs, they all lose their expression of collagen, tenomodulin and mechanosensitive integrin receptors. These changes do not seem to be compensated for by the excess amount of growth factors added (for example, TGF-beta). They indicate that mechanical loading is crucial for stimulation of important proteins for matrix structure formation.

Chronic effect of mechanical loading on matrix cells and tissue

To what extent the adult tendon can adapt to physical training is not fully understood. In cross section studies, it has been shown that endurance runners have thicker Achilles tendon structures than untrained weight matched counterparts. Furthermore, when comparing athletes from different types of sports, it has been found that runners, who repetitively load their calf, and volleyball players, who use explosive jumping activity, display thicker Achilles tendons than kayak rowers, who load their legs less but have a similar athletic status (Magnusson et al., 2010). In elite older runners, the cross sectional area of the patella tendon is larger than in untrained age-matched males. The fibril volume was also larger. This indicates that differences between trained and untrained tendons cannot be explained by water accumulation. This data could, therefore, imply that selection is the cause for these differences. The theory of adaptation being related to training is further supported by research into sports with different loading on two legs, such as fencing and badminton. In these examples, where the quadriceps muscle strength was greater in one leg, it was accompanied by a larger patella tendon cross sectional area (Couppe et al., 2008). To what extent these adaptations of tendon have occurred very early in life or throughout life is not known.

In skeletal muscle, regular training is not associated with any marked increase in collagen content but extreme loading does increase collagen synthesis. This could indicate that collagen degradation increases and that the total collagen content does not, therefore, rise as a result of training. However, this does not indicate to what extent the intramuscular connective tissue will obtain

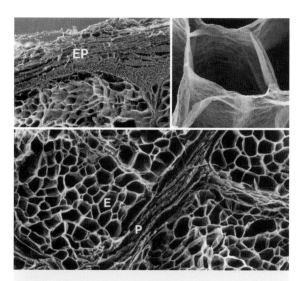

Figure 5.1

Scanning electron micrographs of intramuscular connective tissues (bovine semitendinosus muscle after removal of skeletal muscle protein). Upper left: epimysium (EP); upper right: endomysium surrounding an individual muscle fibre; bottom picture: perimysium (P) plus endomysium (E). Modified from Nishimura et al. (1994) with permission.

altered mechanical properties with training that is unrelated to collagen content but is, rather, related to fibril arrangement or the synthesis of other molecules related to tissue mechanical properties, for example, cross links (see Fig. 5.1).

The borderline between physiological and pathological responses to loading

How much is considered to be adequate loading of connective tissue and how much is too much is an important but, as yet, unresolved question. We do know that appropriate restitution between training bouts will contribute to allow full stimulation of protein synthesis and protein degradation, in order to avoid a gradual net loss of connective tissue over time. Whether this mismatch is the major 'road' leading to matrix tissue overload is not completely clear. The presence of both apoptotic cells, and the release of heat shock proteins and inflammatory substances with heavy tissue loading, could indicate that cells in an overloaded matrix tissue are changing their task from matrix protein production, and adequate maintenance and renewal of tissue, towards a role where the struggle to survive is their primary goal. It may also be that, in the case of tissue overloading, the overloaded cells are shielded from further loading and this will, therefore, result in further degenerative local changes due to a lack of mechanical loading (Arnoczky et al., 2007). Interestingly, the histological and micro-structural changes in early overloading of a tendon, for example, do not mimic the picture of an experimental rupture of a tendon. It must, therefore, represent some other changes behind overuse of connective tissue. It is known that in some tissues, like tendons, the overuse of the tissue is associated with occurrence of neo-vascularisation and the ingrowth of nerve structures that will result in painful symptoms from the overloaded tissue (Magnusson et al., 2010).

Clinical summary

The mechanical loading of connective tissue is important for the maintenance and adaptation of the matrix in regards to its composition, structure and passive mechanical properties. The question that remains, however, is what the cells in the connective tissue will sense. Is it strain or is it other types of stress? There is, though, no doubt that connective tissue will respond to mechanical loading but that the response is very varied dependent upon the magnitude of the load, the type of matrix tissue and the characteristics of the individual. Clinical work suggests that the overloading of tissue in relation to sports, for example, represents a challenge in understanding what signs and markers will provide the 'warning sign' for overloading. Having said that, it is also clear that in many clinical situations, the connective tissue is subjected to far too low a mechanical load. From the data present today, it is clear that mechanical loading provides one of the strongest stimuli, if not the strongest, towards an adaptation of matrix tissue that becomes stronger and, in an injury recovery situation, heals faster and better than if no loading were present.

References

Arnoczky, S.P., Lavagnino, M. & Egerbacher, M. (2007) The mechanobiological aetiopathogenesis of tendinopathy: is it the over-stimulation or the under-stimulation of tendon cells? *Int J Exp Pathol.* 88: 217–226.

Couppe, C., Kongsgaard, M., Aagaard, P., Hansen, P., Bojsen-Moller, J., Kjaer, M. & Magnusson, S.P. (2008) Habitual loading results in tendon hypertrophy and increased stiffness of the human patellar tendon. *J Appl Physiol.* 105: 805–810.

Heinemeier, K.M., Olesen, J.L., Haddad, F., Langberg, H., Kjaer, M., Baldwin, K.M. & Schjerling, P. (2007) Expression of collagen and related growth factors in rat tendon and skeletal muscle in response to specific contraction types. *J Physiol.* 582: 1303–1316.

Heinemeier, K.M., Schjerling, P., Heinemeier, J., Magnusson, S.P. & Kjaer, M. (2013) Lack of tissue renewal in human adult Achilles tendon is revealed by nuclear bomb 14C. *FASEB J.*

Kjaer, M. (2004) Role of extracellular matrix in adaptation of tendon and skeletal muscle to mechanical loading. *Physiol Rev.* 84: 649–698.

Magnusson, S.P., Langberg, H. & Kjaer, M. (2010) The pathogenesis of tendinopathy: balancing the response to loading. *Nat Rev Rheumatol.* 6: 262–268.

Miller, BF., Olesen, J.L., Hansen, M., Dossing, S., Crameri, R.M., Welling, R.J., Langberg, H., Flyvbjerg, A., Kjaer, M., Babraj, J.A., Smith, K. & Rennie, M.J. (2005) Coordinated collagen and muscle protein synthesis in human patella tendon and quadriceps muscle after exercise. *J Physiol.* 567: 1021–1033.

Nishimura, T., Hattori, A. & Takahashi, K. (1994) Ultrastructure of the intramuscular connective tissue in bovine skeletal muscle. A demonstration using the cell-maceration/scanning electron microscope method. *Acta Anat.* 151:250–257.

CHAPTER 6

Anatomy trains in motion

Thomas Myers

Given the new understanding of what Schleip has termed the 'neuro-myo-fascial web' (Schleip, 2003) (Chapter 1), let us now turn our attention to functional chains of myofascia, known as 'myofascial meridians' or, the Anatomy Trains, to explore some implications of this point of view for movement training (Myers 2001, 2009, 2013).

'Muscle' limitations

For the last four hundred years, our guiding light in understanding movement has been the concept of 'a muscle' (Vesalius, 1548). Movement has been understood to be an interplay between the forces in the surrounding universe – gravity, inertia, friction, momentum, etc. – and the force generated by the approximately 600 named muscles working in concentric, eccentric, or static contraction across joints limited by bone shape and ligamentous restriction (Hamilton, 2011). Muscle actions have been principally defined in terms of their origin to insertion on bony attachments (Muscolino, 2002).

Thinking more systemically, in the light of recent research, (Vleeming, 2007) (Barker, 2004) the concept of 'a muscle' working only to draw together its ends looks to be a more limited metaphor: useful to get here but now so outdated as to require many asterisks and caveats. It is now clear, as an example, that muscles also attach to other muscles along their sides (Huijing, 2007). The far-reaching implications to force transmission and muscle mechanics are just being explored (Maas, 2009). The elasticity of large connective structures, such as tendons, changes our thinking about force transmission and efficient movement (Kawakami, 2002). Muscles also attach to and affect nearby ligaments (Van der Wal, 2009). The epimysium also attaches to nerves and neurovascular bundles that serve that muscular tissue (Shacklock, 2005).

Thus, the origin-to-insertion standard theory of muscle action misses out on, at least, the following four aspects which we now know need active consideration:

1. Force transmission via intermuscular fascia to nearby muscles

2. The ability of muscle tension to reinforce nearby ligaments

3. The pull on nearby neurovascular bundles, and

4. (The subject of this chapter) force transmission from segment to segment via fascial continuities spanning the joints (Franklyn-Miller, 2009) (Tietze, 1921).

Fascial neurology

On the neurological side, the nervous system seems to be around six times more sensorially interested in what goes on in the fascial matrix than it does in detecting changes in the muscle itself (Van der Wal, 2009). In other words, there are multiple stretch receptors which, depending on their arrangement, can detect stretch, vibration, pressure, shear, or convey pain, for each muscle spindle detecting length changes.

Furthermore, no representation of individual muscles has been found within the sensory or motor cortex of the brain. The nervous system works in terms of a cybernetic, or self-regulatory system, managing individual neuromotor units governing on the order of 10–100 muscle cells within a muscle (Williams, 1995). The brain organises movement in terms of coordinating these individual units, not, as our anatomy books do, in terms of individual named muscles. This means that the topology of contraction and fascial plane movement within muscles (perimysium) and between them (intermuscular septa) during any motion are far more complex than we have previously assumed (Fukunaga, 2010).

Biotensegrity

Another limitation in our current thinking is suggested by the 'bio-tensegrity' model, which has been applied to the whole body (Fuller, 1975) (Levin, 2003) (Myers, 2009) (Scarr, 2008) and to cellular structure and peri-cellular mechanotransduction (Ingber, 1998) (Horowitz, 1999). This engineering model allows us to go beyond the usual Newtonian thinking in terms of forces and vectors of muscles on joints. This enables us to see how our 70 trillion cells hang together in one organism as an 'adhesome', (Zaidel-Bar et al., 2007), (Zamir & Geiger 2001) and how the 'neuromyofascial web' accommodates movement as a self-adjusting whole. The Anatomy Trains map out an actual set of connected tissues in the parietal myofascia that essentially form the outer tensional network that pulls in on the skeleton to help keep it erect and in the proper relationship: or not, in dysfunction.

In summary, from either a fascial, neurological or biomechanical point of view, the ubiquitous concept of 'a distinct muscle' turns out to be an artifact of our common dissection method, and is neither a biomechanical nor a neurological reality. This idea has yet to penetrate the professional populace working with the public in either rehabilitative or training terms.

Once we reject the old idea, the significance of all these new findings taken together can be summed up in one word: Resilience. All the factors named above contribute to the resilience of human tissue and to rapid global and local distribution of strain and differentiated response of the organism as a whole. The 'isolated muscle theory' that has predominated our thinking has limited our perception of this body-wide 'give' that is essential to resilience.

Anatomy Trains

The Anatomy Trains myofascial meridians map is one small aspect of this larger vision, and concerns consistent longitudinal connections within the singular fascial webbing. It posits myofascial force transmission, at the very least in the stabilising of movement and in postural compensation, from one myofascial unit to another along these lines. To construct the Anatomy Trains map, we look for consistent fibre direction and fascial plane level. In this light, 12 myofascial meridians of at least three muscles each have been described.

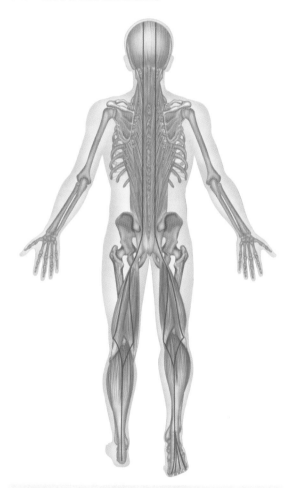

Figure 6.1

Superficial Back Line

The Superficial Back Line, which traverses the posterior aspect of the body from toes to nose, operates functionally to bring our eyes up to positions that satisfy our curiosity, and lifts our body upright and keeps it posturally stable.

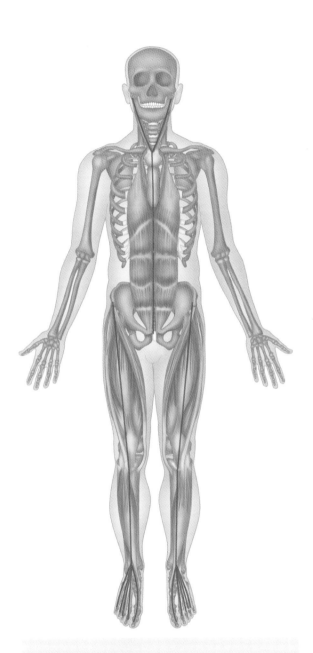

Figure 6.2
Superficial Front Line

The Superficial Front Line, which traverses the anterior surface of the body, protects the ventral cavity and is thus associated with the Startle Response, and creates trunk flexion with leg extension.

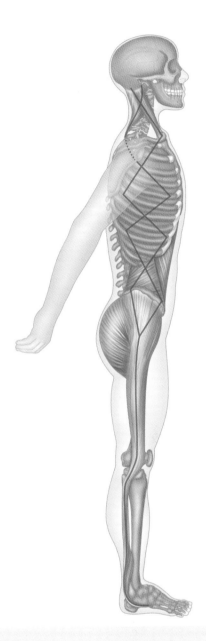

Figure 6.3
Lateral Line

The Lateral Line, which runs from outer arch to ear, operates to create lateral bends or to prevent lateral bends to the opposite side. Thus, the Lateral Line operates to maintain stability during locomotion.

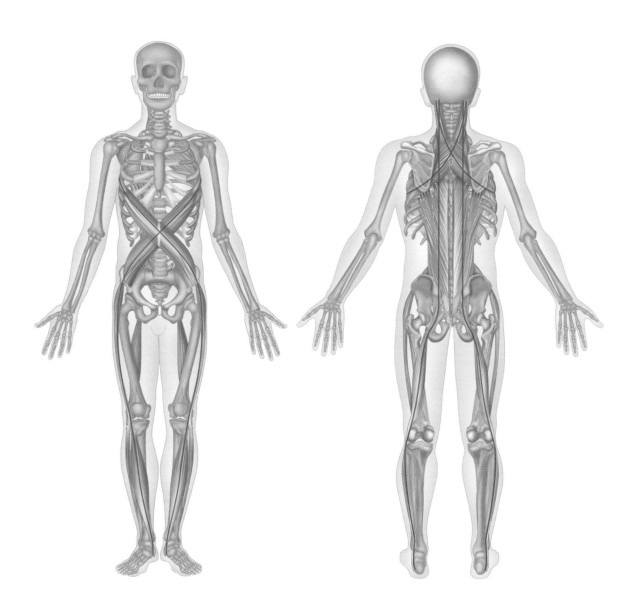

Figure 6.4
Spiral Line: (front and back view)

The Spiral Line winds around the body through the previous three cardinal lines, creating and modulating rotational and oblique movements in gait and sport.

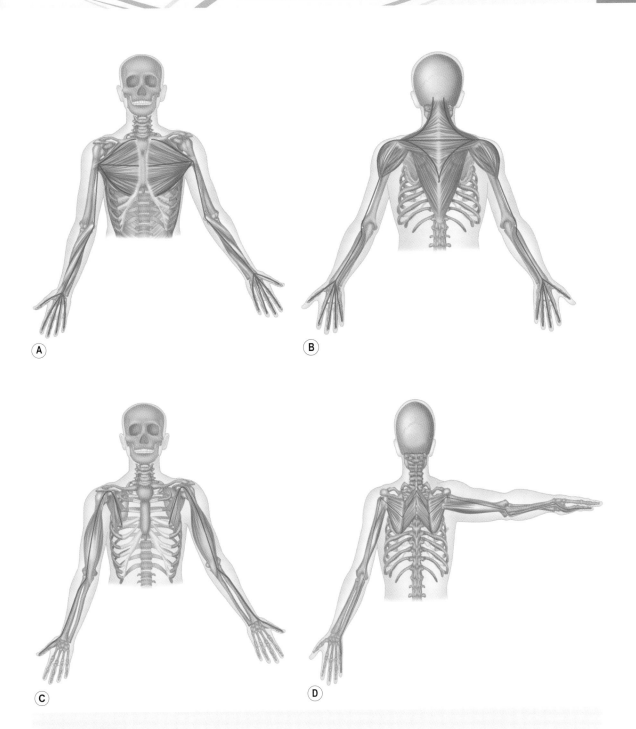

Figure 6.5 ABCD

Arm Lines

The four Arm Lines stabilise and move the arms and shoulders through their wide range of motion.

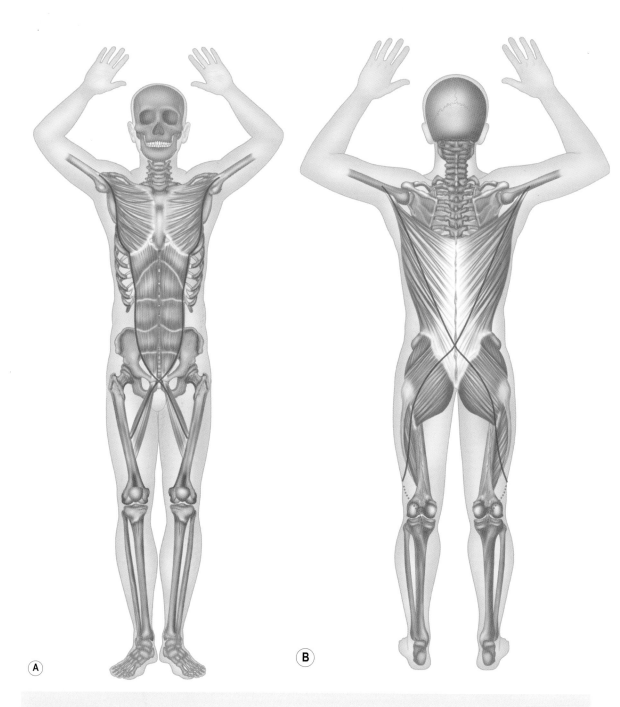

Ⓐ   Ⓑ

Figure 6.6 A & B
Functional Lines

The three Functional Lines stabilise the shoulders to the contralateral and ipsilateral legs, extending the lever arms of the limbs through the trunk.

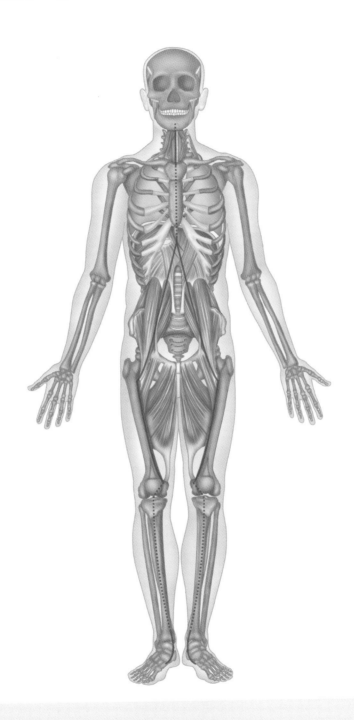

Figure 6.7
Deep Front Line

The Deep Front Line, which runs from the inner arch to the underside of the skull and includes all of what could be termed the body's 'core', supports the stability and axial-appendicular extension in all our movements.

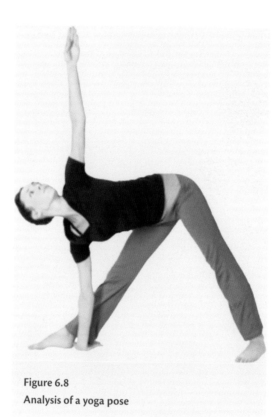

Figure 6.8
Analysis of a yoga pose

Trikonasana

Although difficult on the printed page, let us put the Anatomy Trains map into motion, by looking at a common but complex yoga pose Trikonasana or triangle pose in terms of the Anatomy Trains lines. A good analysis would require seeing the pose executed to both right and left, to see the differences from right to left. Based on this one photo, we can see good form in the legs, with the Lateral Line on the left side being evenly elongated from the outer ankle to the hip, and the Deep Front Line up the inside-back of the right leg up to the pelvic floor on that side.

In the upper body, we see more compensation, not in the upper Lateral Line, but in the upper Spiral Line. From her right ASIS (anterior superior iliac spine), the internal and contralateral external oblique and the serratus anterior on the left rib cage is sufficiently short to pull the left rib cage forward so the breastbone faces down towards the ground. The extra twist is required as compensation in the neck and in resisting the left shoulder coming forward.

Conversely, the left Spiral Line, from the left ASIS passing down and under her right rib cage to the right scapula and on to the left side of the head, could be considered to be too weak and in need of some strengthening to bring the right ribs further forward and allow the twist in the torso to straighten. We can wager that, if it is an imbalance in the Spiral Line, the pose would look significantly different on the other side.

Perhaps our premise is wrong and the inability to rotate the torso is not due to an imbalance in the Spiral Line but in the rotational muscles closer to the spine, perhaps the psoas complex in the front or the multifidus complex in the back. We would test this with palpatory or movement assessments to isolate whether the restriction was in either the neuromotor patterning or the fascia connected to the Spiral Line, Superficial Back Line or the Deep Front Line. Any or all of these together could be the 'cause' of this apparent limitation in movement. Of course, it is possible that the compensation is due to a structural anomaly within the spine, which we could detect by 'end-feel' in the movement assessment.

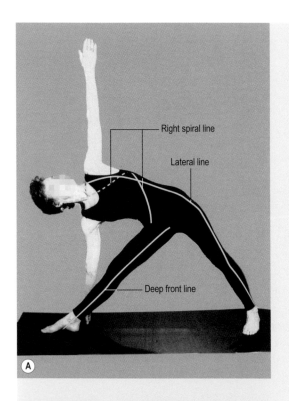

A

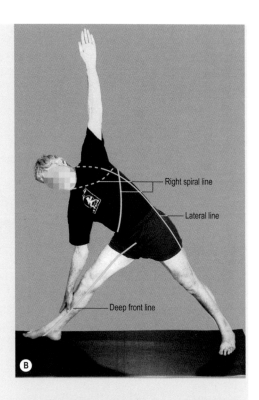

B

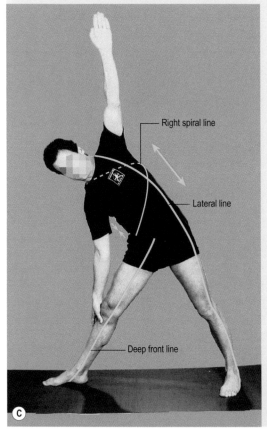

C

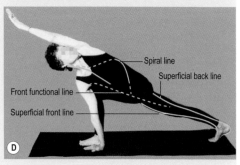

D

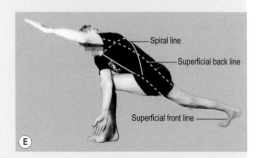

E

(Continued)

(Continued)

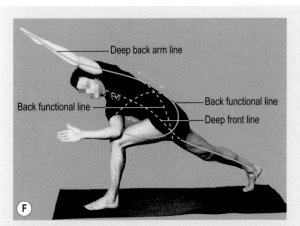

Figures 6.9

A–F Yoga photos from Anatomy Trains (Reproduced with kind permission from Lotus Publishing.)

Putting our hands just below the bra line on either side and encouraging the rib cage toward a left rotation will reveal which tissues are restraining the motion, so that specific and appropriate movement cues or manual therapy may be applied to create even tone along the line.

In the pictures below, we can see a teacher, an experienced student, and a neophyte all doing the same pose. We can readily see how the lines become straighter and more even in tone with developing practice. This palintonicity is a hallmark of elongated and balanced posture, stabilised functional movement, and provides the greatest access to resilience along and deep to the lines.

The author makes no claim as to the exclusive nature of the Anatomy Trains. For one, those with significant deviance from the usual structure, as in a significant scoliosis or alteration from trauma, may create their own fascial 'lines of transmission'. Secondly, the actuality of force transmission along the Anatomy Trains is strongly suggested by some literature (Franklin-Miller et al., 2009) (Vleeming & Stoeckart, 2007) but is yet to be proven by scientific research. The author is confident that something of this nature will prove to be the case but meantime *caveat lector* (reader beware).

Proportional movement

In the stability/mobility (stiffness/control) modeling of human movement, the Anatomy Trains contribute to both. The key to the difference can be summed up as 'proportional movement'.

All biological structures are granted a bit of 'give'. Even living bone demonstrates resilience, though it reduces as the body grows older, and every softer tissue, from cartilage to ligament to tendon to fascia to nerve to every other named tissue, will bend or stretch or deform either a little or a lot before it tears or breaks.

In movement, tissues are commonly taken beyond their resting length into a process of stretch. The stretch is translated into both the cells, of all tissues along the line, and the fibres and mucous (GAGs) of the interstitia (Ingber, 2006) (Langevin et al., 2006).

Given that the bearing point between the bones, at any given moment, constitutes the fulcrum for such tissue stretch, and given that the exogenous forces bearing on the tissues are within that tissue's ability to stay intact, then we can logically conclude that the largest movement will be near the skin, farthest away from that axial point. The rim of the wheel moves more than the hub. Therefore the sensory endings in the skin will be most sensitive to initiated movement.

Secondly, if we accept the notion that the body will distribute such strain both laterally and longitudinally, then there must be a slight 'give' or resilience in the tissues around the joints.

These tissues are called 'muscle attachments' in classical theory, or more generally 'peri-articular tissues'. In the Anatomy Trains metaphor we call them 'stations' to indicate that, even though the connective tissues in those areas are stuck down to the underlying joint capsule or periostea, there is a fundamental continuity of the connective tissue fibres in both direction and plane into the next segment and often onto a different muscle.

Resilience

For instance, the Spiral Line posits a continuity from the tibialis anterior of the anterior crural compartment with the anterior portion of the iliotibial tract, which in turn connects to the tensor fasciae latae and thus to the anterior superior iliac spine.

The Lateral Line suggests a connection from the long fibularis muscle (peroneus longus) across the fibular head at the superior end of the lateral compartment onto the central part of the iliotibial tract and up via the aponeurosis of gluteus medius to a wide attachment on the iliac crest. Deep to this line would be the lateral collateral ligament (LCL), connecting the fibular head to the lateral condyle of the femur just above the joint capsule. Deep to the lateral collateral ligament (LCL) would be the joint capsule itself, which includes the cruciate ligaments.

Although these fascial structures are identified separately, the outside of the knee is a fascial continuity from skin to bone, so all of these structures are connected. There is no discontinuity in the tissue (Guimberteau, 2004). So the question arises: in day-to-day functional movement, or in more strenuous high-performance movement occasioned by sport, dance, or an impending injury, can the tissue 'give' enough to allow the force to be distributed more widely or will all the force be focused on a particular structure, which is then more likely to fail?

Obviously, too much 'give' in these structures would contribute to joint instability and those with 'ligamentous laxity' can experience joint subluxation or malalignment fairly easily (Milhorat et al., 2007). Less obviously, too much stiffness means more strain localisation, which can contribute to local structures, the lateral

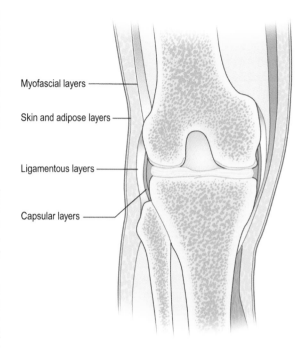

Myofascial layers

Skin and adipose layers

Ligamentous layers

Capsular layers

Figure 6.10

Tissue resilience

collateral ligament (LCL), medial collateral ligament (MCL), or anterior cruciate ligament (ACL) for instance, being strained to the point of tearing.

The ideal lies somewhere in the middle: enough give to allow for strain distribution but not enough to allow for too much joint play. The factors involved in where that ideal set point would be depend on the genetic predisposition to fascial build-up within the person, as well as their training and performance demands.

If we could magically observe, in a healthy living body, a cross-layer slice from the skin down to the outside of the knee capsule during a long lateral reach, like the top of a tennis serve, we would see each successive layer moving on the one below from the surface down to the nearly immoveable bone-to-bone layer. This resilience, or lack thereof, can be felt when placing the hands inside and outside a knee when such a movement is performed. By doing this, with a number of different subjects, it is easy to tell where the resilience is too 'tough', so non-compliant as to lead to a tearing injury in extremis, or too 'tender', overly compliant and likely to lead to joint displacement in extremis.

In the case of 'too tough', specified sustained precise stretching or manual work is called for to increase the resilience across these Anatomy Trains 'stations' that link the muscles across the joints. Cases that show 'too compliant' tissues would require increased muscle tone in the myofascial 'tracks' that support the 'stations', in this case the extensions of the abductors and the fibular muscles. This serves simply as an example of a process going on throughout the body. We could imagine a vertical view from the gluteus maximus to the deepest part of the sacrotuberous ligament in a forward bend or the ubiquitous yoga asana, 'Downward Dog'. We would expect:

- the gluteus to give way easily into an elastic stretch
- the superficial part of the sacrotuberous ligament to link and distribute strain from the hamstrings to the back 'myofascialature' of the thoracolumbar area, and
- the deep portion to maintain the necessary relationship between the sacrum and ischium, allowing only a little give in the sacroiliac joint for the couple of degrees of movement required.

Excess chronic muscle tension or fascial adhesion anywhere in this linked chain could skew the distribution of these forces, creating the conditions for injury, postural compensation, known to trainers as 'bad form', or chronic overuse of tissues leading to pain.

As another example, in a side bend can you see or palpate the progressive movement from the lateral abdominal obliques through lateral edge of the iliocostalis lumborum and the lateral raphé of the abdominals through the quadratus lumborum to the intertransversarii to the intertransverse ligaments near the spine? Lack of resilience in any of these structures will create functional aberrations. The skilled practitioner will apply manual or movement therapy to the precise structures needing either more resilience or more tone.

Give a little

Small movements in the profound tissues allow the big movements closer to the surface. The movement of the dural membranes commonly palpated in cranial osteopathy (Sutherland, 1990) or the mobility of the organs assessed in visceral manipulation (Barrall et al., 1988) are other common examples of small inner movements that have significant effect on the large outer movements if they are missing or aberrated.

In the parietal myofascia, that is the domain of the Anatomy Trains and most trainers, physiotherapists, and manual therapists, we see this in the tiny adjustments in the sacroiliac joints, which have such wide effects on larger movement of the body as a whole. With too little sacroiliac movement, there is a large compensatory pattern in the gait and the tendency to 'export' the problems to the lumbar spine. With laxity and too much sacroiliac movement, the outer body strives to compensate for too much inner movement by using the outer 'myofascialature' as straps.

Across the entire body, from the spine to the limbs and across all the Anatomy Trains lines, we are looking for the 'Goldilocks' feeling of 'just right'. This varies between subjects depending on natural fascial tone. It requires on-the-job training in accurate palpation of the Anatomy Trains 'stations' in the relative movement of inner structures to set the stage for the proper movement of the outer structures.

Turning back to our knee example, soccer/football players, require stability generation on the inside and outside of the 'postural' leg when planting it preparatory to a kick with the opposite foot. As that foot lands, and the player seeks stability, differences in the turf or the player's angle require near instantaneous adjustability in the foot, ankle, knee and hip.

As a test for this adjustability and resilience through the knee, have the player stand in front of you as you kneel and cup your hands around the inside and outside of the knee, covering the Lateral Line tissues on the outside and the Deep Front Line tissues (from the pes anserinus down to the medial collateral ligament) on the inside. Have your client, using the other foot or a handhold for balance and keeping the planted foot on the ground, slowly translate his pelvis laterally from

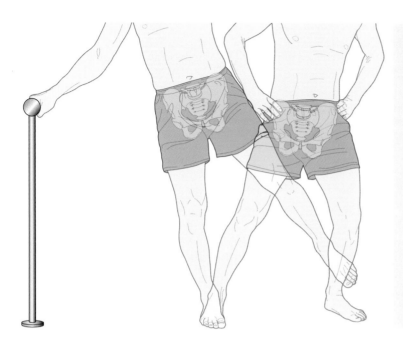

Figure 6.11

Hands on knee

left to right. This will naturally create ab- and adduction at the hip, and inversion and eversion at the subtalar joint at the ankle.

The knee is supposedly simply maintaining its extension between these two lateral movements at the joints above and below. But what do you feel inside and outside the knee in between as they do this movement? In a resilient body, you will feel a slight give in the tissues under your hand. In a healthy body, the skin will move the most, the underlying tissues of the Anatomy Trains (parietal myofasciae) will manifest some give, and at the ligamentous level a very slight give can be felt. With a little practice, you will be able to tell where there is too much give in the tissues and where there is too little, and with a little more practice you will be able to identify which layer within the leg is not coordinating with the rest, and apply to those tissues whatever treatment form is at your disposal.

Clinical summary

The new research on the properties of fascial tissues, the cybernetic nature of neural plasticity and the bio-tensegrity model of the actual engineering relationship between the soft and bony tissues, all suggest that holistic modeling of training results is required to supplement the individual structure model used for the last few centuries. The Anatomy Trains myofascial meridians map provides a model for measuring resilience and total body participation in movement that leads to long-term health. Learning to measure resilience and to recognise where tissue 'give' is not occurring will allow the trainer to make adjustments, often at some distance from the site of stress or pain, that will promote maximum performance with minimum injury.

References

Barker, P.J., Briggs, C.A. & Bogeski, G. (2004) Tensile transmission across the lumbar fascia in unembalmed cadavers: effects of tension to various muscular attachments *Spine* 29(2): 129–138.

Barrall, J.P. & Mercier, P. (1988) *Visceral Manipulation.* Seattle: Eastland Press.
Earls, J. & Myers, T. (2010) *Fascial Release for Structural Balance.* Chichester, Lotus Publishing.

Franklyn-Miller, A., et al. (2009) *The Strain Patterns of the Deep fascia of the Lower Limb*, In: Fascial Research II: Basic Science and Implications for Conventional and Complementary Health Care Munich: Elsevier GmbH.

Fukunaga, T., Kawakami, Y., Kubo, K. & Kanehisa, H. (2002) Muscle and tendon interaction during human movements. *Exerc Sport Sci Rev* 30(3): 106–110.

Fuller, B. (1975) *Synergetics.* Macmillian, New York, Ch 7.

Guimberteau, J.C. (2004) *Strolling under the skin*, Paris: Elsevier.

Hamilton, N., Weimar, W. & Luttgens, K. (2011) *Kinesiology: Scientific Basis of Human Motion*, 12th ed. NY: McGraw-Hill.

Horwitz, A. (1997) Integrins and health. *Scientific American*; May: 68–75.

Huijing, P. (2007) Epimuscular myofascial force transmission between antagonistic and synergistic muscles can explain movement limitation in spastic paresis *J Biomech.* 17(6): 708–724.

Ingber, D. (1998) The architecture of life. *Scientific American* January: 48–57.

Ingber, D. (2006) Mechanical control of tissue morphogenesis during embryological development. *International Journal of Developmental Biology* 50: 255–266.

Kawakami, Y., Muraoka, T., Ito, S., Kanehisa, H. & Fukunaga, T. (2002) In vivo muscle fibre behaviour during countermovement exercise in humans reveals a significant role for tendon elasticity. *J Physiol* 540(2): 635–646.

Langevin, H.M., Bouffard, N.A. & Badger, G.J. (2006) Subcutaneous tissue fibroblast cytoskeletal remodeling induced by acupuncture: evidence for a mechanotransduction-based mechanism. *J of Cell Bio* 207(3): 767–744.

Levin, S. (2003) The Tensegrity-truss as a model for spine mechanics. *J. of Mechanics in Medicine and Biology* 2(3): 374–388.

Maas, H. & Huijing, P. (2009) Synergoistic and antagonistic interaction in the rat forelimb: acute after-effects of coactivation. *J. Applied Physiology* 107: 1453–1462.

Milhorat, T.H., Bolognese, P.A., Nishikawa, M., McDonnell, N.B. & Francomano, C.A. (2007) "Syndrome of occipitoatlantoaxial hypermobility, cranial settling, and chiari malformation type I in patients with hereditary disorders of connective tissue". *Journal of Neurosurgery Spine* 7(6): 601–609.

Muscolino, J. (2002) *The muscular system manual.* Redding CT: JEM Pub.

Myers, T. (2001, 2009, 2013) *Anatomy Trains.* Edinburgh: Churchill Livingstone.

Scarr, G. (2008) A model of the cranial vault as a tensegrity structure, and its significance to normal and abnormal cranial development, *International Journal of Osteopathic Medicine* 11: 80–89.

Schleip, R. (2003) Fascial plasticity - a new neurobiological explanation. *J Bodyw Mov Ther.* 7(1): 11–19, 7(2): 104–116

Shacklock, M. (2005) *Clinical Neurodynamics.* Burlington MA: Butterworth-Heinemann.

Sutherland, W.G. (1990) *Teachings in the Science of Osteopathy.* Portland OR: Rudra Press.

Tietze, A. (1921) Concerning the Architectural Structure of the Connective Tissues of the Human Sole. Bruns' Beitrage zur Klinischen Chirurgie 123: 493–506.

Van der Wal, J. (2009) *The architecture of connective tissue in the musculoskeletal system* in Huijing et al. eds: Fascia Research II, Basic Science and Implications Munich: Elsevier GmbH.

Vesalius, A. (1548) De fabrici corporis humani pub in 1973. NY: Dover Publications.

Vleeming, A. & Stoeckart, R. (2007) The role of the pelvic girdle in coupling the spine and the legs: a clinical-anatomical perspective on pelvic anatomy, Ch 8 in *Movement, stability and lumbo-pelvic pain*, Eds: Vleeming, A., Mooney, V., Stoeckart, R., Edinburgh: Elsevier.

Williams, P., ed (1995) *Gray's Anatomy 38th ed*: The Anatomical Basis of Medicine and Surgery, Edinburgh, Churchill Livingstone. 753.

Zaidel-Bar, R., Itzkovitz, S., Ma'ayan, A., Iyengar, R. & Geiger, B. (2007) Functional atlas of the integrin adhesome. *Nat Cell Biol.* 2007 August; 9(8): 858–867.

Zamir, E. & Geiger, B. (2001) Molecular complexity and dynamics of cell-matrix adhesions. *J. Cell Sci.* 114, 3583–3590.

CHAPTER 7

Purposeful movements as a result of coordinated myofascial chain activity, represented by the models of Kurt Tittel and Leopold Busquet

Philipp Richter

Dancing, figure skating, golf, tennis and even boxing have one thing in common: if performed or played by accomplished people, the movements involved appear simple, fluid and elegant.

The apparent simplicity and elegance are the result of coordinated and well-balanced movements, due to years of intensive and purposeful training. Beside talent, hard work and endurance, a fit and optimally working musculoskeletal system is necessary. The elegance and the precision of the movements results from the fine adjustment of muscle chain movements. The muscles can be seen as an organ of the axial and extremity fasciae. The fasciae link the muscles and form myofascial slings. This chapter examines muscle chains or muscle slings. Using the muscle chain models of Leopold Busquet and Dr Kurt Tittel, it is shown, in some activities, which myofascial chains could underlie the movement patterns. First, the myofascial system will be briefly explained.

The myofascial system

The myofascial system consists of approximately 430 skeletal muscles, which are wrapped by fasciae. Making up more than 40% of the whole body weight, for an average person of 70 kg, it is the biggest organ of the body.

The fasciae connect the muscles with each other and with the skeleton. They also provide the wrapping for the organs, the vessels and the nervous system.

Anatomically, the fasciae can be divided into four groups (Willard et al., 2011):

1. Pannicular fascia: superficial fascia, beneath the skin, which covers the whole body except the orifices of the body.

2. Axial and appendicular fascia: This fascial layer represents the fasciae of the musculoskeletal system, which build the myofascial chains.

3. Visceral fascia: The visceral fasciae is the wrapping of the organs. They are fixed at the cranial base, around the pharingeal tubercel, and throughout the whole spinal column down to the sacrum. In the thorax, this fixing consists of the thoracic mediastinum and in the abdomen the abdominal mediastinal fascia. The organs are provided with nerves and vessels by these structures.

4. Meningeal fascia: They consist of the three meninges: dura mater, arachnoidea, and pia mater. The three meninges represent a continuum and are linked via the Dura mater with the periost.

The four fascial layers represent a unity and are all connected to the spinal column except the fascia superficialis. About 80% of all the afferent fibres of a peripheral nerve come from the myofascial tissue (Schleip, 2003). This is a clear illustration of the importance of the myofascial system for the organism. The continuity of the fasciae, as well as their rich nerval supply, means that the myofascial system is a sensitive and highly efficient organ. It is not only important for mobility and the stability but also for the respiration, the venolymphatic circulation and the mobilisation of the organs (Finet & Williame, 2013). If there are functional or structural disturbances, the fascial continuity can have a negative effect on the musculoskeletal system. Muscle contractions, adhesions or retractions have an impact on the whole myfoascial system. Scars from an operation, or an injury, lead to tensions in the myofascial network.

The musculature can be divided into the appendicular muscles and trunk muscles. Here, it has to be considered that there is also an appropriate force transmission that enables a chain activity.

The trunk muscles can be divided in two groups (Bergmark, 1989):

1. The deep, stabilising system or the local muscles. These include the diaphragm, the pelvic floor, the transversus abdominis and the obliquus internus as well as the multifidi. At the thoracic level there are the intercostal muscles.

2. The superficial system or the global muscles. These include muscles which either have no direct muscular insertion on the spinal column or which link the extremities to the spinal column.

The myofascial chains (Busquet, 1992) or muscular slings (Tittel, 2003) are mainly formed by the superficial muscles.

To allow the myofascial chains to work in the best possible way and enable movement, the trunk must be stabilised. This task is done by the deep stabilising system. Tests have shown that to allow movements of the extremities, the deep muscles contract by fractions of a second earlier than the extremity musculature (Cresswell et al., 1992) (Hodges et al., 1997). The conclusion is that the deep muscles stabilise the trunk in order to give the appendicular muscles a stable hold.

If one considers the fibre direction of the musculature and the collagen fibres in the connective tissue, one can recognise clear fibre lines that can be seen as adaptations of the tissue to strains. Diagonal and longitudinal fibre lines are seen as well as ventral and dorsal, which can be assigned to movement patterns. Indeed, both Busquet and Tittel describe oblique or diagonal chains and straight chains. The straight chains serve symmetric movements like bending or jumping.

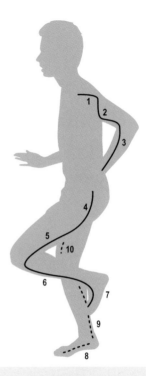

Figure 7.1

Muscle chains of the limbs during running or walking:

Note the alternation of flexion and extension at every joint!

Upper extremity:
1. Shoulder extension,
2. Elbow flexion,
3. Hand extension.

Lower extremity:
4. Hip flexion,
5. Knee flexion,
6. Foot dorsiflexion.
7. Toe flexion,
8. Toe plantar flexion,
9. Ankle extension,
10. Knee extension

4-5-6-7: Flexion chain of the lower limb during the swing phase of gait;
8-9-10: Extension chain of the lower limb during the stance phase of gait.

In contrast, walking and running are activities where a diagonal pattern is obvious. There are also many other activities by which different

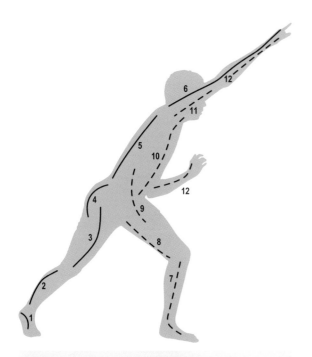

Figure 7.2

Flexion and extension chains:

Extension chain (continuous line):
1. Plantar flexors of the foot,
2. M. triceps surae,
3. M. quadriceps femoris,
4. M. glutaeus maximus,
5. Mm. erector spinae,
6. Extensors of shoulder, elbow, and hand

Flexion chain (dotted line):
7. Dorsal flexors of the foot,
8. Hamstrings,
9. M. iliopsoas,
10. M. rectus abdominis,
11. Mm. pectoralis major and minor,
12. Hand and finger flexors

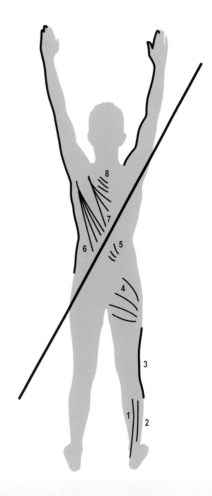

Figure 7.3

Posterior diagonal chain left:
1. M. tibialis posterior,
2. M. triceps surae,
3. Iliotibial tract,
4. M. glutaeus maximus,
5. Iliotransversal fibres of the right M. quadratus lumborum,
6. Left M. latissimus dorsi,
7. Left M. trapezius, ascending part
8. Left Mm. rhomboïdei

patterns of the upper and lower extremities can be recognised, for example, lifting an object from the ground. Here, one can recognise an extension pattern of the lower extremities and the back and a flexion pattern of the arms (Figure 7.6).

A similar pattern can be seen in rowing. While the upper extremities make flexion movements, the lower extremities make extension movements and the other way around. It is different again when a footballer kicks a ball. Here, we have a contraction of the dorsiflexors of the foot, the knee extensors and the hip flexors (Figure 7.6).

The same is true for a tennis player when they hit the ball with a forehand or a backhand.

The following pictures show the muscle chains for three selected activities:

– Throwing
– Kicking a ball
– Lifting a weight from the floor

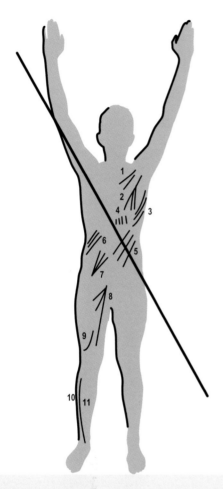

Figure 7.4

Anterior diagonal chain right:

1. Left M. pectoralis minor,
2. Left M. pectoralis major,
3. Left M. serratus anterior,
4. Left Mm. intercostali externi,
5. Left M. obliquus abdominis externus,
6. Right M. obliquus abdominis internus,
7. Right M. iliopsoas,
8. Right Mm. adductorii,
9. Right M. vastus medialis,
10. Right M. peronei,
11. Right M. tibialis anterior

This change of flexion and extension in the articulations of hand, elbow and shoulder cannot be detected (see Figure 7.2).

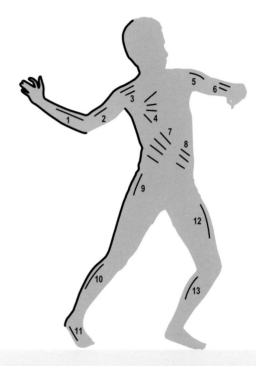

Figure 7.5

Starting position for throwing with the right hand:

Note: Weight distributed on both legs, trunk bent and rotated right, left arm stretched forward for balance. This position allows for pretension on the left anterior diagonal muscle chain.

1. Right flexors of the hand,
2. Right elbow flexors,
3. Right M. deltoideus, anterior part,
4. Right M. pectoralis major,
5. Left M. deltoideus,
6. Left elbow flexors,
7. Right M. obliquus abdominis externus,
8. Left M. obliquus abdominis internus,
9. Right M. glutaeus maximus,
10. Right M. triceps surae,
11. Right plantar flexors,
12. Left M. quadriceps femoris,
13. Left M. triceps surae

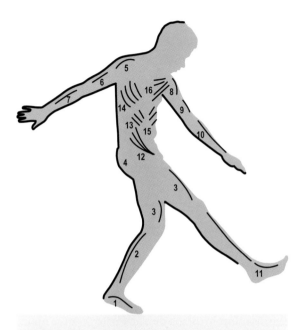

Figure 7. 6

Kicking a ball with the right foot:

Note: There is hip flexion and flexion of the foot (flexion chain) and knee extension (extension chain). Weight is on the left foot (extension chain) and opposite rotation of the shoulder girdle and the pelvis (left anterior diagonal chain).

1. Left plantar flexors,
2. Left M. triceps surae,
3. Left and right M. quadriceps femoris,
4. Left M. glutaeus maximus,
5. Left M. deltoideus, posterior part,
6. Left extensors of the elbow,
7 Left extensors of the hand,
8. Right M. deltoideus, anterior part,
9. Right extensors of the forearm,
10. Right extensors of the hand,
11. Right dorsiflexors of the foot,
12. Right M. iliopsoas,
13. Right M. obliquus abdominis externus,
14. Right M. pectoralis major,
15. Left M. serratus anterior,
16. Left M. pectoralis major

The movement is made with a straight arm. These different examples clearly highlight that the organism uses different strategies to work optimally. Stereotypical patterns exist but they can be changed, if necessary, in order to cope with the demands of the particular activity.

The nervous system plays a crucial role in the improvement of activities. This is known not only from competitive athletes but also from great musicians. The frequency of their training and movement patterns facilitates reflex arcs which finally lead to a most perfect execution of the action. This works due to the plasticity of the nervous system. The sensory receptors of the human organism play an important function in this process. They deliver the necessary information to the central nervous system, which is needed to achieve the requested action. Next to the organs of perception there are the receptors of the musculoskeletal system, which constantly deliver data to the central nervous system. These indicate that the quality of the movements depends on three factors:

1. The optimal function of the organs of perception and of the receptors

2. The capacity of the central nervous system to transform the delivered information into motor components

3. The condition of the musculoskeletal system and of the myofascial chains or slings which should carry out the activity.

Proprioceptive deficiencies, as well as functional or structural disturbances of the myofascial tissue, have a negative impact on the motor functions. It is vital to remember that movements are always the result of myofascial chains. Every dysfunction of a single member of these chains has a negative effect on the overall movement pattern.

When we talk about muscle chains, we need to know the origin, or the starting point, of the movement. A muscle needs a stable hold in order to make a movement. Is it the contact of the foot with the floor while walking or running and the grip of the hands while climbing which count as starting or fixed point? What enables gymnasts or acrobats to perform amazing feats in the air?

Many factors indicate that the trunk is the starting point for movement. This could explain why a movement of the extremities seems to be preceded by a contraction of the trunk stabilisers (Hodges et al., 1999). A stable trunk enables the muscles of the lower extremity to move the body forwards and simultaneously enables the muscles of both arms to swing. Studies seem to verify that dysfunctions of the local trunk stabilisers have a negative impact on the superficial muscles. (Keifer et al., 1997).

During dynamic activities, the myofascial chains have several tasks:

1. To guarantee the stability of the musculoskeletal system, the trunk and articulations of the extremities.

   Lifting heavy weights requires greater stability. The global muscles are contracted to help the local muscles with their stabilising task. Lumbar or pelvic instability clearly demonstrate this. The superficial muscles (M. longissimus and M. iliocostalis) are recruited to ensure stability.

2. To carry out the movement: i.e. to coordinate precision, speed and force.

   When a tennis player executes a strong serve or a javelin thrower has to throw the javelin a great distance, both the force, that the participatory muscles generate, and the speed, with which the service or the throw are executed, are important.

   To do this, first, the muscles are brought into an optimally stretched position to pretension the muscle fibres. This allows the movements to be executed with verve. The acceleration improves the intensity of the throw considerably. In general, this is found in all dynamic movements: before the muscle group becomes active, it is brought into a slightly stretched position to 'carve' the movement (Chapter 10).

3. To maintain the respiration function, as well as bladder and bowel continence.

   The rhythm of respiration is closely linked with movement. This is highlighted in several studies (Hodges et al. 2001, 1997, 2001). Furthermore, it seems logical that for all activities the efficiency of the sphincters has to be assured as well. Some studies suggest that an increase of intra abdominal tension results in a rise of tonus of the sphincters of the pelvic floor as well as of the M. gluteus maximus.

4. Maintenance of equilibrium

   If one considers the starting position of someone throwing a ball, throwing with his right arm, he stands on his right foot and his trunk is leaned to the right and turned. He has lifted his right arm and keeps it stretched before the throw. In order to leave the centre of gravity over his right foot, he stretches his left arm forwards and flexes his left hip. The whole trunk is also turned to the right so that the equilibrium of the trunk is shifted to the pivot leg.

For the efficiency of the action, to throw a ball far, precisely and strongly, it is important that the 'secondary' functions are not overly energy consuming. The body must be brought into a position where the muscles that carry out the action are in an optimal state. All this is enabled by the central nervous system. The muscle slings are activated in the momentum of the movement in order to maintain equilibrium, to stabilise the trunk and the articulations and in order to carry out the actual movement (Figure 7.5).

It is also worth considering the following: given the plethora of movement possibilities of the four extremities and that the trunk is the starting point for the movements of the extremities, wouldn't it be useful to consider the muscle slings of each extremity that could be combined with one another if required?

In the following section, the muscle chains of Leopold Busquet and the muscle slings of Kurt Tittel are represented in a table (Table 7.1). For further detail of the muscles, which create the particular chain or sling, it is worth referring to the original works of the two authors (see bibliography).

In both cases the models are theoretical and represent a global behaviour in a particular situation.

The muscle chains of Leopold Busquet

Leopold Busquet describes five chains: one static chain and four dynamic ones. Two are vertical and two are diagonal dynamic chains.

1. Static posterior chain: This consists of the meninges and the ligaments of the vertebral arches.

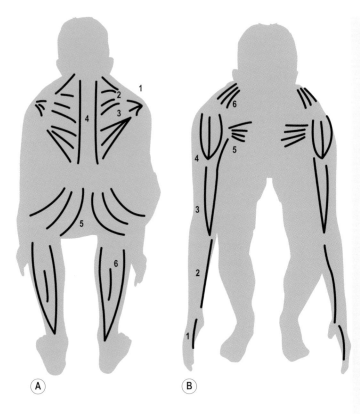

Figure 7.7

Starting position of lifting; back view and front view:

Note: There is activation of the extension chain of the back and lower extremities and of the flexion chain of the upper extremities as well as participation of the Trapezius – Pectoralis sling (muscle sling of Kurt Tittel in static motion.)

A: Back view:
1. Mm. supraspinatus and infraspinatus,
2. M. trapezius, upper part,
3. M. latissimus dorsi,
4. Mm. erector spinae,
5. M. glutaeus maximus,
6. M. triceps surae

B: Front view:
1. Finger flexors,
2. Hand flexors,
3. Mm. biceps brachii and coracobrachialis,
4. M. deltoideus,
5. M. pectoralis major and minor,
6. M. trapezius, upper part

At the pelvis, this chain goes via the gluteal fascia to the iliotibial tract and links the fibula with the membrana interossea.

2. Flexion chain: This chain causes a 'rolling' of the trunk as well as flexion and an internal rotation of the extremities.

3. Extension chain: This chain creates extension of the spinal column as well as extension and an external rotation of the extremities.

4. Anterior diagonal chain: (right) This consists of the ventral diagonal muscles which approach the left shoulder and the right pelvis. It creates flexion, internal rotation and adduction in the left upper extremity and the right lower extremity.

5. Posterior diagonal chain: (right) The muscles of this chain approach the left shoulder and the right ilium from the dorsal. The left arm and the right leg do an extension with abduction and external rotation.

The muscle slings of Kurt Tittel

In his book, *Beschreibende und funktionelle Anatomie des Menschen*, Kurt Tittel describes a multitude of muscle slings, which he represents very memorably with pictures of different sports activities. These slings can be divided into four groups:

1. Extension slings
2. Flexion slings
3. Muscle slings in side bending and rotation of the trunk
4. Muscle slings in static motion pattern.

The flexion and extension slings are very similar to the flexion and extension chains of Leopold Busquet. This also partially applies to the muscle slings in side bending and rotation of the trunk, which have certain similarities with the diagonal chains of Leopold Busquet. The last of the four groups of muscle slings however is not mentioned by Busquet.

Table 7.1

Comparison of the two muscle chain models

L Busquet 5 myofascial chains	K Tittel 5 muscle slings and 3 muscle slings in static motion pattern
1. Static posterior chain: Ligamentus apparatus of the spine including the meninges; gluteal and piriformis sheat; tensor fascia lata and fibula with the interosseal membrane. 2. Flexion chain: Extremities: - foot, knee and hip flexors - arm flexors Trunk: - primary system connecting the pelvis to the head: e.g. M. rectus abdominis - secondary system connecting the pelvis with the limbs: - lower limb: e.g. M. psoas major - shoulder blade: e.g. M. pectoralis minor - arm: e.g. M. pectoralis major 3. Extension chain: Extremities: - foot, knee and hip extensors - arm extensors Trunk: - primary system: Mm. erector spinae - secondary system connecting the trunk with the limbs: - lower limb: e.g. M. glutaeus maximus - shoulder blade: e.g. M. trapezius - arm: e.g. M. latissimus dorsi 4. Diagonal posterior chain (left or right): Muscles connecting the shoulder blade and arm of one side with the pelvis and hip of the other side; e.g.: right M. latissimus dorsi – left M. glutaeus maximus 5. Diagonal anterior chain (left or right): The same arrangement on the anterior body side; e.g. right M. pectoralis major – left M. obliquus internus **Special emphasis** **L. Busquet** - Emphasises visceral and cranial dysfunctions as possible causes for dominating muscle chains - Claims that imbalances of muscle chains may cause spinal troubles, like scoliosis or kypholordosis, and joint disorders like the Osgood-Schlatter disease	1.Extension sling: Extremities: - lower limb: foot, knee and hip extensors - upper limb: arm, elbow and wrist extensors - trunk: Mm. erector trunci 2. Flexion sling: Extremities: - lower limb: foot, knee and hip flexors - upper limb: arm, elbow and wrist flexors - trunk: abdominals and intercostal muscles 3. Muscle slings in sidebending and rotation: a) anteriorly connecting the shoulder blade with the opposite leg: Mm. rhomboidei – M. serratus anterior – M. obliquus externus abdominis – Mm. adductorii of the other side – M. biceps femoris (short head) – Mm. peronei b) anteriorly connecting the arm with the opposite leg: M. pectoralis major – M. obliquus internus abdominis – M. tensor fascia lata – M. tibialis anterior c) posteriorly connecting the arm with the opposite leg: M. latissimus dorsi – M. glutaeus maximus – Tractus iliotibialis– M. tibialis anterior 4. Muscle slings in static motion pattern: Aim: stabilising the shoulder girdle - M. levator – M. trapezius – M. serratus anterior sling - M. trapezius – M. pectoralis sling - Mm. rhomboidei – M. serratus anterior sling **K. Tittel** - Portrays the muscle slings which are active in several sports activities - Presents special muscle slings aimed to stabilise the shoulder girdle

Muscle slings in static motion pattern

These are muscle slings of the trunk, which help to stabilise the shoulder girdle:

- Levator – trapezius sling: cranio caudal stabilisation of the scapula

- Trapezius – pectoralis sling: external-internal rotation of the scapula
- Trapezius – serratus sling: abduction-adduction of the scapula.

These three slings stabilise the shoulder through isometric contractions, when holding a shoulder position. For shoulder movements in this particular level they can also become active in a concentric or eccentric way. To perform arm movements, the shoulder must be stabilised in order to give a fixed point to the arm muscles that perform the arm movement. This is realised by the aforementioned muscle slings.

Comparison of the two muscle chain models

1. The two cranio caudal chains for flexion and extension are identical.

2. As are the diagonal chains of the trunk. In these chains there are slight differences for the muscle slings of the lower extremities. However, both models are easily comprehensible and very complementary.

3. Neither of the models details the muscle slings of the upper extremities. The extreme diversity of the movements of the hands and the fingers, as well as the extent of the movements of the shoulder complex, make it difficult to describe simple and clear patterns. This is why the authors have limited themselves to the flexion and extension patterns.

4. Unlike Leopold Busquet, Kurt Tittel describes special muscle slings for the shoulder complex. This is useful because of the diverse movement possibilities of the upper extremity and the fact that shoulder articulations are mainly stabilised muscularly.

Critical considerations

As mentioned previously, the two models are very alike. They both allow explanation of stereotypical movement patterns.

It is worth noting that there are rare occasions when the diversity of the movements and the different capacities are carried out by one muscle chain alone. For example, lifting an object from the ground: picking up the object requires a flexion chain activity of the upper extremities, whereas the actual lift is performed by an extension chain of the back and the lower extremities. In contrast jumping with both feet simultaneously is performed by the extension chain alone. These symmetric motions are fairly rare. There are also times when many muscle groups are active in order to stabilise and to maintain equilibrium in dynamic activities. In these instances, different chains are often used simultaneously to carry out the actual activity.

For example:

1. Flexion chain of the upper extremities simultaneously with the extension chain of the lower while rowing.

2. Pulling (flexion) with the arms and stretching (extension) of the legs during a tug-of-war.

The action, the aim that the musculoskeletal system wants to achieve, is at the fore. The central nervous system assists the muscle chains in order to fulfil this aim in an energy saving, precise way. When considering different movements, often realised by the four extremities at the same time, one question arises: Should one talk about continuous chains, which link the upper and lower extremities to one another, or would it be wiser to talk about the chains of single extremities, which have their origin in the trunk?

Clinical Summary

*   All body motions are performed by myofascial chains which are probably 'whole body chains'. If there is muscle weakness one should always consider the whole myofascial chain.

*   To be efficient, muscles need a stable hold. This is done by other muscles and the skeleton. Trunk stability seems to be the pre-requisite for this task. The trunk, therefore, plays a major role in muscle performance.

*   As most activities are performed by more than one myofascial chain, which work together simultaneously to optimise the movement, this must also be taken into account in rehabilitation.

*   When we speak about myofascial chains we speak about muscle and fascia. These are two different tissues with different properties but which act together. If there is myofascial dysfunction one should treat both tissues accordingly.

References

Bergmark, A. (1989) Stability of the lumbar spine. A study in mechanical engineering. *Acta Orthopaedica Scandinavica* 230: 20–24.

Busquet, L. (1992) *Les chaînes musculaires, Tome I*. Paris: Editions Frison – Roche.

Busquet, L. (1993) *Les chaînes musculaires, Tome III*. Paris: Editions Frison – Roche.

Busquet, L. (1995) *Les chaînes musculaires, Tome IV*. Paris: Editions Frison – Roche.

Cresswell, A.G., Grundstrom, A. & Thorstensson, A. (1992) Observations on intra-abdominal pressure and patterns of abdominal intra-muscular activity in man. *Acta Physiologica Scandinavica* 144: 409–418.

Finet, G. & Williame, C. (2013) *Viszerale Osteopathie*. Privatverlag der Autoren.

Hodges, P.W. & Richardson, C.A. (1997) Contraction of the abdominal muscles associated with movement of the lower limb. *Phy Ther.* 77: 132–144.

Hodges, P.W., Butler, J.E., Mc Kenzie, D. & Gandevia, S.C. (1997) Contraction of the human diaphragm during postural adjustments. *J Physiol.* 505: 239–548.

Hodges, P.W. & Saunders, S. (2001) *Coordination of the respiratory and locomotor activities of the abdominal muscles during walking in humans*. Christchurch, New Zealand: IUPS Press.

Hodges, P.W., Cresswell, A.G. & Thorstensson, A. (1999) Preparatory trunk motion accompanies rapid upper limb movement. *Exp Brain Res.* 124: 69–79.

Hodges, P.W., Heijnen, I. & Gandevia, S.C. (2001) Reduced postural activity of the diaphragm in humans when respiratory demand is increased. *J Physiol.* 537: 999–1008.

Keiffer, A., Shirazi-Adl, A. & Parnianpour, M. (1997) Stability of the human spine in neutral postures. *Eur Spine J.* 6: 45–53.

Richardson, C., Hodges, P. & Hides, J. (2009) *Segmentale Stabilisation im LWS- und Beckenbereich*. Elsevier Urban & Fischer.

Schleip, R. (2003) Fascial plasticity – a new neurobiological explanation : Part I and II. *J Bodyw Mov Ther.* January.

Tittel, K. (2003) *Beschreibende und funktionelle Anatomie des Menschen*. 14. Ausgabe: Elsevier Urban & Fischer.

Willard, F.H., Fossum, C. & Standley, P.R. (2011) *Foundations of Osteopathic Medicine*. 3. Ed., 74–92. Wolters Kluwer/Lippincott Williams & Wilkinson.

Further reading

Busquet, L. (1992) *Les chaînes musculaires*, Tome II. Paris: Editions Frison-Roche Busquet L. (2004) *Les chaînes musculaires*, Tome V. Editions Busquet.

Busquet-Vanderheyden, M. (2004) *Les chaînes musculaires*, Tome VI. Editions Busquet.

Chauffour, P. & Guillot, J.M. (1985) *Le lien mécanique ostéopathique*. Paris: Edition Maloine.

Richardson, C., Hodges, P. & Hides, J. (2009) *Segmentale Stabilisation im LWS- und Beckenbereich*. 1. Auflage: Elsevier Urban & Fischer.

Richter, P. & Hebgen, E. (2011) *Triggerpunkt und Muskelfunktionsketten*. 3., Auflage: Karl F. Haug Verlag. Stuttgart.

Schleip, R., Findley, T.W., Chaitow, L. & Huijing, P.A. (2012) *Fascia, the tensional network of the human body*. Churchill Livingstone Elsevier.

Vleeming, A., Mooney, V. & Stoeckart, R. (2007) *Movement, stability & lumbopelvic pain*. 2nd edition: Churchill Livingstone Elsevier.

CHAPTER 8

Hyper- and hypomobility of the joints: Consequences for function, activities and participation

Lars Remvig, Birgit Juul-Kristensen and Raoul Engelbert

Introduction

Hypermobility, or joint hypermobility, is a condition in which one or more joints can be moved beyond normal limits. The condition can be caused by hereditary, constitutional, structural, or functional changes in the joint and/or the surrounding connective tissue. Hypermobility has been known for centuries, and the first known description dates back to Hippocrates' observation of it in the limbs of the Scythians, a former central European population.

Nowadays, joint hypermobility is part of the diagnostic criteria for some rare hereditary disorders of connective tissue, such as Ehlers-Danlos Syndrome (EDS) (Beighton et al., 1998), Marfan Syndrom (Loeys et al., 2010) and Osteogenesis Imperfecta (Van Dijk et al., 2010). However, joint hypermobility is also part of the diagnostic criteria for Hypermobility Syndrome (Grahame et al., 2000) a condition that may be part of Ehlers-Danlos syndrome or an ordinary pain syndrome related to abnormal joint mobility.

Abbreviations

EDS	Ehlers-Danlos syndrome
EDS-HT	Ehlers-Danlos syndrome, hypermobile type
GJH	Generalised joint hypermobility
JHS	Joint hypermobility syndrome

Normal/abnormal joint mobility

According to the American Academy of Orthopedic Surgeons it is not possible to precisely determine normal mean joint mobility throughout the body (Surgeons, 1965). Consequently, the American Academy of Orthopedic Surgeons developed consensus-based estimates in degrees derived from statistical means based on reports from four committees of experts.

In general, joint mobility is regarded as a graded phenomenon (Wood, 1971), and a consensus has developed that individual joint mobility follows a Gaussian distribution (Allander et al., 1974) (Fairbank et al., 1984). With this in mind, abnormal joint mobility would reflect movements that deviate from the mean with ± two standard deviations. However, for practical purposes range of motion measurements in degrees are not manageable when testing for generalised joint hypermobility (GJH). Instead, the Beighton tests, that apply a dichotomous principle, are widely used (Beighton et al., 1973), even though the Rotès-Quèrol tests (Rotès-Quérol, 1957) are used more in Spanish and French speaking countries. The Beighton tests were described about 40 years ago (Beighton & Horan, 1970), and slightly revised a few years later to the test system used today (Beighton et al., 1973) (Figure 8.1). However, since then there has been a considerable variation in the descriptions in the literature on how to perform the various tests, and maybe more importantly, also a variation in the cut-off level for a positive test and in the definition of GJH, as demonstrated in Table 8.1.

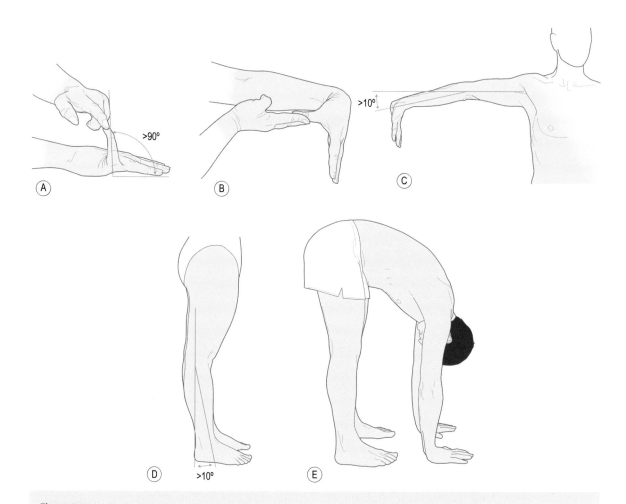

Figure 8.1

The Beighton tests

A. With the client seated, ask them to place their forearm and hand, pronated on the table. Ask them to passively extend the 5th finger. An extension beyond 90° indicates a positive test.

B. With the client seated, arm flexed 90° in shoulder, elbow extended 180° and hand pronated and relaxed, ask them to passively move the first finger to the volar aspect of the forearm. If the forearm is reached the test is positive.

C. With the client standing in front of you, ask them to abduct 90° in the shoulder with relaxed elbow and supinated hand. Support the upper arm with your ipsilateral hand. An extension beyond 10° indicates a positive test.

D. With the client standing in an upright position, turning towards you, ask them to relax and hyperextend their knee. An extension beyond 10° indicates a positive test.

E. From standing position, with their feet slightly apart, ask the client to place their hands on the floor maintaining extended knees. If the palms of the hands can easily be placed on the floor, the test is positive. Tests a. to d. are double-sided giving a total of nine tests.

Method	Tests	Definition	Comments
(Rotes-Querol, 1957)	3 tests	2/3	Adults
(Carter & Wilkinson, 1964)	C&W tests	≥3/5	Children, 6–11 years
(Beighton & Horan, 1969) (5 tests)	Beighton tests	None	Adults
(Rotes-Querol et al., 1972)	R-Q tests	None	Degré I - IV
(Beighton et al., 1973) (9 tests),	Beighton tests	None	Twsana Africans
(Bulbena et al., 1992)Hospital del Mar Criteria, 1992	Del Mar tests	4–5/10	Gender dependent
(Mikkelsson et al., 1996)	Beighton tests	≥6/9	Children, 10–12 years
(Beighton et al., 1998) Villefranche criteria, 1998	Beighton tests	≥5/9	Age, gender, ethnicity!
(Grahame et al., 2000) Brighton criteria, 2000	Beighton tests	≥4/9	Current or historical
(Smits-Engelsman et al., 2011)	Beighton tests	>5/9	Children, 6–12 years

Table 8.1

Various definitions of Generalised Joint Hypermobility

The Beighton tests, as well as the criterion for GJH, have been proven to have high inter-examiner reproducibility in children (Smits-Engelsman et al., 2011) as well as in adults (Bulbena et al., 1992) (Juul-Kristensen et al., 2007), as have the Rotès-Quérol tests (Bulbena et al., 1992). The criterion validity also seems to be high, as a positive Beighton test equals normal mean ROM +3 SD (Fairbank et al., 1984) and as GJH has high correlation to a global joint index (Bulbena et al., 1992).

Prevalence

Information on prevalence of hypermobility varies considerably. This is probably due to the variation in technique and definition, mentioned above, and due to age, gender and ethnicity of the population presented.

For children the cut-off point for defining GJH, using the Beighton scoring, varies from ≥5 to ≥7 positive tests out of nine, depending on the age group studied (Mikkelsson et al., 1996) (Smits-Engelsman et al., 2011). For adults the cut-off point for defining GJH varies between ≥4/9 and ≥5/9 (Beighton et al., 1998) (Grahame et al., 2000).

Information in the literature as to the prevalence of adults with GJH varies considerably, i.e. from 6–57% (Remvig et al., 2007), depending on the population, the diagnostic procedures and cut-off point used.

Pathogenesis

Connective tissue consists of matrix proteins such as proteoglycans and tenascins, and a mixture of various fibrillary components, such as collagen fibres, elastin fibres, fibrillins and fibroblasts. However, there is a multitude of different types of fibres, particularly within the collagenous fibres, and the spatial form and the functionality of the connective tissues in different parts of the body depends on the presence and the mixture of these many different fibre types (Chapter 1).

At least 19 different collagens have been identified, one third being fibrillar (types I, II, III, V and X) and two thirds non-fibrillar collagens (Kuivaniemi et al., 1997). The latter are subdivided into, among others, networking collagens (types IV, VIII and X), fibril associated collagens with interrupted triple helices (types IX, XII, XVI and XIX) and beaded-filament-forming collagens (type VI).

In each collagen type the molecule of a fibrillar collagen is a triple-helix formed by three polypeptide chains, named α-chains, that are wrapped around each other (Mao & Bristow, 2001). This gives rise to the names, for example COL5A1, COL5A2 and COL5A3, signalising collagen type 5, α-helix 1, 2 or 3.

One end of each collagen molecule bears a NH_2-terminal, the other a COOH-terminal, and when fibrils are formed by the collagen molecules these terminals are cleaved by peptidases.

Bearing this in mind, one may better understand why defects in collagen fibres can form so many different clinical phenotypes with varying degrees of hypermobility and other disorders, as we can encounter defects in different types of collagen, in different α-chains and different peptidase deficiency, etc. Some of these changes in the connective tissue may be so serious to the individual that they interact with the functionality and social life of the individuals, i.e. causing a disease, or the changes may even be incompatible with life (Table 8.2).

Recently it was demonstrated that defects in Tenascin-X can be another reason for hypermobility (Schalkwijk et al., 2001). The role of TNX is not fully known, but one of the functions of the protein is probably related to the organisation of collagen fibril deposition.

Pathoanatomy and physiology

Myofibroblasts: Some years ago it was demonstrated that fibroblasts in fascia from the lower leg had an electron microscopic appearance just like heart muscle cells, indicating contractile properties. It was then later demonstrated that they actually had this contractile ability. The content of these myofibroblasts is very high in fascia, in highly trained individuals as well as in certain clinical conditions such as frozen shoulder, Dupuytren's contracture, plantar fibromatosis, etc. (Schleip, 2006). According to these findings one would expect a decreased number of myofibroblasts in fascia from hypermobile patients. However, a recent study on fascia from patients with EDS classical type indicated an *increased* number of myofibroblasts, compared to healthy controls, as well as in individuals with GJH or symptomatic GJH, i.e. joint hypermobility syndrome (personal communication, Wetterslev et al., 2013).

Tendons: Patients with EDS-HT, compared to controls, have a lower passive muscle tension and a lower Achilles tendon stiffness (Rombaut et al., 2012a). Similarly, patients with EDS, classic type, have a 60% reduction in stiffness of the patellar tendon and an increase in elasticity (reduction in Youngs modulus) at maximum force compared to patients with benign JHS and to controls (Nielsen et al., 2012). In contrast there was no difference in tendon dimension based on MRI scan or on tendon elongation (ultrasonography-based) during isometric knee contractions. These results

Type	Notes	Gene(s)	Disorders
I	Scar tissue, tendons, skin, artery walls, endomysium of myofibrils, fibrocartilage, organic parts of bones and teeth	COL1A1 COL1A2	Osteogenesis imperfecta Ehlers-Danlos syndrome IV & V (arthrochalasic, dermatosparaxic) Atypical Marfan syndrome
II	Hyaline cartilage, makes up 50% of all cartilage protein. Vitreous tumour of the eye	COL2A1	Collagenopathy type II and XI
III	Found in artery walls, skin, intestines and the uterus. Is also the fibre type quickly produced by young fibroblasts in granulation tissue before the type I	COL3A1	Ehlers-Danlos syndrome III (vascular)
IV	Basal lamina; eye lens; part of the filtration system in capillaries and in the glomeruli of the kidney	COL4A1 ↓ COL4A6	Alport syndrome Goodpasture syndrome
V	Most interstitial tissue, assoc. with type I, associated with placenta	COL5A1 COL5A2 COL5A3	Ehlers-Danlos syndrome I (classical)

Table 8.2

Location of different collagenous fibres, known gene defects for these fibres and phenotypic presentations/syndromes due to these gene defects

support the general perception that hypermobility is based on changes in the extensibility of the various soft tissue components, i.e. the viscoelastic properties of ligaments, joint capsules, muscle-tendons as well as of fascia, which merge into these structures.

Risk of injuries

Subjects with GJH have an increased risk of injuries, especially in the knee (Stewart & Burden, 2004) (Pacey et al., 2010). Adults with GJH have reduced self-reported knee function (Juul-Kristensen et al., 2012), and the reported functional level corresponds well with the pre-operative functional level in individuals having anterior cruciate ligament injury (Roos et al., 1998).

Today, we have increased knowledge of muscle-tendon strength, strength balance, explosive force, endurance, co-contraction as well as on proprioception, general balance and general physical function:

Strength and strength balance

When measuring knee strength and knee strength balance (hamstring/quadriceps-ratio) in adults, subjects with GJH, JHS, and EDS-HT have lower *isokinetic* knee strength and knee strength balance (Juul-Kristensen et al., 2012) (Rombaut et al., 2012b), whereas *isometric* knee strength and knee strength balance were normal (Jensen et al., 2013) (Mebes et al., 2008).

Ten-year old children with GJH do not have lower isokinetic, or isometric knee strength or knee strength balance (Juul-Kristensen et al., 2012) (Jensen et al., 2013), whereas children with JHS have shown to have lower isometric knee strength (Fatoye et al., 2009), indicating that pain has a role in the ability to develop strength. There might also be a gender effect in performance of muscle strength, since girls and women have lower isokinetic knee extensor strength compared with healthy controls (Juul-Kristensen et al., 2012).

Explosive muscle force

This has been tested in GJH during vertical jump height, where children have increased vertical jump height (Juul-Kristensen et al., 2012) (Remvig et al., 2011), and adults showed the same tendency (Juul-Kristensen et al., 2012) (Mebes et al., 2008).

Endurance

Self-reported muscle endurance in adults with GJH is reduced (Juul-Kristensen et al., 2012), which is also the case when dynamic muscle endurance is measured in adults with either JHS or EDS-HT (Sahin et al., 2008b) (Rombaut et al., 2012b). One study found, in children only, a reduced self-reported activity level, and a greater need for rest (Schubert-Hjalmarsson et al., 2012).

Co-contraction

Muscle activity pattern over the knee is changed in both adults and children with GJH, seen as lower hamstring muscle activity at a submaximal level (Jensen et al., 2013) and increased knee muscle activity, i.e. more co-contraction, in both quadriceps and hamstrings (Jensen et al., 2013) (Greenwood et al., 2011). The adults with GJH also have reduced steadiness (Jensen et al., 2013), indicating a certain degree of knee instability.

Proprioception

Proprioception in adults with JHS is reduced in the knees, fingers and shoulders (Sahin et al., 2008a) (Jeremiah & Alexander, 2010), especially in combination with pain. Likewise in adults with EDS-HT, proprioception in the knees was reduced (Rombaut et al., 2010a).

General balance

Balance is reduced in adults with GJH (Falkerslev et al., 2012) (Mebes et al., 2008) and in EDS-HT (Rombaut et al., 2011b), whereas several studies have found balance to be increased in 8–10 year old children with GJH (Juul-Kristensen et al., 2009) (Remvig et al., 2011). However, when both pain and hypermobility are present as in children with JHS or EDS-HT, balance is significantly reduced (Schubert-Hjalmarsson et al., 2012).

General physical function

The general physical function is reduced in adults with EDS-HT (measured by chair-rise test) in addition to decreased self-reported physical activity/fitness (Rombaut et al., 2010b). The general physical function of 8–10 year-old children with GJH shows an improved fine coordination pattern, i.e. faster reaction time (Juul-Kristensen et al., 2009) and improved precision (Remvig et al., 2011). For children with JHS the motor control is reduced (Schubert-Hjalmarsson et al., 2012), along with a potential reduced motor development (Bird, 2005) (Adib et al., 2005).

All the above-mentioned signs of reduced function may be a possible explanation of the increased risk of injuries.

Symptom development

Several studies have anticipated that GJH is a predictor for development of osteoarthritis over time (Murray, 2006) (Remvig et al., 2007) but no longitudinal studies have so far confirmed this standpoint.

Self-reported knee function in adults with GJH, having at least one hypermobile knee, and adults with knee osteoarthritis, is very similar. Both groups show increased knee pain and reduced function and reduced Active Daily Living compared to a healthy population (Roos et al., 1998) (Juul-Kristensen et al., 2012).

Furthermore, when looking at gait patterns, adults with GJH have changes very similar to adults with knee osteoarthritis, and to adults with anterior cruciate ligament injuries. They also walk with increased knee flexion (Simonsen et al., 2012). Adults with EDS-HT walk with a gait pattern that is poorer and more unsecure than a healthy control group (Rombaut et al., 2011b) (Galli et al., 2011).

Ten-year-old children with GJH have a normal gait pattern (Nikolajsen et al., 2011) but children with JHS walk with stiffer knees (Fatoye et al., 2011). Whether there is a symptom development ranging from childhood to adulthood along with a development from GJH to JHS/EDS-HT has not been confirmed but can be anticipated.

Pain development

Cross-sectional studies have shown that pain is not more frequent in children of 8–10 years old with GJH compared to those without GJH (Juul-Kristensen et al., 2009) (Remvig et al., 2011). However, longitudinal studies have shown that the combination of GJH6 (i.e. GJH with six positive out of nine Beighton tests) and pain at 10 years of age is a predictor for pain recurrence and persistence at 14 years of age in both neck and lower limbs (El-Metwally et al., 2005), in contrast to GJH6 at 10 years of age without pain (El-Metwally et al., 2007) (McCluskey et al., 2012). Recently it was shown, that GJH6 at age14 is a predictor for general pain at 18 years of age (Tobias et al., 2013).

Treatment effect

Several studies have analysed the effect of treatment on subjects with JHS. Proprioceptive training has been successful (Sahin et al., 2008a) but specific or frequent training in children had no extra effect (Kemp et al., 2010, Mintz-Itkin et al., 2009). Uncontrolled studies showed stabilisation exercises to have a positive effect on adults and adolescents with JHS (Ferrell et al., 2004) (Gyldenkerne et al., 2006), and joint protection and advice of non contact-sporting activities are recommended, although the effect has not been scientifically verified (Keer & Simmonds, 2011, Pacey et al., 2010). 'Trial and error' is the most frequent approach in treatment, and has often shown limited effect in adults with EDS-HT (medication, surgery, physiotherapy) (Rombaut et al., 2011a).

Although there is no evidence for any specific treatment, active modes of physiotherapy are still the first choice, as in similar musculoskeletal conditions, such as fibromyalgia and chronic fatigue/pain, for example. This will often include a variety of elements like muscle strength, endurance, proprioception, coordination, balance, general neuromuscular training with low loads, cardiovascular and physical fitness training, in addition to pain management education.

A recent study on children with GJH and osteogenesis imperfecta showed successful effects of progressive training (Van Brussel et al., 2008). This corresponds with recommendations for adults from American College of Sports Medicine (Garber et al., 2011) and the recommendations from the National Strength and Conditioning Association for Children (Faigenbaum et al., 1999). In general neuromotor exercise training must be performed beyond the normal daily activity level. For these connective tissue conditions it must be stressed that the activity or training level must not be too intense. Overtraining should be avoided as this may result in a corresponding loss of confidence in treatment. The treatment approach will often benefit from both a mono and a multidisciplinary approach.

Hypomobility

Hypomobility can be defined as decreased joint mobility due to inherited or acquired structural changes in the joint and/or the surrounding connective tissue (Table 8.3). The range of joint motion is determined by the interaction between the extra-articular (neurological system, muscles) and the intra-articular structures (Hogeweg et al., 1994). The inherited form of hypomobility is probably due to a genetically determined change in the stiffness of the joint ligaments. As the collagen network determines most of the biomechanical properties of ligaments, the molecular defect involved in the pathogenesis of hypomobility may reside within these proteins.

Normal/abnormal joint mobility

As mentioned previously, population studies revealed that inter-individual variation in joint mobility fits into a – more or less skewed – Gaussian distribution. Joint **hyper**mobility at one end of this distribution, has been described above. Remarkably, joint **hypo**mobility, at the other end of the distribution, has, with or without specific musculoskeletal complaints, only been described in the literature as a separate entity since 2004, and no articles regarding (symptomatic) generalised joint hypomobility have been published since 2006.

Local joint hypomobility has been defined as range of motion in that particular joint lower than mean range of motion –1 standard deviation of the control group (Engelbert et al., 2004) (Engelbert

Table 8.3

Conditions with hypomobility

1. Inherited
   a. Local
      - Congenital talipes equino, talus verticalis, congenital osseous malformations
      - Idiopathic toe walking
      - Arthrogryposis and fetal hypomobility syndrome, amyoplasia, congenital absence of muscles
   b. Generalized
      - Symptomatic generalized hypomobility

1. Acquired
   a. Skin conditions
      - Scleroderma
      - Scar formation
   b. Muscle conditions
      - Duchenne disease
      - Inactivity (postoperative/prolonged bedrest)
   c. Joint conditions
      - Joint/vertebral dysfunctions
      - Degenerative conditions
      - Arthritis (RA, JRA, SLE, reactive, infectious, etc.)
      - Haemophilia arthropathy
   d. Skeletal conditions
      - Fractures
      - Dysplasia
   e. Neurologic conditions
      - Cerebral haemorrhage/thrombosis, etc.
      - Cerebral paresis
      - Peripheral nerve dysfunction with paresis
      - Stiff man syndrome
   f. Psychologic/Psychiatric conditions
      - Conversion disorders

et al., 2006). Until now a scoring system for generalised joint hypomobility has not been available and no national or international definition on generalised joint hypomobility exists.

Prevalence

There is no knowledge of the prevalence of hypomobility with or without musculoskeletal complaints, as no studies unfortunately can be traced regarding these aspects.

The estimated prevalence of local joint hypomobility, as observed in idiopathic toe walking, varies from 5% to 12% in healthy children (Engelbert et al., 2011) (Bernard et al., 2005) and idiopathic toe walking seems to have a higher prevalence in boys than in girls (Sobel et al., 1997). Indeed, the prevalence of the inherited conditions with hypomobility is estimated to be very low.

Pathogenesis and physiology

Congenital talipes equinovarus is caused by genetic factors such as Edwards syndrome, a genetic defect with three copies of chromosome 18.

Idiopathic toe walking. Decreased range of joint motion is frequently observed in the ankle joint, leading to toe walking, a physical sign that can be attributed to an underlying neurological or neuromuscular disease, such as spastic diplegic cerebral palsy (Wren et al., 2010) or Duchenne muscular dystrophy (Hyde et al., 2000) and orthopaedic problems, such as congenital talipes equinus (Caselli et al., 1988). Nevertheless, in some children differential diagnostics provide no pathogenetic or pathophysiologic substrate to explain the toe walking. This is described as 'idiopathic toe walking' (Conrad & Bleck, 1980). Many authors investigated the etiology of idiopathic toe walking. Toe walking may be a hereditary genetic disorder with an autosomal dominant pattern of inheritance with variable expression (Katz & Mubarak, 1984) and it is associated with an increase in the proportion of type I muscle fibres (Eastwood et al., 1997) and with sensory processing dysfunction (Williams et al., 2012).

Arthrogryposis and *foetal hypomobility syndrome* has a multifold etiology. Among these are vascular and environmental causes, but probably more important genetic disorders of both the connective tissue and nervous system (Haliloglu & Topaloglu, 2013).

Symptomatic generalised hypomobility: A group of children with this condition has been described in which the range of joint motion of nearly all joints was decreased compared to a reference group (Engelbert et al., 2004). The primary cause of such a systemic decrease in range of joint motion is likely to be an increased stiffness of joint ligaments and musculo-tendinous structures. Since the collagen network determines the biomechanical properties of these structures, the molecular defect involved in the pathogenesis

of hypomobility may reside within this network (Engelbert et al., 2004). Bone density was significantly lower in these children with symptomatic generalised hypomobility than in the reference group. Also urinary pyridinoline cross-link levels were significantly lower in the children compared to the controls, and in the unaffected skin of three children with symptomatic generalised hypomobility operated upon, substantial amounts of pyridinoline cross-links were present, compared to the skin data from the 10 healthy Caucasians (3.6 times lower). In the hypertrophic scar tissue of a 16-year-old girl with substantial generalised hypomobility, twice as much as the mean values reported for hypertrophic scar tissue or keloid and 20-fold higher than normal skin were found. The collagen cross-link data of the substantial generalised hypomobility skin biopsies and the hypertrophic scar tissue seem to be indicative of an abnormality in collagen processing.

Symptom: inclusive pain – development

Authors agree that idiopathic toe walking is a diagnosis *per exclusionem*. However, they do not all agree on which diseases and disorders should be excluded from this definition. It is generally accepted that idiopathic toe walking is diagnosed when children persist to walk on their toes and when they do not show any signs of neurological, neuromuscular and orthopaedic disorders. Some authors, however, regard 'gastrocnemius soleus muscle equinus' and 'congenital short tendon calcaneus' as primary orthopaedic disorders that cause toe walking (Caselli, 2002) (Furrer & Deonna, 1982). On the contrary, more recently, authors suggested that children with idiopathic toe walking develop a contracture of the Achilles tendon secondary to prolonged toe walking, because contractures were mainly found in older children who toe walked and no evidence was found for contractures to be present at birth (Brunt et al., 2004) (Clark et al., 2010). This is not yet confirmed by longitudinal studies.

The consequences of persistent and untreated toe walking are unclear. Some authors believe that the chance of developing more severe limitations in range of motion of the ankle joint, leading to fixed equinus contractures later in life, is higher than in children who do not walk on their toes (Engelbert et al., 2011) (Hemo et al., 2006). However, no longitudinal studies support this with evidence. Conversely, based on a follow-up study on 80 children (48 untreated), it was concluded that persistent toe walking did not result in significant functional disturbance, foot deformities or pain (Stricker & Angulo, 1998).

Substantial generalised hypomobility was studied in 19 children in whom toe walking was present in 14 (74%), whereas motor performance was normal in 94% (Engelbert et al., 2006) (Engelbert et al., 2004). Exercise-induced pain in calf, knee and/or hip muscles was reported in 13 (68%). Exercise tolerance was normal in 14 children (78%), whereas four children (22%) could not complete the test because of pain in calf, knee and/or hip muscles.

The associated exercise-induced pain is probably caused by a relative overuse of musculo-tendinous structures adjacent to the stiff joints. In children with musculoskeletal pain-related syndromes, particularly in children with (symptomatic) generalised joint hypermobility or hypomobility, maximal exercise capacity is significantly decreased compared to age- and gender-matched control subjects. The most probable explanation for the reduced exercise tolerance was deconditioning (Engelbert et al., 2006).

Treatment effect

The treatment for idiopathic toe walking varies: conservative as well as surgical procedures are advocated in the literature. Young children and children without a limitation in ankle dorsiflexion are often treated by conservative interventions and older, resistant cases with a limitation in ankle dorsiflexion are treated with surgical procedures. Conservative interventions include observation, stretching exercises of the plantar flexors either guided by a physiotherapist or guided by the parents, motor control intervention, auditory feedback, semi-orthopaedic shoes, ankle-foot orthoses and serial casting, as well as the use of botulinum toxin type A. Most interventions aim for at least 10° of dorsiflexion (McMulkin et al., 2006), which is indicated for a mature heel-to-toe walking

pattern. The natural course of idiopathic toe walking remains unclear. It was shown that prolonged toe walking did not result in pain, functional disturbances or foot deformities (Stricker & Angulo, 1998). This is consistent with the findings of Hirsch and Wagner (Hirsch & Wagner, 2004) who studied 14 children with former idiopathic toe walking (follow-up: 7–21 years) and found that three patients still showed some toe walking when they were unobtrusively observed. No fixed contracture was present. These authors concluded that idiopathic toe walking in childhood is a benign condition, which resolves spontaneously in most instances and causes the child little concern while it lasts. Therefore, surgical treatment should be reserved for cases with a fixed contracture of the tendon Achilles. Recently, a systematic review was performed and found that the effects of conservative and surgical interventions for children with idiopathic toe walking remain unclear. Comparisons across studies cannot be made, due to the differences in designs, interventions and definitions for idiopathic toe walking (Bakker et al., 2013).

Acquired hypomobility

The acquired form of hypomobility can be due to inactivity, overuse or trauma, which among other things include age, contractures, various forms of arthritis, osteoarthritis, segmental dysfunction in the vertebral column, luxations, reflex dystrophia (shoulder-hand syndrome) and cerebral palsy. These conditions are described elsewhere.

Clinical summary

Hypermobility

- Subjects with generalised joint hypermobility have an increased risk of joint injuries.
- Subjects with generalised joint hypermobility have symptoms and reduced physical function similar to patients with osteoarthritis.
- Having generalised joint hypermobility as a child is a predictor for general pain in adolescence.

- The scientific evidence for treatment of symptomatic generalised joint hypermobility is very weak.

Hypomobility

- In subjects with local and generalised joint hypomobility differential diagnostics are indicated.
- In local and generalised joint hypomobility muscular overuse lesions can be traced

whereas in generalised joint hypermobility ligamental and articular problems occur.

Hyper- and hypomobility

- Decreased physical fitness in joint hyper- and hypomobility might be caused by deconditioning whereas decreased muscle strength might be due to problems in collagen synthesis.

References

Adib, N., Davies, K., Grahame, R., Woo, P. & Murray, K.J. (2005) Joint hypermobility syndrome in childhood. A not so benign multisystem disorder? *Rheumatology.* (Oxford).

Allander, E., Bjornsson, O.J., Olafsson, O., Sigfusson, N. & Thorsteinsson, J. (1974) Normal range of joint movements in shoulder, hip, wrist and thumb with special reference to side: a comparison between two populations. *Int J Epidemiol.* 3: 253–261.

Bakker, P., Custers, J.W.H., Van Der Schaaf, M., De Wolf, S. & Engelbert, R.H.H. (2013) Effectiveness of conservative and surgical interventions in children with idiopathic toe walking: a systematic review. Submitted.

Barton, L.M. & Bird, H.A. (1996) Improving pain by the stabilization of hyperlax joints. *J Orthop Rheumatol.* 9: 46–51.

Beighton, P., De Paepe, A., Steinmann, B., Tsipouras, P. & Wenstrup, R.J. (1998) Ehlers-Danlos syndromes: revised nosology, Villefranche. (1997) Ehlers-Danlos National Foundation (USA) and Ehlers-Danlos Support Group (UK). *Am J Med Genet.* 77: 31–37.

Beighton, P. & Horan, F.T. (1969) Surgical aspects of the Ehlers-Danlos syndrome. A survey of 100 cass. *Br J Surg.* 56: 255–259.

Beighton, P., Solomon, L. & Soskolne, C.L. (1973) Articular mobility in an African population. *Annals of the Rheumatic Diseases* 32: 413–418.

Beighton, P. H. & Horan, F.T. (1970) Dominant inheritance in familial generalised articular hypermobility. *J Bone Joint Surg Br.* 52: 145–147.

Bernard, M.K., Vogler, L. & Merkenschlager, A. (2005) Prevalence of toe-walking in childhood. *Neuropediatrics.* 36: 116.

Bird, H.A. (2005) Joint hypermobility in children. *Rheumatology* (Oxford).

Blasier, R.B., Carpenter, J.E. & Huston, L.J. (1994) Shoulder proprioception. Effect of joint laxity, joint position, and direction of motion. *Orthopaedic Review* 23: 45–50.

Bridges, A.J., Smith, E. & Reid, J. (1992) Joint hypermobility in adults referred to rheumatology clinics. *Ann Rheum Dis.* 51: 793–796.

Brunt, D., Woo, R., Kim, H.D., Ko, M.S., Senesac, C. & Li, S. (2004) Effect of botulinum toxin type A on gait of children who are idiopathic toe-walkers. *J Surg Orthop Adv.* 13: 49–155.

Bulbena, A., Duro, J.C., Porta, M., Faus, S., Vallescar, R. & Martin-Santos, R. (1992) Clinical assessment of hypermobility of joints: assembling criteria. *J Rheumatol.* 19: 115–122.

Carter, C. & Wilkinson, J. (1964) Persistent joint laxity and congenital dislocation of the hip. *J Bone Joint Surg.* 46B: 40–45.

Caselli, M.A. (2002) Habitual toe walking: Learn to evaluate and treat this idiopathic childhood condition. *Podiatry Manage.* 21: 163.

Caselli, M.A., Rzonca, E.C. & Lue, B.Y. (1988). Habitual toe-walking: evaluation and approach to treatment. *Clin Podiatr Med Surg.* 5: 547–559.

Clark, E., Sweeney, J.K., Yocum, A. & Mccoy, S.W. (2010) Effects of motor control intervention for children with idiopathic toe walking: a 5-case series. *Pediatr Phys Ther.* 22: 417–426.

Conrad, L. & Bleck, E.E. (1980) Augmented auditory feed back in the treatment of equinus gait in children. *Dev Med Child Neurol.* 22: 713–718.

Eastwood, D.M., Dennett, X., Shield, L.K. & Dickens, D.R. (1997) Muscle abnormalities in idiopathic toe-walkers. *J Pediatr Orthoped.* Part B, 6: 215–218.

El-Metwally, A., Salminen, J.J., Auvinen, A., Kautiainen, H. & Mikkelsson, M. (2004) Prognosis of non-specific musculoskeletal pain in preadolescents: a prospective 4-year follow-up study till adolescence. *Pain* 110: 550–559.

El-Metwally, A., Salminen, J.J., Auvinen, A., Kautiainen, H. & Mikkelsson, M. (2005) Lower limb pain in a preadolescent population: prognosis and risk factors for chronicity – a prospective 1- and 4-year follow-up study. *Pediatric* 116: 673–681.

El-Metwally, A., Salminen, J.J., Auvinen, A., Macfarlane, G. & Mikkelsson, M. (2007) Risk factors for development of non-specific musculoskeletal pain in preteens and early adolescents: a prospective 1-year follow-up study. *BMC Musculoskelet Disord.* 8: 46.

Engelbert, R.H.H., Uiterwaal, C.S.P.M., Sakkers, R.J.B., Van Tintelen, J.P., Helders, P.J.M. & Bank, R.A. (2004)

Benign generalised hypomobility of the joints; a new clinical entity? - clinical, biochemical and osseal characteristics. *Pediatrics* 113: 714–719.

Engelbert, R.H., Van, B.M., Henneken, T., Helders, P.J. & Takken, T. (2006) Exercise tolerance in children and adolescents with musculoskeletal pain in joint hypermobility and joint hypomobility syndrome. *Pediatrics* 118: e690–e696.

Engelbert, R., Gorter, J.W., Uiterwaal, C., Van De Putte, E. & Helders, P. (2011) Idiopathic toe-walking in children, adolescents and young adults: a matter of local or generalised stiffness? *BMC Musculoskelet Disord.* 12: 61.

Faigenbaum, A.D., Westcott, W.L., Loud, R.L. & Long, C. (1999) The effects of different resistance training protocols on muscular strength and endurance development in children. *Pediatrics* 104: e5.

Fairbank, J.C., Pynsent, P.B. & Phillips, H. (1984) Quantitative measurements of joint mobility in adolescents. *Ann Rheum Dis.* 43: 288–294.

Falkerslev, S., Baagø, C., Alkjær, T., Remvig, L., Kristensen, J.H., Larsen, P.K., Juul-Kristensen, B. & Simonsen, E. (2012) Dynamic balance during gait in children and adults with generalised joint hypermobility. *Clin biomech.* Submitted after revision.

Fatoye, F., Palmer, S., Macmillan, F., Rowe, P. & van der Linden, M. (2009) Proprioception and muscle torque deficits in children with hypermobility syndrome. *Rheumatology* (Oxford). 48: 152–157.

Fatoye, F. A., Palmer, S., van der Linden, M. L., Rowe, P. J. & Macmillan, F. (2011) Gait kinematics and passive knee joint range of motion in children with hypermobility syndrome. *Gait Posture* 33: 447–451.

Ferrell, W.R., Tennant, N., Sturrock, R.D., Ashton, L., Creed, G., Brydson, G. & Rafferty, D. (2004) Amelioration of symptoms by enhancement of proprioception in patients with joint hypermobility syndrome. *Arthritis Rheum.* 50: 3323–3328.

Furrer, F. & Deonna, T. (1982) Persistent toe-walking in children. A comprehensive clinical study of 28 cases. *Helvetica Paediatrica Acta.* 37: 301–316.

Galli, M., Cimolin, V., Rigoldi, C., Castori, M., Celletti, C., Albertini, G. & Camerota, F. (2011) Gait strategy in patients with Ehlers-Danlos syndrome hypermobility type: a kinematic and kinetic evaluation using 3D gait analysis. *Res Dev Disabil.* 32: 1663–1668.

Garber, C.E., Blissmer, B., Deschenes, M.R., Franklin, B.A., Lamonte, M.J., Lee, I.M., Nieman, D.C., Swain, D.P. & American College of Sports Medicine (2011) American College of Sports Medicine position stand. Quantity and quality of exercise for developing and maintaining cardiorespiratory, musculoskeletal, and neuromotor fitness in apparently healthy adults: guidance for prescribing exercise. *Med Sci Sports Exerc.* 43: 1334–1359.

Grahame, R., Bird, H.A. & Child, A. (2000) The revised (Brighton 1998) criteria for the diagnosis of benign joint hypermobility syndrome (BJHS). *J Rheumatol.* 27: 1777–1779.

Greenwood, N.L., Duffell, L.D., Alexander, C.M. & Mcgregor, A.H. (2011) Electromyographic activity of pelvic and lower limb muscles during postural tasks in people with benign joint hypermobility syndrome and non hypermobile people. A pilot study. *Man Ther.* 16: 623–628.

Gyldenkerne, B., Iversen, K., Roegind, H., Fastrup, D., Hall, K. & Remvig, L. (2006) Prevalence of general hypermobility in 12–13-year-old school children and impact of an intervention against injury and pain incidence. *Adv Physiother.* Preview, 1–6.

Haliloglu, G. & Topaloglu, H. (2013) Arthrogryposis and fetal hypomobility syndrome. *Handb Clin Neurol.* 113: 1311–1319.

Hall, M.G., Ferrell, W.R., Sturrock, R.D., Hamblen, D.L. & Baxendale, R.H. (1995) The effect of the hypermobility syndrome on knee joint proprioception. *Br J Rheumatol.* 34: 121–125.

Hemo, Y., Macdessi, S.J., Pierce, R.A., Aiona, M.D. & Sussman, M.D. (2006) Outcome of patients after Achilles tendon lengthening for treatment of idiopathic toe walking. *J Pediatr Orthoped.* 26 (3): 36–40.

Hirsch, G. & Wagner, B. (2004) The natural history of idiopathic toe-walking: a long-term follow-up of fourteen conservatively treated children. *Acta Paediatrica* 93: 196–199.

Hogeweg, J.A., Langereis, M.J., Bernards, A.T.M., Faber, J.A.J. & Helders, P.J.M. (1994) Goniometry – variability in the clinical practice of a conventional goniometer in healthy subjects. *Eur J Phys Med Rehab.* 4: 2–7.

Hyde, S.A., Filytrup, I., Glent, S., Kroksmark, A. K., Salling, B., Steffensen, B. F., Werlauff, U. & Erlandsen, M. (2000) A randomized comparative study of two methods for controlling Tendo Achilles contracture in Duchenne muscular dystrophy. *Neuromuscular Disord.* 10: 257–263.

Jansson, A., Saartok, T., Werner, S. & Renstrom, P. (2004) General joint laxity in 1845 Swedish school children of different ages: age- and gender-specific distributions. *Acta Paediatrica* 93: 1202–1206.

Jensen, B.R., Olesen, A.S., Pedersen, M.T., Kristensen, J.H., Remvig, L., Simonsen, E.B. & Juul-Kristensen, B. (2013) Effect of generalized joint hypermobility on knee function and muscle activation in children and adults. *Muscle Nerve*, accepted, 1–9.

Jeremiah, H.M. & Alexander, C.M. (2010) Do hypermobile subjects without pain have alteration to the feedback mechanism controlling the shoulder? *Musculoskeletal Care*, 157–163.

Jonsson, H. & Valtysdottir, S. T. (1995) Hypermobility features in patients with hand osteoarthritis. *Osteoarthr Cartilage* 3: 1–5.

Jonsson, H., Valtysdottir, S.T., Kjartansson, O. & Brekkan, A. (1996) Hypermobility associated with osteoarthritis of the thumb base: a clinical and radiological subset of hand osteoarthritis. *Ann Rheum Dis.* 55: 540–543.

Juul-Kristensen, B., Hansen, H., Simonsen, E.B., Alkjaer, T., Kristensen, J.H., Jensen, B.R. & Remvig, L. (2012) Knee function in 10-year-old children and adults with Generalised Joint Hypermobility. *Knee* 19: 773–778.

Juul-Kristensen, B., Kristensen, J. H., Frausing, B., Jensen, D. V., Rogind, H. & Remvig, L. (2009) Motor competence and physical activity in 8-year-old school children with generalized joint hypermobility. *Pediatrics*, 124: 1380–1387.

Juul-Kristensen, B., Rogind, H., Jensen, D.V. & Remvig, L. (2007) Inter-examiner reproducibility of tests and criteria for generalized joint hypermobility and benign joint hypermobility syndrome. *Rheumatology* (Oxford). 46: 1835–1841.

Katz, M.M. & Mubarak, S.J. (1984) Hereditary tendo Achillis contractures. *J Pediatr Orthoped*. 4: 711–714.

Keer, R. & Simmonds, J. (2011) Joint protection and physical rehabilitation of the adult with hypermobility syndrome. *Curre Opin Rheumatol*. 23: 131–136.

Kemp, S., Roberts, I., Gamble, C., Wilkinson, S., Davidson, J. E., Baildam, E.M., Cleary, A.G., Mccann, L. J. & Beresford, M.W. (2010) A randomized comparative trial of generalized vs targeted physiotherapy in the management of childhood hypermobility. *Rheumatology* 49: 315–325.

Kerr, A., Macmillan, C., Uttley, W. & Luqmani, R. (2000) Physiotherapy for children with Hypermobility Syndrome. *Physiotherapy* 86: 313–317.

Kraus, V.B., Li, Y.J., Martin, E.R., Jordan, J.M., Renner, J.B., Doherty, M., Wilson, A.G., Moskowitz, R., Hochberg, M., Loeser, R., Hooper, M. & Sundseth, S. (2004) Articular hypermobility is a protective factor for hand osteoarthritis. *Arthritis Rheumatism* 50: 2178–2183.

Kuivaniemi, H., Tromp, G. & Prockop, D.J. (1997) Mutations in fibrillar collagens (types I, II, III, and XI), fibril-associated collagen (type IX), and network-forming collagen (type X) cause a spectrum of diseases of bone, cartilage, and blood vessels. *Human Mutation*. 9: 300–315.

Loeys, B.L., Dietz, H.C., Braverman, A.C., Callewaert, B.L., De Backer, J., Devereux, R.B., Hilhorst-Hofstee, Y., Jondeau, G., Faivre, L., Milewicz, D.M., Pyeritz, R.E., Sponseller, P.D., Wordsworth, P. & De Paepe, A.M. (2010) The revised Ghent nosology for the Marfan syndrome. *J Med Genet*. 47: 476–485.

Mallik, A.K., Ferrell, W.R., Mcdonald, A.G. & Sturrock, R.D. (1994) Impaired proprioceptive acuity at the proximal interphalangeal joint in patients with the hypermobility syndrome. *Br J Rheumatol*. 33: 631–637.

Mao, J.R. & Bristow, J. (2001) The Ehlers-Danlos syndrome: on beyond collagens. *J Clin Invest*. 107: 1063–1069.

Mccluskey, G., O'kane, E., Hann, D., Weekes, J. & Rooney, M. (2012) Hypermobility and musculoskeletal pain in children: a systematic review. *Scand J Rheumatol*. 41: 329–383.

Mcmulkin, M.L., Baird, G.O., Caskey, P.M. & Ferguson, R.L. (2006) Comprehensive outcomes of surgically treated idiopathic toe walkers. *J Pediatri Orthoped*. 26: 606–611.

Mebes, C., Amstutz, A., Luder, G., Ziswiler, H.R., Stettler, M., Villiger, P.M. & Radlinger, L. (2008) Isometric rate of force development, maximum voluntary contraction, and balance in women with and without joint hypermobility. *Arthritis Rheumatism* 59: 665–1669.

Mikkelsson, M., Salminen, J.J. & Kautiainen, H. (1996) Joint hypermobility is not a contributing factor to musculoskeletal pain in pre-adolescents. *J Rheumatol*. 23: 1963–1967.

Mintz-Itkin, R., Lerman-Sagie, T., Zuk, L., Itkin-Webman, T. & Davidovitch, M. (2009) Does physical therapy improve outcome in infants with joint hypermobility and benign hypotonia? *J Child Neurol*. 24: 714–719.

Murray, K.J. (2006) Hypermobility disorders in children and adolescents. *Best Pract Res Clin Rheumatol*. 20: 329–351.

Myer, G.D., Ford, K.R., Paterno, M.V., Nick, T.G. & Hewett, T.E. (2008) The effects of generalized joint laxity on risk of anterior cruciate ligament injury in young female athletes. *Am J Sports Med*. 36: 1073–1080.

Nielsen, R.H., Couppé, C., Olsen, M.R., Jensen, J.K., Svensson, R., Heinemeier, K. M., Magnusson, P., Remvig, L. & Kjaer, M. (2012) Biomechanical properties of the patellar tendon as a possible new diagnostic tool for classic Ehlers-Danlos Syndrome. Lassen day. Copenhagen: unpublished data.

Nikolajsen, H., Larsen, P.K., Simonsen, E.B., Alkjaer, T., Halkjër-Kristensen, J., Jensen, B.R., Remvig, L. & Juul-Kristensen, B. (2011) Altered knee and hip moments in children with generalised joint hypermobility during normal gait. WCPT-congress 2011, Amsterdam.

Pacey, V., Nicholson, L.L., Adams, R.D., Munn, J. & Munns, C.F. (2010) Generalized joint hypermobility and risk of lower limb joint injury during sport: a systematic review with meta-analysis. *Am J Sports Med*. 38: 1487–1497.

Remvig, L., Jensen, D.V. & Ward, R.C. (2007) Epidemiology of general joint hypermobility and basis for the proposed criteria for benign joint hypermobility syndrome: review of the literature. *J Rheumatol*. 34: 804–809.

Remvig, L., Kümmel, C., Kristensen, J.H., Boas, G. & Juul-Kristensen, B. (2011) Prevalence of Generalised Joint Hypermobility, Arthralgia and Motor Competence in 10-year old school children. *Int Musculoskelet Med*. 33: 137–145.

Rombaut, L., De, P.A., Malfait, F., Cools, A. & Calders, P. (2010a) Joint position sense and vibratory perception sense in patients with Ehlers-Danlos syndrome type III (hypermobility type). *Clin. Rheumatol*. 29: 289–295.

Rombaut, L., Malfait, F., Cools, A., De, P.A. & Calders, P. (2010b) Musculoskeletal complaints, physical activity and health-related quality of life among patients with the Ehlers-Danlos syndrome hypermobility type. *Disabil Rehabil*. 32: 1339–1345.

Rombaut, L., Malfait, F., De Wandele, I., Cools, A., Thijs, Y., De Paepe, A. & Calders, P. (2011a) Medication, surgery, and physiotherapy among patients with the hypermobility type of Ehlers-Danlos syndrome. *Arch Phys Med Rehabil.* 92: 1106–1112.

Rombaut, L., Malfait, F., De Wandele, I., Mahieu, N., Thijs, Y., Segers, P., De Paepe, A. & Calders, P. (2012a) Muscle-tendon tissue properties in the hypermobility type of Ehlers-Danlos syndrome. *Arthritis Care Res (Hoboken).* 64: 766–772.

Rombaut, L., Malfait, F., De Wandele, I., Taes, Y., Thijs, Y., De Paepe, A. & Calders, P. (2012b) Muscle mass, muscle strength, functional performance and physical impairment in women with the hypermobility type of Ehlers-Danlos syndrome. *Arthritis Care Res (Hoboken).*

Rombaut, L., Malfait, F., De Wandele, I., Thijs, Y., Palmans, T., De Paepe, A. & Calders, P. (2011b) Balance, gait, falls, and fear of falling in women with the hypermobility type of Ehlers-Danlos syndrome. *Arthritis Care Res (Hoboken).* 63: 1432–1439.

Roos, E.M., Roos, H.P., Ekdahl, C. & Lohmander, L.S. (1998) Knee injury and Osteoarthritis Outcome Score (KOOS) – validation of a Swedish version. *Scand J Med Sci Sports.* 8: 439–448.

Rotés-Quèrol, J. (1957) [Articular laxity considered as factor of changes of the locomotor apparatus]. *Rev Rhum Mal Osteoartic.* 24: 535–539.

Rotes-Querol, J., Duran, J., Subiros, R., Pifferer, J. & Gomez, J. (1972) La laxité articulaire comme facteur d'alterations de l'appareil locomoteur (Nouvelle étude 1971). *Rhumatologie* 24: 179–191.

Sahin, N., Baskent, A., Cakmak, A., Salli, A., Ugurlu, H. & Berker, E. (2008a) Evaluation of knee proprioception and effects of proprioception exercise in patients with benign joint hypermobility syndrome. *Rheumatol Int.* 28: 995–1000.

Sahin, N., Baskent, A., Ugurlu, H. & Berker, E. (2008b) Isokinetic evaluation of knee extensor/flexor muscle strength in patients with hypermobility syndrome. *Rheumatol Int.* 28: 643–648.

Schalkwijk, J., Zweers, M.C., Steijlen, P.M., Dean, W.B., Taylor, G., Van Vlijmen, I.M., Van Haren, B., Miller, W.L. & Bristow, J. (2001) A recessive form of the Ehlers-Danlos syndrome caused by tenascin-X deficiency. *N Engl J Med.* 345: 1167–1175.

Schleip, R. (2006) *Active fascial contractility. Implications for musculoskeletal mechanics.* Dr.biol.hum, University of Ulm.

Schubert-Hjalmarsson, E., Ohman, A., Kyllerman, M. & Beckung, E. (2012) Pain, balance, activity, and participation in children with hypermobility syndrome. *Pediatr Phys Ther.* 24: 339–44.

Scott, D., Bird, H. & Wright, V. (1979) Joint laxity leading to osteoarthrosis. *Rheumatol Rehabil.* 18: 167–169.

Silman, A.J., Haskard, D. & Day, S. (1986) Distribution of joint mobility in a normal population: results of the use of fixed torque measuring devices. *Ann Rheum Dis.* 45: 27–30.

Simmonds, J.V. & Keer, R.J. (2008) Hypermobility and the hypermobility syndrome, part 2: assessment and management of hypermobility syndrome: illustrated via case studies. *Manual Ther.* 13: e1–e11.

Simonsen, E.B., Tegner, H., Alkjaer, T., Larsen, P.K., Kristensen, J.H., Jensen, B. R., Remvig, L. & Juul-Kristensen, B. (2012) Gait analysis of adults with generalised joint hypermobility. *Clin Biomech* (Bristol, Avon), doi, 10.1016/j.clinbiomech.2012.01.008.

Smits-Engelsman, B., Klerks, M. & Kirby, A. (2011) Beighton score: a valid measure for generalized hypermobility in children. *J Pediatr.* 158: 119–123, e1–e4.

Sobel, E., Caselli, M.A. & Velez, Z. (1997) Effect of persistent toe walking on ankle equinus. Analysis of 60 idiopathic toe walkers. *J Am Podiatr Med Assoc.* 87: 17–22.

Stewart, D.R. & Burden, S.B. (2004) Does generalised ligamentous laxity increase seasonal incidence of injuries in male first division club rugby players? *Br J Sports Med.* 38: 457–460.

Stricker, S.J. & Angulo, J.C. (1998) Idiopathic toe walking: a comparison of treatment methods. *J Pediatr Orthoped.* 18: 289–293.

Surgeons, A.A.O.O. (1965) *Joint motion: method of measuring and recording.* Edinburgh: Churchill Livingstone.

Tirosh, E., Jaffe, M., Marmur, R., Taub, Y. & Rosenberg, Z. (1991) Prognosis of motor development and joint hypermobility. *Dis Child.* 66: 931–933.

Tobias, J.H., Deere, K., Palmer, S., Clark, E.M. & Clinch, J. (2013) Hypermobility is a risk factor for musculoskeletal pain in adolescence: Findings from a prospective cohort study. *Arthritis Rheumatism.*

Van Brussel, M., Takken, T., Uiterwaal, C.S., Pruijs, H.J., Van Der Net, J., Helders, P.J. & Engelbert, R.H. (2008) Physical training in children with osteogenesis imperfecta. *J Pediatr.* 152: 111–116.

Van Dijk, F.S., Pals, G., Van Rijn, R.R., Nikkels, P.G. & Cobben, J. M. (2010) Classification of Osteogenesis Imperfecta revisited. *Eur J Med Genet.* 53: 1–5.

Wetterslev, M., Kristensen, J.H., Roennebech, J., Bertelsen, T., Laursen, H., Schleip, R. & Remvig, L. (2013) Myofibroblast content in fascia from patients with Ehlers-Danlos Syndrome, Hypermobile type. – Letter to the Editor. *Rheumatology,* submitted May.

Williams, C.M., Tinley, P., Curtin, M. & Nielsen, S. (2012) Vibration perception thresholds in children with idiopathic toe walking gait. *J Child Neurol.* 27: 1017–1021.

Wood, P. (1971) Is hypermobility a discrete entity? *Proc R Soc Med.* 64: 690–692.

Wren, T. A., Cheatwood, A. P., Rethlefsen, S. A., Hara, R., Perez, F.J. & Kay, R.M. (2010) Achilles tendon length and medial gastrocnemius architecture in children with cerebral palsy and equinus gait. *J Pediatr Orthoped.* 30: 479–484.

Further reading

Visit http://www.ncbi.nlm.nih.gov where you can find updated reviews about the various Hereditary Disorders of Connective Tissue.

Dupuytren's Disease and Related Hyperproliferative Disorders: Principles, Research and Clinical Perspectives. (2012) Editors: Eaton, C., Heinrich Seegenschmiedt, H., Bayat, A., Gabbiani, G., Werker, P. & Wolfgang, W. Berlin, Heidelberg: Springer Verlag.

CHAPTER 9

Human movement performance: Stretching misconceptions and future trends

Eyal Lederman

Introduction

Stretching is the behaviour an individual adopts often with the aim of maintaining agility, improving or recovering range of movement (ROM) in various musculoskeletal conditions. It is also used recreationally and in sports training to enhance movement performance and for prevention of injuries. However, in recent years the value of stretching has been eroded by research and many of the assumptions that are the foundations for these practices have been called into question. This chapter will explore the plausibility of some basic assumptions and how they standup to research findings. Does training that involves stretching have any value for improving ROM and enhancing human movement performance?

Do we need to stretch regularly?

There is an enduring belief that our sedentary lifestyle does not expose us sufficiently to end-range movements, such as we would encounter if we lived in the wilderness. It is assumed that this lack of exposure results in progressive loss of ROM. This in turn would impede normal functional performance in daily or sport activities, increase the likelihood to develop musculoskeletal conditions or even be detrimental to our health. So, the most basic premise is that stretching is essential for maintaining or improving human performance.

As a phenomenon in human behaviour only a relatively small group of individuals stretch regularly. Those who do, often leave out particular parts of the body. For example, hardly anybody stretches their little finger or their forearm into full pronation-supination. So what happens to the majority who do not stretch? Do they gradually stiffen into a solid unyielding dysfunctional mass? What happens to the parts that we never stretch? Do they stand out as being stiff or range-restricted?

Such catastrophic movement outcomes are not evident. It seems that going about our daily activities provides sufficient challenges to maintain functional ranges. Otherwise we would all suffer from some catastrophic progressive stiffening fate. This suggests that stretching is not a biological-physiological necessity but perhaps a socio-cultural construct. Indeed, it seems that only humans engage in regular, systematic stretching.

ROM adaptation, pandiculation and clinical stretching

There is a shared animal and human behaviour of 'having a stretch' and yawning called pandiculation (Bertolucci, 2011) (Campbell & de Waal, 2011). This behaviour is often mistaken for an activity that maintains agility. As discussed above, normal daily activities seem to provide the necessary loading forces required to maintain the functional ROM. Pandiculation is unlikely to play a role in functional ROM. If we observe individuals' pandiculation, it tends to be a stereotypic movement pattern often restricted to particular body areas. For example, a person will often pandiculate with their trunk into extension but rarely into full flexion, side-bending or rotation. If it was important for maintaining agility, we would expect pandiculation to involve every musculoskeletal structure in the body. Again, the question arises what happens to these 'un-pandiculated' movement ranges, do they stand out as being stiffer or less agile? This also raises another question, can pandiculation behaviour provide enough force to maintain functional ROM or increase it?

The pandiculation discussion brings us to another common misunderstanding about stretching and ROM adaptation. To bring about ROM adaptation the individual has to engage in specific behaviour that includes raising the intensity of their physical activity beyond its current level (*overloading*), as well as increasing the training duration (Lederman, 2013). For adaptation to occur the training has to be above a certain *loading threshold* (Lederman, 2013). Often these thresholds are well above the levels experienced during functional daily activities (Figure 9.1) (Arampatzis et al., 2010) (Muijka & Padilla, 2001). If it were otherwise, normal standing would result in complete and permanent flattening of the plantar fascia, the weight of the viscera would result in an epidemic of pelvic floor collapses and office workers who sit all day would end up with extraordinary spinal flexion agility. Loading threshold means that in many areas of the body the loading forces have to be several times above body weight to bring about ROM adaptation. This means that many clinical stretching approaches are unlikely to provide the necessary force levels or are too short in duration to stimulate ROM adaptation. It is of no surprise that a recent systematic review concluded that

clinical stretching (including passive and active approaches) have a low therapeutic value in recovering ROM losses (Katalinic, 2010). As will be discussed below, there is also a problem of specificity and clinical stretching.

Overloading principles and loading thresholds suggest that pandiculation is an unlikely candidate for maintaining functional agility or driving ROM adaptation. For pandiculation to effectively drive ROM adaptation it would have to be repeated hundreds of times per day. It would also require far greater loading forces than those experienced by this gentle activity.

The most important message from the discussion so far is that functional movement, the natural movement repertoire of the individual, is sufficient to maintain the normal ROM (Lederman, 2013) (Figure 9.1). To drive ROM adaptation we have to re-evaluate the current practice of stretching. Research informs us that we need to move towards functional movement approaches that integrate ROM challenges into daily normal daily tasks (Lederman, 2013).

Stretching and human movement performance

Another common belief is that human performance can be enhanced by an acute bout of warm-up stretching before a competition or, in the long-term, by regular stretch training.

If warm-up stretching were beneficial for enhancing performance we would have expected nature to have 'factored-in' stretching as part of animal behaviour. However, with the exception of humans, no other animal seems to perform pre–exertion activities that resemble a stretch warm-up. Lions do not limber up with a stretch before they chase their prey, and, reciprocally, the prey does not halt the chase for the lack of a stretch. The stretch warm-up in humans seems to be largely ceremonial. A person would stretch in the park before a jog but would not consider stretching to be important before sprinting for a bus. A person may stretch before lifting weights in the gym but a builder is unlikely to stretch although they may be lifting and carrying throughout the day. We have evolved to perform

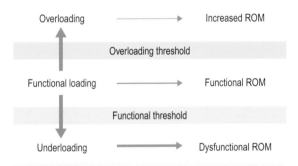

Figure 9.1

Functional ROM is maintained by the forces imposed on the body during daily activities. Greater loading (stretching) forces, beyond a certain loading threshold are needed to increase these ranges. Dysfunctional or reduced ROM may occur when loading forces are too low, below a functional threshold (After Lederman, 2013).

maximally, instantly and without the need to limber up with stretching. It does not seem to confer any biological advantage nor is it physiologically essential to performance.

This observation is reflected in research that looks at stretching in sports. Stretching as a warm-up before and after exercising has failed to show any benefit for alleviating muscle soreness, it provides no protection against sports injuries and vigorous stretching before an event may even reduce sports performance (Andersen, 2005) (Herbert et al., 2011) (Simic et al., 2012). It was demonstrated that strength performance can be reduced by between 4.5% to 28%, irrespective of the stretching technique used (Rubini et al., 2007) (Young & Behm, 2002).

However, that still leaves us with the question about long-term stretching. Can such training provide some adaptive musculoskeletal changes that would result in improved performance? If we accept the assumption that stretch training improves sports performance it would suggest that humans have cracked what nature has never been able to do: create a universal exercise that will have a positive impact on the performance of all other tasks and activities. Is there any evidence for this elsewhere in animal behaviour?

It seems that animals do what they do without having to use training that is outside their movement repertoire (Lederman, 2013). They develop their functional movement repertoire by simply doing their species-specific activities and nothing more. Birds learn to fly by flying and optimise flying by more flying. This behaviour is called task-specific practice or functional training (Lederman, 2013). They don't do wing press-ups or stretching, termed here extra-functional training.

If regular stretching could improve a wide range of unrelated activities it would mean that a very agile individual, such as a ballerina, would excel in all sports activities. But how likely is a ballerina to exhibit high levels of performance in running, swimming, cycling, football or weight training, activities for which stretching is often recommended? Why don't we see ballerinas and yoga instructors winning medals in the Olympics? To answer these questions we need to look at an adaptation phenomenon called specificity.

Specificity in adaptation

When we learn a new skill, the motor, tissue and physiological adaptation is specific for that task (specificity), (DeAnna et al., 2006) (Haga et al., 2008) (Millet et al., 2009). This allows the task to be performed optimally with minimal energy expenditure, physical stress and error. This adaptation is profoundly unique, optimised for that particular activity but often unsuitable for a different activity (Osgood, 1949) (Henry, 1958) (Holding, 1965) (van Ingen Schenau et al., 1994). This means that training gains are task-specific. They do not seem to carry over or transfer to an activity which is dissimilar. Even activities that look identical, such as sprinting and distance-running each have their unique, biomechanical and physiological non-transferable adaptation. The knee force-angle profile is different between these activities, and the leg muscles in sprinters have greater fascicle length and lesser pennation angle than in distance runners (Abe et al., 2000). Furthermore, studies in motor control over the period of a century have also demonstrated that such task specific adaption takes place in the central nervous system including the spinal cord and brain centres (Lederman, 2010). So, sports specific adaptation is a whole body phenomenon that includes peripheral musculoskeletal and central control changes. That is why sprinters don't make great marathon runners and vice-versa.

Specificity and transfer has been studied extensively in sports with the aim of identifying training methods that could improve sport performance. Overall, most studies show a lack of transfer and, on the occasion when it is demonstrated, it seems to be of marginal effect and unpredictable. For example, sprinting performance was shown to improve by single-leg horizontal jumps but not by vertical jumps using both limbs, such as jump squats (Young, 2006). Vertical jumps are improved by training in vertical but not by training in sideways jumps (King & Cipriani, 2010). Transfer may fail to occur even in training systems that closely resemble the task. For example, resistance sprint training using a towing device fails to improve sprint performance. Similarly, off-ice skating exercises do not improve on-ice performance in speed skaters.

Resistance training in swimming results in a different swimming style using large amplitude trunk movement that may not be beneficial for free, unrestricted swimming (Maglischo, 2003). Core stability exercises fail to improve sports performance (Hibbs et al., 2008) (Parkhouse & Ball, 2010) (Okada et al., 2011). Different forms of resistance exercise have failed to improve sports-specific activities such as football kicks (Young & Rath, 2011), sprinting, netball, hockey (Farlinger & Fowles, 2008), throwing velocity in water polo (Bloomfield et al., 1990) and rowing (Bell et al., 1989). Even resistance training in one particular posture may not transfer force gains to other postures (Wilson et al., 1996). Cross-training by cycling does not improve running and may even reduce running economy (Mutton et al., 1993) (Pizza et al., 1995). Training in isolated tasks, such as hip flexibility or trunk strengthening activities, does not improve the economy of walking or running (Godges et al., 1993). Upper limb resistance exercises do not improve arm coordination (Krzystof et al., 2000), and so on.

From a specificity perspective, regular stretching is unlikely to improve the performance of a dissimilar task. Indeed, to date, the evidence suggests that regular stretch training does not improve sports performance and may even be reduced by acute bouts of stretching (Behm, 2004) (Kay & Blazevich, 2012). The sport specific adaptation is likely to be very different from the musculoskeletal adaptation induced by stretch training. It is, therefore, unlikely to meet the physiological demands of the particular sport activity. At best stretching may have no effect but at worst, it may introduce a 'competition in adaptation' if the individual is excessively focusing on their extra-functional stretching rather than their sports specific training (Lederman, 2010 & 2013). Under these circumstances stretching is very likely to have a negative effect on performance.

The question that is often raised at this point is: what about sports activities which require agility? For example, martial arts, dance and gymnastic activities. Is stretching in any form useful? A high-kick in martial arts is one example. The active end-range of movement, in this particular task, is determined by the decline in force of the agonists, i.e. hip flexors, versus rise in passive tension in the antagonistic tissues. To increase this range, it is not unusual for a martial art expert to focus on hip flexor strength and stretch the passive antagonistic tissues (say, hamstrings or posterior fascial chain). This form of training contains several commonly expressed basic assumptions: that performance can be enhanced by fragmenting whole movement to smaller units, that focusing on individual tissue is possible and desirable in training and that passive stretching can have an influence on active movement performance. But are any of these assumptions correct?

Goal and whole versus movement fragmentation

When we observe human movement, a large selection of this repertoire is directed towards external goals: to reach for a cup, hit a ball or walk across the room. The intention to attain the goal triggers the execution of the associated movement, including all the anticipatory postural adjustments that precede it (Elsner & Hommel, 2001) (Rosenbaum et al., 2004). This response is a whole body event, it is not specific to a particular joint or muscle (Hughlings-Jackson, 1889).

For an outsider observing a person performing a task, say lifting a cup, the action can be broken into two components: the movement that typifies the task (unique arm movement) and the goal of this movement (to lift the cup). However, this separation is artificial. In most activities, the movement and its goals are a unified response and not separated entities (Hommel & Prinz, 1997). Several studies demonstrated that training that focuses on the outcome of the movement rather than on the body and its workings enables the individual to produce greater peak forces, execute faster movement, and increase joint movement accuracy with less muscular activity (Wulf & Dufek, 2009) (Wulf et al., 2010). External, goal-focused training engages the individual in whole movement patterns, optimises motor learning and promotes movement economy (Totsika & Wulf, 2003) (Wulf et al., 2010) (Lohse et al., 2010).

The organisation of movement around its goals means that any given muscle will participate in many different tasks. In other words, no muscle is designed to carry out a specific task. This means that muscle recruitment is task specific (Doemges & Rack, 1992) (Weiss & Flanders, 2004) (Carpenter et al., 2008). Hence, the recruitment pattern of the lower limb muscles will be very different between activities such as standing, walking, reaching to the sides, forward bending or lifting or any other imaginable movement (Andersson et al., 1996) (Urquhart et al., 2005). Training a specific muscle or muscle chain is unlikely to improve the performance or recover the control of the task. This is because the task determines the muscle's activation pattern and not the other way round. It would be like trying to learn a tennis serve by practicing biceps activation, triceps and then forearm control, and so on. The best way to enhance performance is to practice the task itself, during which the whole recruitment sequence is rehearsed simultaneously. Single muscle or muscle-chain activation simply does not exist in motor organisation or in the physiology of movement. If Aristotle were around now he would have pointed out that, 'The task is different from the sum of its muscles and joints.'

Training practices that favour movement fragmentation are more likely to improve the specific fragmented activity but not the whole movement (Krakauer et al., 2006). For example, training that improves the local power at the ankle or ankle and knee fails to transfer to gains in vertical jumping, although this task depends on these neuromuscular components. Likewise, exercises that isolate parts of the kicking action are not recommended because these do not appear to transfer well to kicking performance. Training should be of the whole kicking action (Young & Rath, 2011). Similarly, training in isolated tasks, such as hip flexibility or trunk strengthening activities does not improve the economy of walking or running (Godges et al., 1993).

Using the high-kick example, we can see two potential training approaches here. One is to fragment the movement of kicking and then integrate it later. The other approach is the 'whole and goal' task specific approach: just train by performing a lot of high-kicks. The problem with the fragmented approach is that it will fail to capture the complex intermuscular coordination of the limb's synergists – the explosive contraction of the hip flexors with a simultaneous 'explosive relaxation' of the extensors. The pattern of hip flexors recruitment during specific strength training is profoundly dissimilar to the kicking task. It is, therefore, unlikely to transfer any gains to the kicking action. However, and more simply, by practicing the task itself specific adaptation occurs spontaneously throughout the body centrally, as motor control changes, and peripherally, by musculoskeletal adaptation. It is a far more economical and effective method of training. But what about a passive stretching component, can it help to improve the high-kick?

Passive stretching and movement performance

If we observe human movement it is mostly active. Passive movement is a rare event in this repertoire. It is well established that being active is essential for motor learning or improving movement performance (Lederman, 2010). Hence, to improve performance or recover motor control, an active form of ROM training or rehabilitation is likely to be more effective than passive movement which includes many forms of stretching approaches.

The dominance of active over passive movement for motor learning and recovery is related to several factors. Movement is organised as sequences that involve sensory component, central integration and an efferent motor output (Schmidt & Lee, 2005). Only during active movement are the efferent, motor recruitment sequences generated, which is essential for encoding the movement (with the exception of motor visualisation) (Lederman, 2005). For that simple reason passive stretching cannot improve active control as it only engages the sensory component of the system.

During motor learning a unique sensory image is created centrally for that particular movement. We become familiar with what the task 'feels like'. However, changing the sensory experience within the same task may affect its performance; for example, subjects were trained to walk across a balance beam either with or without vision. It was found that the participants improved their balance more in the sensory condition for which they trained (Robertson & Elliott, 1996) (Proteau et al., 1998). Furthermore, sensory experiences may not transfer well between tasks. Learning tactile discrimination of a particular texture may fail to improve tactile discrimination of an unfamiliar texture. Such sensory specificity was demonstrated in blind Braille readers (Grant et al., 2000). They outperformed sighted individuals on palpation tasks that use Braille-like dot patterns (a familiar pattern). However, they did not differ from sighted individuals when presented with a novel palpation discrimination task (a surface with ridges of different widths and orientations). This implies that the sensory experience during passive or even active stretching is unlikely to transfer performance gains to a dissimilar active functional daily or sport task.

Another difference is that it is only during active movement that the sensory experience (afferent) is coupled with motor processes (efferent). This sensory-motor coupling has an important implication for correcting movement errors and consequently for enhancing motor learning and skill performance (Paillard & Brouchon, 1968) (Laszlo & Bairstow, 1971) (McCloskey & Gandevia, 1978).

So, from a motor control point of view, passive stretching is unlikely to improve high-kick performance. However, there is still a niggling question about passive stretching and extreme movement ranges. In many joints, such as the hip, passive movement range is greater than the active one (Lederman, 2013). However, the active range limitation can be overcome by an explosive flexion, such as in a high-kick. In this situation, the extra range is attained by the momentum of the leg mass and counteracted by the passive tension in the antagonistic tissues. (That is why the range would be smaller if the kick were performed slowly.) So perhaps, for extreme movement ranges, passive stretching may be

necessary to 'eliminate' the passive antagonistic limitations. This may explain why dancers and martial art practitioners spend so much training effort in passive stretching. However, we don't know if that is necessary, i.e. is practicing a high-kick sufficient to attain the range requirements for this task or is it essential to add passive stretching? Would a dancer be less agile in their active performance if they eliminated all passive stretching from their training programme? This is an area of training where more research is urgently needed and one which we will be exploring in our research centre at University College London (UCL).

Towards a functional approach

Training research in stretching suggests that stretching in all its forms is not a physiological necessity nor does it confer any obvious benefits to human performance. The specificity principle suggests that physical tasks can be improved by simply practicing the task itself. For increasing range of movement it might be sufficient to actively practice the task at end range, e.g. to increase stride length in sprinting just sprint with a wider stride or to increase an overhead pitching ROM practice pitching at end-range (Lederman, 2013). Such task-specific training contains all the essential components for enhancing performance. It is actively performed, goal orientated and practiced as a whole. This form of training encourages concomitant peripheral and central adaptation that is specific for the particular task. Traditional stretching, as well as other forms of extra-functional training, might be superfluous to the functional needs of the person. The exception, perhaps, are individuals who require extraordinary flexibility.

In the last two decades there has also been an erosion in the therapeutic value of stretching in recovering ROM in various musculoskeletal conditions. A recent Cochrane systematic review reported that in the short term, stretching provides 3° improvements, 1° in the medium-term and no influence in the long-term (up to seven months), regardless of the type of stretching used (Katalinic et al., 2010). Perhaps we should consider applying the task-specific functional

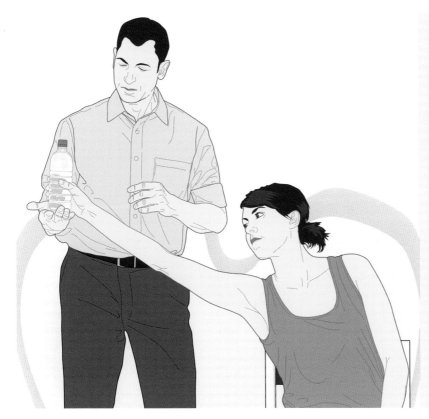

Figure 9.2

A functional approach in stretching

This form of rehabilitation encourages the patient to perform daily tasks at their end range of movement. In this example the patient who has a restricted abduction ROM is encouraged to reach into full abduction. They are then instructed to perform a functional task such as placing a bottle on a shelf at that end range. This approach uses the training/rehabilitation principles of specificity, overloading and exposure as well as promoting whole and goal movement.

principles to rehabilitation of ROM. A person with contractures of the hip should be rehabilitated by walking with a wide stride length, a person suffering from the stiff phase of frozen shoulder, who can't reach overhead, should be encouraged to simply reach overhead (Figure 9.2), frequently throughout the day, and so on. The rationale and evidence for a functional approach is discussed in Lederman E 2013 *Therapeutic Stretching: Towards a Functional Approach* (Lederman, 2013).

Clinical Summary

- Functional daily activities maintain and normalise functional ROM. Stretching is likely to be superfluous.
- Training promotes whole body adaptation which is unique to that activity (specificity) and may not transfer to another task/activity.

- Stretching is likely to promote specific adaptation which is unlikely to transfer gains to sports performance.
- Performance is enhanced by goal-orientated and whole movement. Stretching practices, which focus internally on specific tissues, may degrade performance.
- Fragmenting movement into smaller anatomical units is likely to degrade movement performance.
- Task performance is unlikely to be improved by passive stretching approaches. There is no motor efferent activity during passive movement and an absence of sensory-motor coupling.
- Range of movement is likely to be enhanced by practice of the task at end-ranges. This is a functional behaviourally driven approach for enhancing and recovering ROM.

References

Abe, T., Kumagai, K. & Brechue, W.F. (2000) Fascicle length of leg muscles is greater in sprinters than distance runners. *Med Sci Sports Exerc.* 32(6): 1125–1129.

Andersen, J.C. (2005) Stretching before and after exercise: effect on muscle soreness and injury risk. *Journal of Athletic Training.* 40(3): 218–220.

Andersson, E.A., Oddsson, L.I., Grundstrom, H. et al. (1996) EMG activities of the quadratus lumborum and erector spinae muscles during flexion-relaxation and other motor tasks. *Clin Biomech* (Bristol, Avon) 11: 392–400.

Arampatzis, A., Peper, A., Bierbaum, S., et al. (2010) Plasticity of human Achilles tendon mechanical and morphological properties in response to cyclic strain. *J Biomech.* 43(6): 3073–3079.

Behm, D.G. (2004) Effect of acute static stretching on force, balance, reaction time, and movement time. *Med. Sci. Sports Exerc.* 36: 1397–1402.

Bell, G.J., Petersen, S.R, Quinney, H.A. & Wenger, H.A. (1989) The effect of velocity-specific strength training on peak torque and anaerobic rowing power. *J Sports Sci.* 7(3): 205–214.

Bertolucci, L.F. (2011) Pandiculation: nature's way of maintaining the functional integrity of the myofascial system? *J Bodyw Mov Ther.* 15(3): 268–280.

Bloomfield, J., Blanksby, B.A., Ackland, T.R. & Allison, G.T. (1990) The influence of strength training on overhead throwing velocity of elite water polo players. *Australian Journal of Since and Medicine in Sport.* 22(3): 63–67.

Campbell, M.W. & de Waal, F.B.M. (2011) Ingroup-outgroup bias in contagious yawning by chimpanzees supports link to empathy. *PLoS ONE.* 6(4): e18283.

Carpenter, M.G., Tokuno, C.D., Thorstensson, A., et al. (2008) Differential control of abdominal muscles during multi-directional support-surface translations in man. *Exp Brain Res.* Apr 29.

DeAnna, L.A., Boychuk, J., Remple, M.S., et al. (2006) Motor training induces experience-specific patterns of plasticity across motor cortex and spinal cord. *J Appl Physiol.* 101: 1776–1782.

Doemges, F. & Rack, P.M.H. (1992) (B) Changes in the stretch reflex of the human first interosseous muscle during different tasks. *J of Physiol.* 447: 563–573.

Elsner, B. & Hommel, B. (2001) Effect anticipation and action control. *J Exp Psychol Hum Percept Perform.* Feb; 27(1): 229–240.

Farlinger, C.M. & Fowles, J.R. (2008) The effect of sequence of skating-specific training on skating performance. *Int J Sports Physiol Perform.* Jun; 3(2): 185–198.

Godges, J.J., MacRae, P.G. & Engelke, K.A. (1993) Effects of exercise on hip range of motion, trunk muscle performance, and gait economy. *Phys Ther.* Jul 73(7): 468–477.

Grant, A.C., Thiagarajah, M.C. & Sathian, K. (2000) Tactile perception in blind Braille readers: a psychophysical study of acuity and hyperacuity using gratings and dot patterns. *Percept Psychophys.* Feb; 62(2): 301–312.

Haga, M., Pedersen, A.V.H. & Sigmundsson, H. (2008) Interrelationship among selected measures of motor skills Child: *Care, Health and Development.* 34(2): 245–248.

Henry, F. (1958) Specificity vs. generality in learning motor skills. In 61st Annual Proceedings of the College of the Physical Education Association. Santa Monica, CA.

Herbert, R.D, et al. (2011) Stretching to prevent or reduce muscle soreness after exercise. *Cochrane Database Syst Rev.* Jul 6(7). CD004577.

Hibbs, A.E., et al. (2008) Optimizing performance by improving core stability and core strength. *Sports Med.* 38(12): 995–1008.

Holding, D.H. (1965) *Principles of training.* Oxford: Pergamon.

Hommel, B. & Prinz, W. (1997) Toward an action-concept model of stimulus–response compatibility. In: Hommel, B, Prinz, W, Eds. *Theoretical issues in stimulus–response compatibility.* Amsterdam: Elsevier.

Hughlings-Jackson, J. (1889) On the comparative study of disease of the nervous system. *Brit Med J.* Aug. 17: 55–62.

Katalinic, O.M., Harvey, L.A., Herbert, R.D., et al. (2010) Stretch for the treatment and prevention of contractures. *Cochrane Database Syst Rev.* Sept 8(9). CD007455.

Kay, A.D. & Blazevich, A.J. (2012) Effect of acute static stretch on maximal muscle performance: a systematic review. *Med Sci Sports Exerc.* Jan, 44(1): 154–164.

King, J.A. & Cipriani, D.J. (2010) Comparing preseason frontal and sagittal plane plyometric programs on within-task-task jump height in high-school basketball players. *J Strength Cond Res.* Aug; 24(8): 2109–2114.

Krakauer, J.W., Mazzoni, P., Ghazizadeh, A., Ravindran, R. & Shadmehr, R. (2006) Generalization of motor learning depends on the history of prior action. *PLoS Biol.* 4 (10). e316. DOI: 10.1371/journal.pbio.0040316.

Krzysztzof, N., Waskiewicz, Z., Zajac, A. & Goralczyk, R. (2000) The effects of exhaustive bench press on bimanual coordination. In, C.P. Lee (Ed.) *Proceedings of 2nd International Conference on Weightlifting and Strength Training.* p. 86.

Laszlo, J.I. & Bairstow, P.J. (1971) Accuracy of movement, peripheral feedback and efferent copy. *Journal of Motor Behaviour.* 3: 241–252.

Lederman, E. (2005) *The science and practice of manual therapy.* Elsevier.

Lederman, E. (2010) *Neuromuscular rehabilitation in manual and physical therapies.* Elsevier.

Lederman, E. (2013) *Therapeutic stretching: towards a functional approach.* Elsevier.

Lohse, K.R., Sherwood D.E. & Healy A.F. (2010) How changing the focus of attention affects performance, kinematics, and electromyography in dart throwing. *Hum Mov Sci.* Aug, 29(4): 542–555.

Maglischo, E.W. (2003) *Swimming fastest.* Human Kinetics.

McCloskey, D.I. & Gandevia, S.C. (1978) Role of inputs from skin, joints and muscles and of corollary discharges, in human discriminatory tasks. In: Gordon G (Ed) *Active touch*. Oxford: Pergamon Press, 177–188.

Millet, G.P., Vleck, V.E. & Bentley, D.J. (2009) Physiological differences between cycling and running: lessons from triathletes. *Sports Med*. 39(3): 179–206.

Mujika, M. & Padilla, S. (2001) Muscular characteristics of detraining in humans. *Med Sci Sports Exerc*. 333: 1297–1303.

Mutton, D.L, Loy, S.F, Rogers, D.M, et al. (1993) Effect of run vs combined cycle/run training on VO2max and running performance. *Med Sci Sports Exerc*. Dec; 25(12): 1393–1397.

Okada, T, Huxel, K.C. & Nesser, T.W. (2011) Relationship between core stability, functional movement, and performance. *J Strength Cond Res*. Jan 25(1): 252–261.

Osgood, C.E. (1949) The similarity paradox in human learning: a resolution. *Psychol Rev*. 56: 132–143.

Paillard, J. & Brouchon, M. (1968) Active and passive movements in the calibration of position sense. In: **Freedman**, S.J. (ed) *The neuropsychology of spatially oriented behavior*. Homewood, IL: Dorsey Press, 37–55.

Parkhouse, K.L. & Ball, N. (2010) Influence of dynamic versus static core exercises on performance in field based fitness tests. *JBMT*. In Press Dec.

Pizza, F.X., Flynn, M.G., Starling, R.D., et al. (1995) Run training vs cross training: influence of increased training on running economy, foot impact shock and run performance. *Int J Sports Med*. Apr; 16(3): 180–184.

Proteau, L., Tremblay, L. & Dejaeger, D. (1998) Practice does not diminish the role of visual information in on-line control of a precision walking task: support for the specificity of practice hypothesis. *J Mot Behav*. Jun; 30(2): 143–150.

Robertson, S. & Elliott, D. (1996) Specificity of learning and dynamic balance. *Res Q Exerc Sport*. Mar; 67(1): 69–75.

Rosenbaum, D.A., Meulenbroek, R.G.J & Vaughan, J. (2004) What is the point of motor planning? Int. *Journal of Sport and Exercise Psychology*. 2: 439–469.

Rubini, E.C., Costa, A.L. & Gomes, P.S. (2007) The effects of stretching on strength performance. *Sports Med*. 37: 213–224.

Schmidt, R.A. & Lee, T.D. (2005.) *Motor control and learning*. Fourth Edition. UK: Human Kinetics.

Simic, L., Sarabon, N. & Markovic, G. (2012) Does pre-exercise static stretching inhibit maximal muscular performance? A meta-analytical review. *Scand J Med Sci Sports*. Feb 8. doi: 10.1111/j.1600–0838.2012.01444.x. [Epub ahead of print]

Totsika, V. & Wulf, G. (2003) The influence of external and internal foci of attention on transfer to novel situations and skills. *Res Q Exerc Sport*. Jun; 74(2): 220–225.

Urquhart, D.M., Hodges, P.W. & Story, I.H. (2005) Postural activity of the abdominal muscles varies between regions of these muscles and between body positions. *Gait Posture*. Dec; 22(4): 295–301.

van Ingen Schenau, G.J., de Koning, J.J. & de Groot, G. (1994) Optimisation of sprinting performance in running, cycling and speed skating. *Sports Med*. Apr; 17(4): 259–275.

Weiss, E.J. & Flanders, M. (2004) Muscular and postural synergies of the human hand. J *Neurophysiol*. Jul; 92(1): 523–535.

Wilson, G.J., Murphy, A.J. & Walshe, A. (1996) The specificity of strength training: the effect of posture. *Eur J Appl Physiol Occup Physiol*. 73(3–4): 346–352.

Wulf, G. & Dufek, J.S. (2009) Increased jump height with an external focus due to enhanced lower extremity joint kinetics. *J Mot Behav*. Oct; 41(5): 401–409.

Wulf, G., Dufek, J.S., Lozano, L. & Pettigrew, C. (2010) Increased jump height and reduced EMG activity with an external focus. *Hum Mov Sci*. Jun; 29(3): 440–448. Epub 2010 Apr 21.

Young, W.B. (2006) Transfer of strength and power training to sports performance. *Int J Sports Physiol Perform*. 1(2): 74–83.

Young, W.B. & Behm, D.G. (2002) Should static stretching be used during a warm-up for strength and power activities? *Strength Conditioning J*. 24: 33–37.

Young, W.B. & Rath, D.A. (2011) Enhancing foot velocity in football kicking: the role of strength training. *J Strength Cond Res*. Feb; 25(2): 561–566.

CHAPTER 10

Fascial tissues in motion: Elastic storage and recoil dynamics

Robert Schleip

The catapult mechanism: Elastic recoil of fascial tissues

During the 1980s those studying the field of muscular physiology were intrigued by the capacity of kangaroos to perform powerful jumps, ranging up to 13 metres in length. Since these animals do not have bulky leg muscles, the general assumption was that their leg musculature would contain some unusual muscle fibres that enabled them to perform explosive contractions. In fact, some researchers were convinced that they would find 'super-fast twitch fibres' in the kangaroos' hind limbs. However, no matter how hard the researchers looked, they could not find any unusual muscle fibres. This left them puzzled: if muscles create the force for these impressive jumps, why do these animals contain the same muscle fibres as a koala? Eventually, they looked for the answer where nobody had looked previously, in the properties of the tendons. It was here that they found an amazing capacity, which was subsequently called the 'catapult effect'. Similar to an elastic spring of stainless steel, the long tendons were able to store and release kinetic energy with amazing efficiency (Kram & Dawson, 1998).

When the kangaroo hits the ground their tendons, as well as the fascial aponeuroses of their hind legs, are tensioned like elastic bands. The subsequent release of this stored energy is what makes these amazing jumps possible. Soon afterwards the same mechanism was also discovered in gazelles. These animals are capable of impressive leaping as well as running, although their musculature is not particularly strong. Since gazelles are generally considered to be rather delicate, it made the elastic springiness all the more interesting. Similar impressive elastic storage capacities were later confirmed to exist in horses.

Homo sapiens: The elastic 'gazelle' within the primate family

It was only when the technology of high-resolution ultrasound examination achieved a high-enough level of resolution to observe single sarcomeres in muscles, that a similar orchestration of loading between muscle and fascia was discovered in human locomotion. In fact it was found, rather surprisingly, that human fasciae have a similar kinetic storage capacity to that of kangaroos and gazelles (Sawicki et al., 2009). This capacity is not only used when we run or jump but also when walking, as a significant part of the energy of the movement comes from the same elastic springiness of the collagenous tissues described above. Neither chimpanzees, bonobos, orangutans or any other primate seems to have developed a similar elastic storage capacity within the fascial tissues of their legs, compared with their long legged homo sapiens relatives. This is reflected in the shorter muscle fascicles and thinner tendons in the distal legs of humans compared with non-human primates, making them much better adapted to the elastic storage and release of kinetic energy (Alexander, 1991).

This recent discovery has led to an active revision of long-accepted principles in the field of movement science. According to the previously unquestioned classical model of muscular dynamics, it was assumed that in a muscular joint movement, the skeletal muscle fibres involved shorten. This energy then passes through passive tendons, resulting in the movement (see Figure 10.1). This classic form of energy transfer is still true, according to these recent measurements, for slow as well as more rapid movements with a steady limb speed, such as cycling. Here, the muscle fibres actively change their length, while the tendons and aponeuroses scarcely lengthen. The fascial elements mostly fulfil a passive role in this movement orchestration. This is in contrast to oscillatory movement with an elastic spring quality, such as hopping, running or skipping, in which the length of the muscle fibres scarcely changes. While the muscle fibres contract in an almost isometric fashion, they stiffen temporarily without any significant change of their length, the fascial elements function in an elastic way with a movement similar to that of a resonating elastic spring made of stainless steel (Figure 10.2). It is mainly this lengthening

and shortening of the fascial elements that 'produces' the actual movement. Think of a catapult: the person putting their muscular energy into the tensioning of the elastic band is like the muscle fibres, which stores the kinetic energy in the fascial tissues. Usually the direction of the muscular preparatory work goes into an opposite orientation to the intended explosive power movement. For an archer, this would mean that his muscles pull backwards on the bow in order to increase the potential movement energy. When the force is released, it is the collagen (or elastic band) that propels the object (or arrow) into the intended direction, while the muscular elements step out of the way and take a rest. Imagine an archer, who tries to shoot faster by propelling the arrow forward with his muscles. This would be too slow. When properly

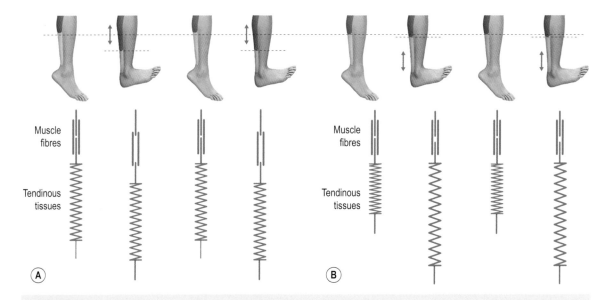

Figure 10.1

Comparison of length changes of muscular and collagenous elements in conventional 'muscle training' (A) and in a more fascially oriented movement with elastic recoil properties (B)

The elastic tendinous (or fascial) elements are shown as springs, the muscle fibre as straight lines. Note that during a conventional movement **A** the elastic collagenous elements do not change their length significantly while the contractile muscle fibres change their length significantly. **B** However, during rhythmically oscillatory movements, like running or hopping, the muscle fibres contract almost isometrically while the fascial collagenous elements lengthen and shorten like an elastic yo-yo spring. (Illustration adapted from Kawakami et al. (2002). reproduced with kind permission of www.fascialnet.com)

few cycles most people intuitively figure out the optimal resonant frequency of the system. This is usually achieved when finding a rhythm in which a tiny lift action of the holding finger, starting just a split second before the turning point, increases the stretch loading of the elastic spring. Interestingly, in a completely elastic system, the ideal resonant frequency depends mostly on two factors: (1) the length of the swinging element and (2) the stiffness of the strained tissues. When trying to dance or bounce on wet sand, most people will find that slower music is more suitable, whereas a more rapid rhythm tends to suit dancing barefoot with the forefeet on a hard dance floor with tightly contracted calf muscles.

For rhythmic movements that involve temporarily leaving the ground with both feet, such as running, hopping, skipping, etc. rhythms between 150 and 170 beats per minute (BPM) usually work best. When trying to find music to support effortless swinging and bouncing movements that do not involve leaving the ground, most people find that a slower rhythm between 120 and 140 BPM is optimum (Table 10.1). But what do you do if the music is too slow or too fast? Excluding options such as only choosing every second beat, it may work to change the length of the swinging body portion and/or to adapt the stiffness of the loaded fascial tissues by increasing or decreasing the active tonus of some of the attached muscle portions.

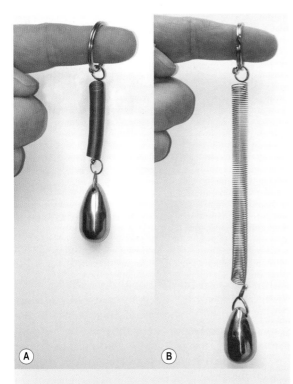

Figure 10.2 A & B
Experimenting with elastic recoil properties

When finding the ideal resonance frequency of an elastically swinging system a repetitively applied minute finger movement (possibly less than 1 mm in amplitude) may provide sufficient muscular contribution for achieving a large harmonic swinging movement. Photos courtesy of fascialnet.com

Kangaroo hopping versus frog jumping

In elastically oscillating movements, such as hopping in kangaroos, the energy production of the involved muscles are mainly concerned with pacing the best rhythm. This is comparable to the movements of a conductor's baton or the sticks of a slalom skier. It is, therefore, not surprising that the muscles involved when a kangaroo hops generate the same force at all speeds (Kram & Dawson, 1998). Similarly, a study examining the gait of women of the African Luo and Kikuyu tribes carrying loads of up to 20% of their body weight on their heads, found that their oxygen consumption was largely independent of the weight, provided they were allowed to walk at a speed comfortable

loaded, collagen can shorten at a much faster speed than any muscle fibre could contract. However, this only works if the loaded collagen tissue has a high elastic storage capacity. Imagine an archer trying to shoot with a bow made of concrete and a non-elastic rope.

Resonant frequency: Length and stiffness as crucial factors

In order to understand fascial recoil, try experimenting with a weight that is suspended on an elastic band or stainless steel spring (see Figure 10.2). With eyes open or closed, within a

Rhythmic activity		BPMt
Walking		**100–135**
	Slow pedestrian gait	100–120
	Rapid walking	120–135
Free dancing		**120–155**
	Swinging/rocking motions	120–130
	Bouncing (knee bends, etc.)	130–140
	Hopping/jumping	140–155
Running		**150–170**
	Slow running (6–8 kmh)	150–158
	Medium speed running (8–10 kmh)	158–163
	Sprinting (10–15 kmh)	163–170

Table 10.1

Resonant frequencies of different human rhythmic movement activities

Note that swinging movements, which involve gravity driven pendulum dynamics, do not usually involve the elastic stretch-recoil properties of fascial tissues. Whilst they offer other benefits, they should not, therefore, be considered as a specific training of fascial elasticity.

for them. When well-trained British soldiers were examined, carrying up to 20% of their body weight on their backpacks, their energy consumption increased in proportion to the weight carried. Interestingly, when the African women were asked to walk at an uncomfortably faster or slower pace, they exhibited the same weight dependent (and probably more muscular driven) pattern in their energy expenditure as the soldiers (Alexander, 1986; Zorn & Hodeck, 2011) (Chapter 17).

Compared with these rhythmically oscillating movements, a different orchestration between muscles and elastic tissue properties is at work during single explosive movements. For example, when a frog leaps, sometimes up to 10 metres, it also utilises the elastic recoil properties in its leg fasciae. However, here the contraction speed of the muscle fibres is of prime importance. The orchestration between muscular contractile dynamics and the rebound dynamics of collagenous tissues is similar to casting a long elastic fishing rod. A rapid muscular motion then starts to exert a strong pulling force on the distal limb as well as on related collagenous tissues. While initially some of that force seems 'lost' in the elastic compliance of tendons and aponeuroses, these tissues subsequently release the stored muscular energy via a rapidly accelerating motion, the speed of which surpasses the potential maximal muscle contraction velocity by several times. Note that in such 'singular' motions, a sense of rhythm or

resonant frequencies is not as crucially involved as in oscillatory rhythmic motions. In addition, the magnitude of the initial muscular contraction is of major importance: the more rapidly and strongly the muscles start to contract, the more powerful the resulting elastic recoil action of the fascial tissues will become.

Of course various complex combinations may exist between these two extremes. For example, throwing a baseball or a javelin has been shown to exert acceleration speeds that significantly surpass those of all other primates (Rouch et al., 2013). This is partly accomplished by a muscularly driven 'stretching backwards' motion (i.e. in the opposite direction to the intended forward throwing motion) in which kinetic energy is stored in various collagenous membranes and tendons. This initial phase simulates some of the hopping kangaroo dynamics, explored earlier, in which a sense of rhythm and resonant frequencies play important roles. The subsequent phase, consisting of a forward swinging motion, then utilises similar storage and release dynamics as are found in the powerful frog jump.

Plyometrics: Two different mechanisms

For competitive athletes, plyometric training is considered old hat. The field of plyometrics (Chapter 22), also known as jump training, was first introduced to the Western sports scene in the early 1980s. It involves training routines that move the total length of a 'muscle-tendon complex' from a state of extension to a shortened state in a rapid or 'explosive' way, such as in repetitive jumping. This is also called the 'stretch-shortening cycle'. The eccentric contraction of involved muscle fibres during the initial lengthening phase has been shown to play an essential role: the more rapid and powerful these preparatory eccentric contractions are, the more force is subsequently exerted in the final contraction phase. Plyometric training has been shown to increase jumping height, as well as many other athletic performance outcomes (Fig. 10.3).

The general explanation for the proposed mechanism is a combination of two factors: (1) a change in mechanical properties, here understood as an elastic energy storage-recoil process within the muscle-tendon unit; and (2) an optimisation of neural properties in the form of an augmented stretch reflex and the resulting activation of an increased number of motor units within the involved muscle fibre bundles (Kubo et al., 2007). While it was unclear to what respective degree each of those very different mechanisms are involved in the total outcome, most authors, and athletes, considered the improved neuromuscular orchestration and the assumed augmentation of myogenic contraction power as the dominant player. In contrast, the proposed utilisation of passive biomechanical storage and release properties was considered to play a secondary 'supporting role', compared with the active muscular contraction component.

Modern ultrasound technology allowed a team of French sports scientists to investigate the relative proportion of those two mechanisms (Fouré et al., 2011). By measuring length changes in the triceps surae muscles and the Achilles tendon, they observed that plyometric training, consisting of 34 sessions of one hour over 14 weeks, resulted in an *increased* utilisation of passive tissue properties and a *decreased* utilisation of active contractile muscular elements. After this systematic training process, the increased acceleration and jumping performance was accompanied by more 'lazy' muscle fibres during the shortening phase but with an increased passive 'elastic recoil property' of

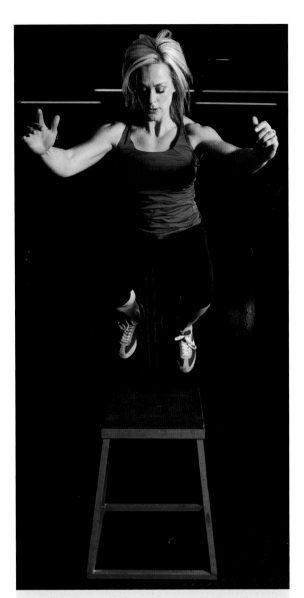

Figure 10.3

Plyometric training, if done properly, can increase jumping height and induce a gradual remodeling of tendinous tissues towards an increased kinetic storage capacity. Recent investigations revealed that the performance improvement goes along with a 'lazier' muscle activation in trained jumpers together with an augmented use of passive elastic recoil properties (Fouré, 2011). © iStock.com/jason_v

the spring-loaded elements within the muscle-tendon unit.

If the storage-release mechanism is occurring 'somewhere' within the total muscle-tendon complex, then the question is worth exploring, whether it happens mostly within the collagenous elements (the tendon, epimysium and intramuscular connective tissues) or whether it also occurs within the muscle fibres themselves. Muscle fibres are composed of smaller tubular myofibrils, the basic functional unit of which is called a sarcomere. Several sarcomeres arranged in series constitute a myofibril. The most appealing candidates for elastic energy storage within the sarcomeres are the titin proteins (Linke, 2000). These are the largest known proteins in the human body and form a more recently discovered third filament system within a sarcomere, apart from the previously known thick (mostly myosin) and thin (mostly actin) filaments. While these unique proteins are capable of impressive elastic recoil properties, their contribution to the stretch-shortening cycle in rapidly accelerating single movements, such as in jumping or throwing, constituted a matter of dispute. However, a detailed examination with isolated myofibres from frogs revealed that the potential elastic recoil power of these titin proteins tends to be considerably dampened by other intramuscular contraction dynamics. They may, therefore, be prevented from contributing to the elastic recoil properties in a significant manner. The researchers concluded that titin elastic recoil is able to support the active muscular shortening under low load only or during prolonged shortening from greater physiological sarcomere lengths (Minajeva, 2002). In other words, with the high loads applied during most plyometric training routines, the intramuscular titin elements seem to play only a minor role in the passive recoil dynamics of the total muscle-tendon complex. While the suggested conclusions of this animal study need to be validated with more detailed research, including human skeletal muscle tissues, these current results suggest that the collagenous (i.e. fascial) tissues are, most likely, providing the main energy storage and release mechanism that is synonymous with the increased athletic performance achieved using plyometric exercise training.

But what about the potential contribution of the intramuscular titin elements to oscillatory rhythmic recoil movements such as in kangaroo hopping and human running? Here, the length changes of the affected myofascial tissues involve only minor length changes within the muscular sarcomeres, in contrast to the collagenous tendinous elements (Figure 10.1). Since the titin elements are embedded within the sarcomeres this clearly suggests that most of the elastic recoil dynamics in such movements are achieved within the collagenous elements and not within the muscular titin components. In other words: training of elastic storage capacities, whether in single motions such as throwing or in oscillatory movements such as jogging, mainly involves an increase of collagenous elastic properties, rather than intramuscular sarcomeric adaptations.

Clinical Summary

- Fascial tissues are capable of storing and releasing kinetic energy similar to an elastic spring.
- While this 'catapult mechanism' was first examined in a detailed manner in Australian kangaroos, subsequent research revealed that it also plays a major role in human oscillatory movements such as running, hopping or walking.
- As was examined in the energy efficient gait of some African women, there are significant inter-individual differences as to how much this elastic recoil mechanism is utilised.
- Adequate training can enhance the capacity to utilize less muscular energy and more fascial elasticity in rapid accelerating movements.
- A key factor in the orchestration is adequate timing: the precise matching of the muscular activations with the resonant frequency of the swinging system.

References

Alexander, R.M. (1986) Human energetics: Making headway in Africa. *Nature*. 319: 623–624.

Alexander, R.M. (1991) Elastic mechanisms in primate locomotion. *Z Morphol Anthropol*. 78(3): 315–320.

Fouré, A., Nordez, A., McNair P.J. & Cornu, C. (2011) Effects of plyometric training on both active and passive parts of the plantarflexors series elastic component stiffness of muscle–tendon complex. *Eur J Appl Physiol*. 111: 539–548.

Kawakami, Y., Muraoka, T., Ito, S., Kanehisa, H. & Fukunaga, T. (2002) In vivo muscle fibre behaviour during countermovement exercise in humans reveals a significant role for tendon elasticity. *J Physiol*. 540: 635–646.

Kubo, K., Morimoto, M., Komuro, T. et al. (2007) Effects of plyometric and weight training on muscle-tendon complex and jump performance. *Med Sci Sports Exerc* 39: 1801–1810.

Kram, R. & Dawson, T.J. (1998) Energetics and biomechanics of locomotion by red kangaroos (Macropus rufus). *Comparat Biochem Physiol*. B120: 41–49.

Linke, W.A. (2000) Titin elasticity in the context of the sarcomere: force and extensibility measurements on single myofibrils. *Adv Exp Med Biol*. 481: 179–202.

Minajeva, A., Neagoe, C., Kulke, M. & Linke, W.A. (2002) Titin-based contribution to shortening velocity of rabbit skeletal myofibrils. *J Physiol*. 540 (Pt 1): 177–188.

Roach, N.T., Venkadesan, M., Rainbow, M.J. & Lieberman. D.E. (2013) Elastic energy storage in the shoulder and the evolution of high-speed throwing in Homo. *Nature* 498(7455): 483–486.

Sawicki, G.S., Lewis, C.L. & Ferris, D.P. (2009) It pays to have a spring in your step. *Exercise Sport Sci R*. 37: 130–138.

Zorn, A. & Hodeck, K. (2011) Walk with elastic fascia. In: Erik Dalton: *Dynamic body – Exploring form, expanding function*. Freedom From Pain Institute, Oklahoma. 96–123.

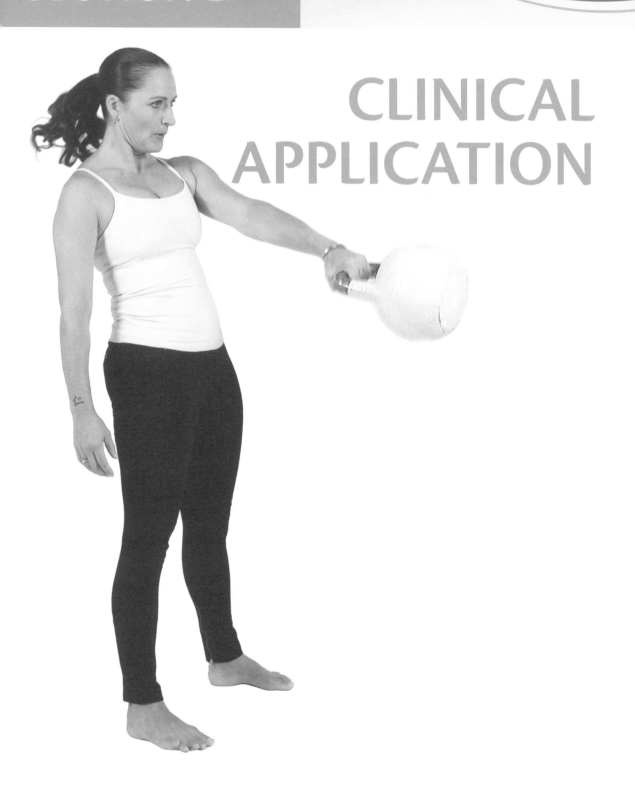

CLINICAL
APPLICATION

CHAPTER 11

Fascial Fitness

Robert Schleip and Divo Müller

How to build a youthful, resilient fascial body

The elegant movements of a dancer, the impressive perfomance of a circus artist, the powerful goal-striking shot of a soccer star is not only a question of muscular strength, good cardiovascular condition, neuromuscular coordination (Jenkins, 2005) and good luck in genetics. According to findings in the international field of fascia research, the muscular connective tissues, called myofasciae, have more meaning for 'a body in motion', than was ever considered decades ago. Recent research findings prove that the body-wide fascial network plays a significant role in force transmission, hydration (fluid dynamic) and proprioception (Chapter 4).

A specific training, focusing on the question of how to build a strong and flexible fascial body, could be of great importance for athletes, dancers, martial arts students and somatic oriented movement advocates. The optimal fascial body is both elastic and resilient and can, therefore, be relied upon to respond effectively in a variety of challenges and circumstances thereby providing a high degree of injury prevention (Kjaer et al., 2009) (Chapter 5).

This chapter mainly focuses on one main specific aspect of Fascial Fitness: the elastic recoil capacity of the collagenous tissues. It explores the question of how to stimulate the fibroblasts to lay down new collagenous fibres in a healthy and youthful network architecture. The physiological and biomechanical foundations that underly the following training principles are described in Chapters 1 and 10.

Fascial Fitness practical application to enhance elastic recoil

1. Preparatory counter movement

To increase the dynamic of elastic recoil and the catapult effect, the movement is first initiated with a pre-tensioning in the opposite direction, followed by the actual movement. A suitable metaphor would be the archer who prestretches the tendon of his bow in the opposite direction before shooting the arrow in the desired direction. Applying muscular effort in pushing the arrow forward would be of no sense or comparable effectiveness (Chapter 10).

Frontal leg

Standing with feet hip-width apart, shift the weight onto one leg (Figure 11.1 A and B). In the beginning, to aid balance, hold on to the back of a chair. To progress, you may later remove the balance aid, once the movement is familiar and fluent.

- Start with easy swings of the free leg, swinging backwards and forwards, like a pendulum. In such swinging motion kinetic energy is rhythmically stored and released; however, the storage of kinetic energy occurs in the spatial relation of the swinging weight towards gravity, whereas the fascial tissues are not – or not yet – stretch-loaded.

- Increase the loading by deliberately pre-stretching in the opposite direction (backwards), followed by releasing the stored energy through the frontal swing. Here, the kinetic energy is also stored and released, although this time the storage involves an elastic elongation (stretch) of collageneous tissues within the body.

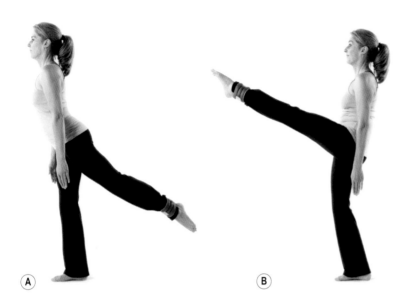

A   B

Figure 11.1 A & B
Leg swing

A The leg is first extended backwards in such a way that a pre-stretch is created in the front.

B The stored tension is then suddenly released and the leg is accelerated forward like a swinging pendulum.

- To further enhance the 'catapult effect', initiate the frontal leg swing proximally, from your pubic bone or sternum, immediately followed by the distal end, via the pre-stretched leg and foot.
- To load the tissues even more effectively and enhance proprioceptive refinement, use ankle weights.

Fascial effects: The frontal leg swings are optimal to increase elasticity in short hip flexors and to lengthen hamstrings.

2. The Ninja principle

This principle uses the metaphor of the legendary Japanese warriors, who reputedly moved as silently as cats leaving no trace. When engaging fascial elements in bouncy movements, such as jumping, running or dancing, the quality of motion should be as smooth and quiet as possible. A change in direction is preceded by a gradual deceleration of the movement before the turning point and a gradual acceleration afterwards. Any harsh, jerky or noisy movement would be counterproductive. The sensed benefits could be a perception of fluid, elegant and effective movement, like a cat in a dynamic leap or stalking while hunting.

Daily fascial training: Stair Dancing

Walking up and down stairs can become an instant fascial recoil training, when the Ninja principle is applied. A variation of easy bounces in stepping is suggested with the focus of making as little noise as possible. The 'no sound parameter' provides useful feedback to engage the fascial springiness: the quieter and gentler the better. Dancing fascially up and down the stairs would be of additional benefit using a 'barefoot like' plantar-foot contact with the ground (Chapter 18).

Fascial fitness: Basic elastic recoil exercise – Flying Sword

The Fascial Fitness exercise called 'the Flying Sword' is one of the core exercises to train elastic recoil, especially in the lumbodorsal fascia. Beginners start with steps 1 to 3, subsequently adopting the more refined aspects presented in steps 4 and 5 once the earlier steps have been mastered. Most important is the orchestration of the movement, without muscular effort or strain and optimally performed: fast, fluid and powerful.

Three basic steps to enhance elastic recoil

1. Preparatory countermovement
2. Proximal initiation of the power motion
3. Sequential delay of more distal body parts in following this movement.

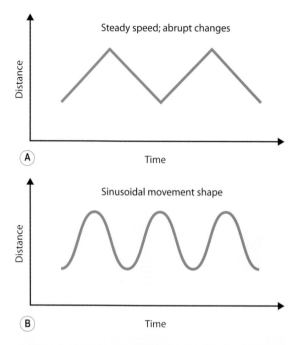

Figure 11.2 A & B

Movement quality in change of direction: jerky versus elegant turns

When a dynamic arm movement (e.g. forward and back), is performed with lack of proprioceptive refinement, the tendency is to use sudden turns and provoke abrupt loading patterns (see graph above). In contrast, when the same movements are conducted, with an internal search for elegance, then a more sinusoidal movement directional change can be observed. This is characterised by a gradual deceleration before the turning point, which is followed by a subsequent gradual acceleration. In this pattern, the loaded tissues are less prone to injuries, and the movements appear fluid and graceful.

Equipment: Weight, dumbbell, kettle bell, swing dumbbell

Stand with feet a little wider than hip width apart, so the weight can easily be moved between your knees.

Step 1: Preparatory countermovement

Hold the weight with both hands and lift your arms up above your head. Pre-tensioning is achieved, while bending the body's axis slightly backward and extending it in an upward lengthening at the same time (Figure 11.3A). This increases the elastic tension in the front fascial 'body suit'.

Bring the weight down, by releasing the pre-tension through the upper body and arms. This allows them to spring forward and down like a catapult, allowing the weight to 'fly' like a sword between your knees (Figures 11.3B & 11.3C).

Then reverse this process. Here, the catapult capacity of the fascia is activated by an active pre-tensioning of the posterior fascia by directing the weight further backwards. Before moving from the forward bending position, the flexor muscles on the front of the body are first, briefly, activated. This momentarily pulls the body even further back and down and at the same time the fascia on the back of the body is loaded with greater tension. The kinetic energy, which is stored on the posterior side of the fascial net, is dynamically released via a passive recoil effect as the upper body flies back to the original upright position.

Rhythm is it

A feeling of rhythm is required to ensure that the individual is not relying on muscle work of their back muscles but rather on the dynamic recoil activity of the fascia, in addition to the preparatory countermovement. This is similar to the timing necessary when playing with a yo-yo. If the inherent rhythm is met, it swings with almost effortless ease and flow (Chapter 10).

Step 2: Proximal initiation to perform the actual motion

From the pre-tensed backward bending position, the forward movement is initated by a proximal pull of the sternum followed by the distal parts of the body (Figure 11.4). In this exercise, the sternum or pubic bone initates the release forwards and downwards.

Step 3: Sequential delay of more distal body parts following this movement

The proximal initiation of Step 2 is immediately followed by a sequential delay of the more distal

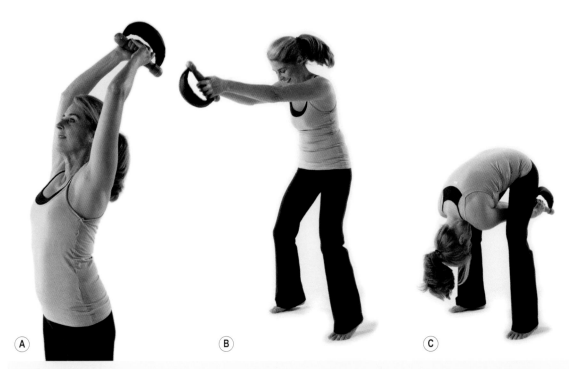

Figure 11.3 A B C
Flying Sword

A The principle of preparatory countermovement is an effective way to load the fascial tissues, before performing the actual movement in the desired direction. For example, in this exercise we start the movement with a pre-stretch into the opposite direction, slightly bending backwards.

B Releasing down: The stored energy in the connective tissues allow a dynamic end efficient movement performance. In this phase we 'fly' down, with hardly any muscular effort, but counting instead on the capacity of fascia to store kinetic energy and release it.

C At the turning point: pull the weight and the upper body slightly more backwards into the preparatory counter-movement. To increase the catapult effect and loading of the fascia of the back, briefly activate the flexor muscles on the front of the body first, before releasing the stored energy in flying up into the starting position.

body parts. In this exercise, the arms and hands holding the weight, follow behind creating a 'wave like' movement. By using the proximal initiation and sequential delay of the distal parts, the pre-tension of the body is further increased and dynamic power and acceleration is enhanced.

Two advanced steps to enhance elastic recoil

Having mastered these basic steps in a recoil movement exercise, add these two more advanced steps to refine the movements' orchestration.

The following two steps are practised immediately prior to the basic three steps described before:

Advanced step 1: Increase of sensory awareness – proprioceptive refinement

One of the big surprises in recent fascial findings was the discovery that fascia contains a rich supply of sensory nerves, including proprioceptive receptors, multimodal receptors and nociceptive nerve endings. This means that fascia is alive (Chapter 4)!

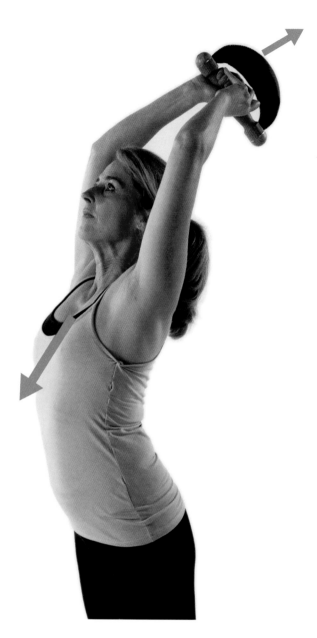

Figure 11.4
Proximal initiation and distal delay

To increase the catapult effect and its power in action, we initiate the movement by the proximal pull of the sternum, followed by a distal delay of the upper body, in this example by the arms and the hands, creating a flowing whip like movement and thereby increasing the catapult and its powerful effect.

Recent findings indicate that the superficial fascial layers of the body are, in fact, much more densely populated with sensory nerve endings than the connective tissues situated internally (Benetazzo et al., 2011) (Tesarz et al., 2011). In particular, the transition zone between the fascia profunda and the subdermal loose connective tissue seems to have the highest sensorial innervation (Tesarz et al., 2011). The body wide connective tissue network is certainly our most important organ for proprioception (Schleip, 2003).

For a long time, proprioception shared a similar history as fascia and, at the turn of this century was rediscovered as our main movement sense. In a movement training, there are a variety of ways to train and stimulate sensory or proprioceptive refinement. Common and effective ways *before* the actual movement include rubbing, tapping, rolling, brushing or kinesio-taping specific bodyparts to stimulate the receptors of the superficial fascial layers.

In a more refined preparation, mindfulness and the benefits of conscious attention focus may be used (Moseley et al., 2008). For example, by focusing on the natural expansive wave of inhalation to expand from within into the surrounding space or by sensing the slightest touch of the air on the skin (Chapter 4).

Advanced step 2: Tensegral expansion

Tensegrity (Chapter 1) and the essential role that fascial membranes play in the structural well-being of the body, is used in this principle. *Before* we move into action, we first engage a 360° body-wide spacious expansion. This can be achieved by an all over pre-tensioning of the superficial fascia, which envelopes the body as a whole. In Fascial Fitness training, we describe this as 'tensing the tiger body suit'. Recent findings show that this kind of 'tensegral' pre-tension is a substitute for a 'power pose' known from the animal kingdom. This has instant positive effects by dropping endocrine stress levels (Carney et al., 2010).

In the Flying Sword exercise, this would be 'created' by bringing attention to the body's 'poles', engaging a slight bi-directional movement apart, from top to toe. In fascial terms, from the plantar fascia to the galea aponeurotica, as well as a widening from front to back. The same kind of attention is added while bending backwards, to load the fascial chain of the front. Here, the tensegral expansion between the vertebrae is enhanced, to avoid any buckling and, therefore, straining in the cervicals or the lumbars.

Fascial stretching

In Fascial Fitness, both dynamic and slow stretching applications are used. Instead of stretching isolated muscle groups, the aim is finding body movements that engage the longest possible myofascial chains (Chapter 6). In the slower stretches, this is not done by passively waiting as in a lengthening classical Hatha yoga pose, or in a conventional isolated muscle stretch. Since the majority of the human fascial net is composed of membranous sheets, rather than long narrow stripes, multidirectional angular variations are frequently explored during stretching. This might include sideways or diagonal movement variations as well as spiralling rotations. With this method, large areas of the fascial network are simultaneously involved.

The dynamic stretching variation may be familiar to many readers as it was part of the physical education in the first half of the last century. During recent decades, such bouncing stretches were considered to be generally harmful to the tissue but more contemporary research has confirmed the method's merits. While stretching immediately before athletic performance (e.g. 5 minutes before a competitive run) can be counterproductive (Chapter 9), long-term and regular use of such dynamic stretching, when correctly performed, can positively influence the architecture of the connective tissue in that it becomes more elastic (Decoster et al., 2005). For dynamic stretching, the muscles and tissue should be warmed up first and any jerking or abrupt movements should be avoided. The aforementioned principles of elastic recoil can often be applied, including the proprioceptive refinement, using a sinusoidal deceleration and the preparatory counter movement.

When the elongated myofibres are in a relaxed condition then a slow stretching approach is sufficient to reach many intramuscular fascial tissues. However, it does not reach the tendinous tissues since these are arranged in series with the relaxed and soft myofibres (see Fig. 11.5C). In order to stimulate these tendinous and aponeurotic tissues, more dynamically swinging stretch movements are recommended, similar to the elegant and fluid extensional movements of rhythmic gymnasts. The same tissues can also be targeted by muscular activation (e.g. against resistance) in a lengthened position, similar to how a cat sometimes enjoys pulling his front claws towards the trunk when stretching (Fig. 11.5D). Finally, so-called 'mini-bounces' can also be employed as soft and playful explorations in the lengthened stretch position.

Fascial training guidelines

One main intention of a connective tissue oriented training is to influence the matrix remodelling via specific training activities which may, after

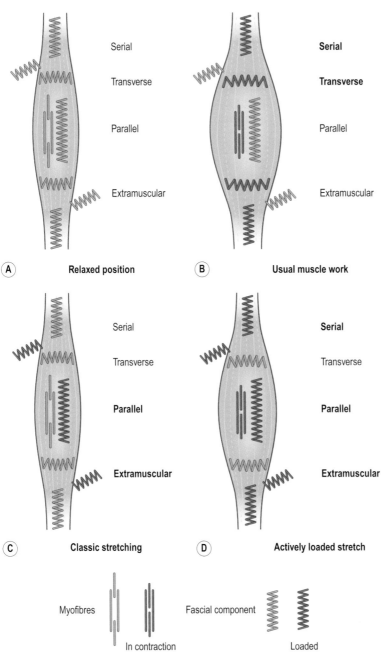

Figure 11.5

Loading of different fascial components

A Muscle in relaxed position: The tissue muscle is at normal length and the myofibres are relaxed. Here none of the fascial elements is being stretched.

B Usual muscle work: The myofibres are actively contracted while the muscle is at normal length range. Those fascial tissues are loaded which are either arranged in series with the myofibres or which run transverse to them.

C Classic stretching: The muscle is elongated and its contractile myofibres are relaxed. Here fascial tissues are being stretched which are oriented parallel to the myofibres, as well as extramuscular connections. However, fascial tissues oriented in series with the myofibres are not sufficiently loaded, since most of the elongation in that serially arranged force chain is taken up by the relaxed myofibres.

D Actively loaded stretch: The muscle is activated in long end range positions. Most of the fascial components are being stretched and stimulated in that loading pattern. Note that various mixtures and combinations between the four different fascial components exist. This simplified abstraction therefore serves as a basic orientation only.

6–24 months, result in a more resilient 'silk-like body suit'. This creates a strong and elastic fibrous network that is at the same time flexible, allowing smooth gliding joint mobility over wide angular ranges. A few Fascial Fitness training guidelines to support optimal results are listed below.

Low loading

Inclusion of fascial rebound and long myofascial chains often triggers an exhilarating sense of playfulness, fun and adventure orientation. However, if untamed this can also lead to more frequent injuries than standard muscle training which features monotonous repetitions. Start with much lower loads and repetitions than usual. Increase load only if a sense of elegance can be maintained, particularly during the elastic rebound phase.

Low frequency

The examination of collagen turnover in a tendon after exercise has shown that collagen synthesis is, indeed, increased after exercise. Yet the fibroblasts also break collagen down at the same time. Furthermore 24–48 hours after exercise, collagen degradation is greater than collagen synthesis. After 48 hours and thereafter this situation is reversed. Therefore, it is suggested that this appropriate tissue stimulation only occurs one to two times per week (Magnusson et al., 2010) (Chapter 1).

Long lasting effect

In contrast to muscular strength training, in which big gains occur rapidly in only a few weeks, fascia renewal is much slower (Chapter 1). Therefore, the improvements during the first few weeks may be small and less obvious on the outside. It usually takes 3–9 months to see tissue remodelling effects from the outside as well as 'feel' them in palpation. In muscular training, a plateau is reached relatively quickly with further increase hard to gain. However, fascial improvements have a cumulative effect and will not be lost as quickly (for example, when training is stopped because of health or work related reasons) and are, therefore, of a more sustainable quality (Kjaer et al., 2009) (Chapter 5). Regular application over two or three years will definitely be expected to yield long-lasting tissue improvements in the form of an improved strength and elasticity of the global fascial net.

Clinical summary

Fascial Fitness training does not seek to compete with neuromuscular or cardiovascular training, both of which can have very important health effects that are not possible with fascial training alone. On the contrary, fascial training is suggested as either a sporadic or more regular addition to comprehensive movement training. It promises to lead towards remodelling of the body-wide fascial network in such a way that it works with increased effectiveness and refinement in terms of its kinetic storage capacity, as well as a sensory organ for proprioception. Further research is required to validate whether it does, indeed, fullfil its basic promise of an increased protection against repetitive strain injuries in sports medicine.

References

Benetazzo, L., Bizzego, A., De Caro, R., Frigo, G., Guidolin, D. & Stecco, C. (2011). 3D reconstruction of the crural and thoracolumbar fasciae. *Surg Radio Anat.* 33: 855–862.

Carney, D.R., Cuddy, A.J. & Yap, A. (2010). Power posing: brief nonverbal displays affect neuroendocrine levels and risk tolerance. *J Psychol Sci.* Oct; 21(10): 1363–1368.

Decoster, L.C., Cleland, J., Altieri, C. & Russell, P. (2005). The effects of hamstring stretching on range of motion: a systematic literature review. *J Orthopedi Sports Phy Ther.* 35: 377–387.

Jenkins, S. (2005). Sports Science Handbook. In: *The Essential Guide to Kinesiology, Sport & Exercise Science, vol. 1.* Multi-science Publishing Co. Ltd., Essex, UK.

Kjaer, M., Langberg, H., Heinemeier, K., Bayer, M.L., Hansen, M., Holm, L., Doessing, S., Kongsgaard, M., Krogsgaard, M.R. & Magnusson, S.P. (2009). From mechanical loading to collagen synthesis, structural changes and function in human tendon. *Scand J Med Sci Sports* 19: 500–510.

Magnusson, S.P., Langberg, H. & Kjaer, M. (2010). The pathogenesis of tendinopathy: balancing the response to loading. *Nat Rev Rheumatol.* 6: 262–268.

Moseley, G.L., Zalucki, N.M. & Wiech, K. (2008). Tactile discrimination, but not tactile stimulation alone, reduces chronic limb pain. *Pain* 137: 600–608.

Schleip, R. (2003). Fascial plasticity- a new neurobiological explanation. Part 1. *J Bodyw Mov Ther.* 7: 11–19.

Tesarz, J., Hoheisel, U., Wiedenhofer, B. & Mense, S. (2011). Sensory innervation of the thoracolumbar fascia in rats and humans. *Neuroscience* 194: 302–308.

Bibliography

Bertolucci, L.F. (2011). Pandiculation: nature's way of maintaining the functional integrity of the myofascial system? *J Bodyw Move Ther.* 5: 268–280.

Pollack, G.H. (2001). *Cells, gels and the engines of life. A new, unifying approach to cell function.* Ebner and Sons Publishers, Seattle, Washington.

Schleip R. & Müller D.G. (2013). Training principles for fascial connective tissues: scientific foundation and suggested practical applications. *J Bodyw Mov Ther.* Jan; 17(1): 103–115.

CHAPTER 12

Fascial form in yoga

Joanne Avison

Yoga is not about stretching (Chapter 9). Yoga is about fostering balance in the length and tension relationships in the body. This preserves one of the most valuable features of the fascial matrix – its elasticity. Stretching is but one aspect of promoting elasticity. We are, essentially, designed for storing the potential energy of recoil (Chapter 10). In practice, stretching is not always the way to do that.

Certain body types, or body histories, can mean that stretching-for-length is the last thing some people need. The kind of stretching that simply pulls on the tissues (Richards, 2012), can be potentially harmful rather than healing. Yoga and fascia are both beautifully designed to honour any and everybody's ability to manage movement forces, not necessarily *forced movements*.

True elasticity is one of several fundamental principles of the fascial matrix profoundly enhanced by the practice of yoga. It is a reciprocal relationship because the growing understanding of the fascial tensional network makes sense of yoga, in all its potential for health and vitality. The optimisation of tensional integrity of the tissues and the whole architecture can be depleted by over stretching, just as appropriate stretching can invigorate and strengthen it.

The unifying experience

Yoga did not develop under the laws of Cartesian Reductionist theory that have dominated Western anatomy, physiology, biomechanics and psychology for centuries. As an art and a science it was only ever based in the unifying experience of mind, body and being. Its ancient wisdom had no history of treating these aspects of 'humans being' and 'humans doing' separately.

Reducing 'human doing' to functions and actions of muscles, bones, nerves and linear theories of biomechanical levers sits awkwardly with our fully animated and instinctive experience on the yoga mat. The properties of the fascia, as a ubiquitous sensory tensional network of tissues, make perfect sense of it.

The postures (asanas) in all their rich variety of shape and position, range and dynamics, are a means to explore balance and restore energy to those tissues, if we remain awake to their tensional integrity. Therein lies the *containment* of energy, the natural elasticity of compliance and our vitality. Even in Corpse Pose (*Shivasana*), the body rests under tension. We don't turn into an amoebic puddle on the mat when we are not moving, nor do we take the shape of the postures. Yoga, fascia and elasticity make very practical and palpable sense of each other.

'A recognised characteristic of connective tissue is its impressive adaptability. When regularly put under increasing physiological strain, it changes its architectural properties to meet the increasing demand.'
Robert Schleip (2011)

We have considerable power over the nature of the demand we put on the tissues. If we place no strain on them at all, it is the demand for inertia that effectively causes its own 'lack-of' strain patterns. This can lead to a requirement to tension the tensional network rather than stretch a relatively untensioned one. That isn't to say certain types of stretching are not valuable to all bodies. Consider Instinctive Stretching or Pandiculation (see Instinctive Stretching). This can wake up sedentary tissues and relieve tight ones. However, it is distinct from the kind of stretching for which yoga sometimes has a reputation.

Some yoga practices are dedicated to long sequences, which suit the development of 'elastic momentum'. However there is a caveat under

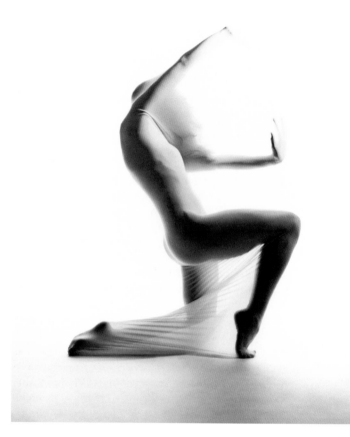

Figure 12.1

Tensional Integrity in movement and stillness, moment-by-moment and move-ment-by-movement. (Model: Samira Schmidli, reproduced with kind permission from David Woolley, photographer.)

the 'Fascialogical' theme of tensional integrity. If a dynamic series is repeated at very regular and frequent intervals all in one direction of strain, for example, flexion biased, it is likely to have a cumulative effect that can cost elasticity in the longer term, potentially encouraging a particular strain pattern. However, if it is regularly coun-terbalanced with a series that is, for example, extension biased then this pattern can be bal-anced and more beneficial. The fascial matrix is a refined force transmission system (Langevin, 2006) and will respond according to the forces put through it.

It is possible to ensure an equally refined balance of forces to optimise the elastic capacity and recoil facility of the body (Chapter 10), without over straining it in one particular direction. Once we understand the polarities involved and the defini-tion of elasticity, we can accumulate the benefits of increased resilience, compliance and spring load-ing throughout our systems. It gives us moment-to-moment and movement-to-movement balance at naturally instinctive speed.

Three key points

There are three key points that contribute to understanding elasticity and stretching of the fas-cial form in yoga practice.

1. **Terminology:** what exactly is elasticity?

2. **Tensional integrity:** how does this work in the whole body?

3. **Energy storage capacity:** how is it optimised in practice?

Once these points are clarified, we can begin to see the foundation of elasticity as a valuable attribute of the whole tissue matrix. Then the advantages can be suitably derived from all variations of Hatha yoga styles (Ashtanga, Restorative, Vinyasa Flow, Kria, Iyengar, etc).

1. Terminology

Elasticity is the capacity of a material to change shape (deform) under external force and resist internally, thereby returning to previous form (reform). This is measured as the difference between the *stiffness* (resistance to *deformation*) and the elastic return (*reformation*).

A common misunderstanding in the classroom seems to be that

(a) something has to be made of elastic to display elasticity and

(b) when we let go of an elastic band or elasticated fabric, as it lies at rest, we are modelling our body at rest. Both of these ideas are inaccurate.

Stiffness is the *resistance* to deformation but stiff springs, think car parts, can have more *elasticity* than weaker springs, think slinky toy, because they store more energy and rebound more efficiently. Hard steel ball bearings bounce better than rubber balls (Levin, 2013). A material does not have to be made of elastic to show elasticity or have the capacity to store elastic energy.

We rest pre-tensioned, or pre-stiffened, by the architectural design of our bones and soft tissues. Our 'elasticity' does not just refer to the amount we can stretch. It refers to the ability or capacity to restore a change in shape. That is a suitable balance between stiffness (i.e. resistance to deformation) and elasticity (i.e. the ability to reform or restore the original shape). We are poised between the extremes of either *when we are relaxed*. When we take up a yoga pose, to the extent that we can form the shape of the pose (deformation), it is counterbalanced by the ability to release it without imposition. If we force a stretch, then the ability of the tissues to restore (reformation) might be compromised.

The question is of a balance between these two states, rather than a focus on maximum flexibility for its own sake (Chapter 9). Appropriate counter poses, and respect for the elastic limit, invite an overall balance to the whole practice.

When you pull on an elastic band or fabric you are measuring its *stiffness* or *deformation capacity*. When you release the band, the extent to which it immediately restores its original shape is a measure of its *elasticity* or *reformation ability*. In fact our tissues rest pre-stiffened or pre-tensioned, poised for movement. If we go beyond the elastic limit, it is a different state: that of plasticity.

Plasticity: Beyond elasticity is a point where reformation is no longer possible. The so-called stretch is irreversible. The material doesn't spring back when you let it go and retains the shape of the deformation. Between that point, the elastic limit, and the breaking or tearing point, is termed *plasticity*: when the new shape stays there. The subsequent changes are distinguished in terms of malleability and ductility or brittleness. All of these are properties of different types of materials.

Viscoelasticity is a characteristic of the living body: a solid and fluid medium. 'Viscoelasticity is a property of all tensegrity structures. It is a non-linear time dependent deformation. It is called "viscoelastic" because when stressed it first behaves as if it were a liquid, then behaves as an elastic solid, not because it is made up from those two states. When stress is removed, it does it backwards and there is a splashdown (soft landing)' Levin (2013).

Stiffness in liquids is measured by thickness or *viscosity*. The speed and ease with which you can stir water is faster and takes less effort than stirring honey because water has comparatively lower viscosity or stiffness. At the same time, honey could be considered harder to deform than water. They are different values or properties that, in combination within the tissues, make for a variety of tensional possibilities. Car springs have 'dampers' on them to slow down the rate of elastic return. The fluids in our tissues act as dampers and give them viscoelastic properties, which regulate the rate of resistance and reformation (Richards, 2012).

Our entire structural matrix links the proteins, gels, emulsions and the complex components of our tissues and fluids, to integrate these fluid and solid elements together, appropriately *for us*. At every level of detail there is a balance of stiffness and elasticity in response to how we load or use them. All together, this exquisitely detailed matrix forms a *viscoelastic* medium for the tissues, which develop the collagen matrix according to their loading and the timing/frequency of that accumulated history. Habitual or deliberate strain patterns profoundly affect tissue morphology and mobility. Forced stretching can compromise the tissues' innate ability to spring back if it isn't counter balanced, or sufficiently stiffened to optimise elasticity. This ability is expressed on the mat as a balance between strength, length and flexibility.

2. Tensional integrity

One of the main features of our structural balance in motion is based upon the architectural principles of biotensegrity (Levin, 2012).

This is the basis of our architecture. Unlike the elastic band resting on the table, *untensioned*, we remain tensioned all the time, to enclose and occupy space. By the basic laws of biotensegrity every movement affects the whole and is transmitted through it.

'Tensegrity structures are omni-directional, independent of gravity, load distributing and energy efficient, hierarchical and self-generating. They are also ubiquitous in nature, once you know what to look for.'

Stephen Levin (Levin, 2009)

As biotensegrity structures, we have the ability to squeeze and draw in our structure and tissues as a whole, besides being able to stretch and fill or expand them, omnidirectionally, like the bladder or the lungs, for example. The fascial fabric, bones, myofascia, organs, joints, vessels and cavities of our architecture are held together and apart simultaneously. They are globally contained through the tension/compression principles of biotensegrity architecture (Levin, 1990)(Martin, 2012)(Ingber, 1998) (Flemons, 2006).

This is the basis of 'primordial biologic structure' (Levin, 1990). Such a design is organised for stored energy capacity through the balance of stiffness to elasticity in the entire architecture on every scale. It is a foundational principle of human, indeed living, form and one that we naturally explore in every yoga pose (asana). Essentially we seek to preserve and promote elastic integrity.

3. Energy storage capacity

We constantly work under three phases of elastic range, not one. We can stretch and release and we can squeeze and release. The breath is the first place to recognise this law in motion. We breathe in and breathe out in the inhale/exhale rhythm. However, we can then exhale *more* to empty or squeeze and *release by inhaling*. It is a three-phase process and one that yoga is intent to maintain in suitable balance. Dynamic sequences, slower restorative practice and the stillness of meditation are designed to explore this range and accumulate a resource of actively contained energy storage capacity throughout the body. This is enhanced by many of the yogic breathing practices.

For the whole body, over emphasis on softening, stiffening or stretching will not necessarily result in optimum elasticity in movement, whatever the activity (Chapter 9). The focus in yoga is on the refined *transition and continuity* between stretch, release and squeeze through the middle range of resting tension.

While this may seem like an obvious statement shown in diagrammatic form, it is not always understood when applied practically. Even in yoga classes, breathing exercises are often done without the distinctions of their value in preserving and promoting compliance and energy storage ability in the tissues. They have global implications of accumulating and fine-tuning elasticity.

If we train the body in one aspect, i.e. just squeezing (stiffening), just stretching or just softening (releasing), or in one direction (i.e. just flexion) we can compromise elastic integrity. If we counter pose and counteract to maintain that tensional balance, we frequently load the tissues for optimum tensional integrity and range in all degrees of potential. Stretching becomes a feature of balance and suitable control, rather than a purpose for its own sake.

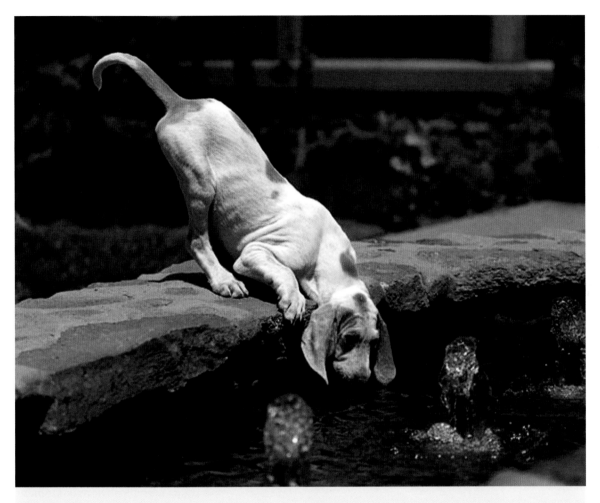

Figure 12.2

The tensional integrity of the whole body can be seen being used for balance. From nose tip to tail tip, this puppy reached out as part of a whole body-balancing act to drink from the pool, extending the tensional integrity to the tip of its tongue. (Reproduced with kind permission from Shane McDermott, www.wildearthilluminations.com)

Instinctive stretching

This is a way of stretching that doesn't seem to compromise the tissues and naturally regulates the dangers of over stretching globally. Animals can provide us with some clues.

Consider the cheetah, for example. Cats can rest and relax, stretch at a suitable time and move at great speed and pounce on prey. At rest, they become languid and serene. When they have rested, they frequently yawn-stretch their whole

body to wake up their tissues after releasing them for a period of time. This particular type of stretching is called pandiculation (Bertolucci, 2010). It is what we call a 'lengthening contraction' in yoga. It is a feature of movement with a purpose in nature, to reactivate the tissues after resting them and reorganise, or prime, the internal bonds and fluids ready for mobility (Chapter 9).

When a cheetah anticipates prey (peak performance), the last thing they do is stretch. They prime their tissues by 'squeezing' or stiffening

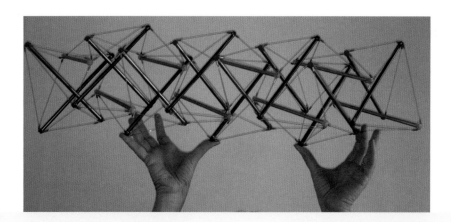

Figure 12.3

A tensegrity mast; originally presented by Kenneth Snelson as a system called 'floating compression' the term 'tensegrity' was coined by Buckminster Fuller as 'tensional integrity' and developed since by Dr Stephen Levin into biotensegrity. (See further information). It is an elastic architecture, balanced between stiffness and elasticity. It bounces and resists deformation, retaining its three-dimensional form. (Model by Bruce Hamilton – see further information.)

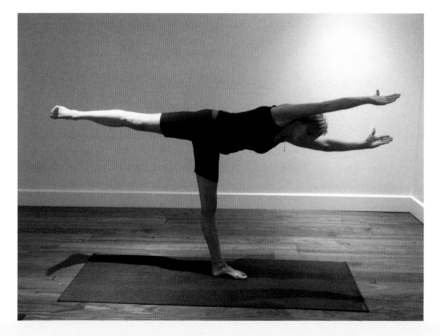

Figure 12.4

A classical model of the spine might suggest that it is a stacked column. This posture would not be possible if that were the case. Nor is it the muscular strength of Katie's standing foot that is holding her up. Her ability to hold and modify this pose is based upon the tensional integrity of her balance as a whole. (Reproduced with kind permission from Katie Courts, www.yoga-nut.co.uk.)

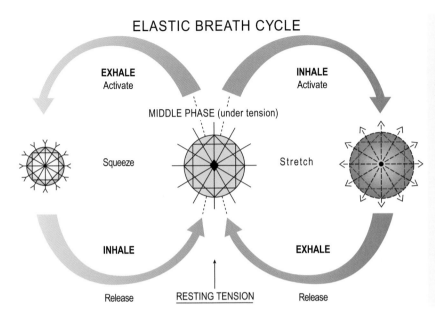

ELASTIC BREATH CYCLE

Figure 12.5

Resting tension is the middle phase, between the breaths. Inhalation is the stretch to expand and exhale restores resting tension. The 'exhale plus' is the ability to squeeze and contain the breath, which restores resting tension by inhaling (Avison, 2014). (Reproduced with kind permission from Art of Contemporary Yoga Ltd.)

them: they stalk. They are ready to deploy the potential to pounce or sprint as required, maximising their catapult capacity by tensioning the global tissue matrix. Even their fur stands on end, perhaps for super-sensitivity to the task. Cheetahs, like many other mammals, focus and draw their tissues *in* to make them fit for purpose, globally. There is a time and a place, a dose and degree, for stretching.

Research in British Columbia, as to how hibernating bears survive a winter of sleep without osteoporosis or degenerative conditions to their muscles after months of inertia, revealed an interesting instinctive habit. They get up around midday every day and do 20–40 minutes of movement. They do gentle yoga-type stretches in all directions, yawning and wriggling and pacing around, reanimating the tissues, before they settle back and sleep and hibernate for the next 24 hours.

Stretching is part of our nature, particularly when accompanied by yawning. This wholeheartedly reflects the 'felt' sense of tension and compression, or biotensegrity, in the system. It facilitates stretch-and-squeeze simultaneously and naturally self-regulates the body sense.

How often do we remember to stretch and yawn after rest? Given the hours we spend in planes, trains and automobiles, not to mention at our desks. Do we counter balance them with yawning stretches? No cat, dog or bear would forget to do this after a period of inertia. It is instinctive to many animals. We, on the other hand, will force-stretch to reach the most extraordinary shapes as if *that* is the purpose of yoga.

The shapes themselves can be valuable because the body responds to variability and range but we need patience and purpose in how we explore their full form over time. Building a repertoire in the body of cumulative 'enquiries' and 'balances' is a clear advantage in improving vitality and may have distinct therapeutic value (Broad, 2012). It also speaks to issues of inertia that recent research shows to play a key role in many degenerative diseases (Henson, 2013). However, it is optimally used in a very instinctive way, in order to *explore* those shapes for a given individual and maintain their value in enhancing elasticity. If someone is super-bendy, or super soft they might find improved elasticity in tensioning, or stiffening, their network, not stretching it.

An example in practice: dog pose

Rather than forcing the stretch, time is taken to tension (stiffen) the body, contain and gather it in, (i.e. 'squeeze') to 'find the ground' or base

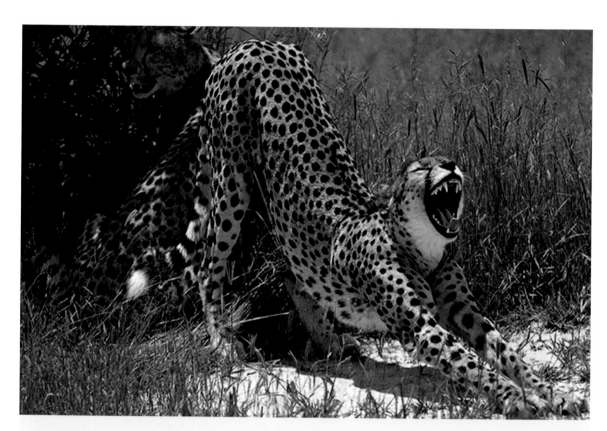

Figure 12.6
Yawning Stretch or pandiculation

A wild cheetah in up-down dog pose, its own version of Adho-Urdhva Muhka Svanasana. (Notice the beautiful side bend of the cheetah in the background). (Reproduced with kind permission from Shane McDermott, www. wildearthilluminations.com).

of support. This allows the heels to explore their tensional relationship throughout the back of the body and invites the movement *towards* the ground. This, in turn, facilitates the knee to be opened naturally, without pushing it back or hyper-extending the joint (Fig. 12.7).

This listening approach ensures that the fold at the hip does not pull the pelvis into a posterior tilt, which would, in turn, compromise the lumbar spine (lordosis), thus pulling on the shoulders or neck and leaving Alexander straining to stretch in order to 'achieve' the pose (Fig. 12.8).

Balancing the *tensional components* includes the whole body at all its folding potentials (joints), gathering in the continuous integrity of the tensional matrix. It naturally facilitates Alexander's ability to squeeze/contain throughout the architecture and then 'fill' the pose in 360 degrees, through an actively loaded stretch (or lengthening contraction), rather than strain for it through pulling on any part of the Superficial Back Line (Myers, 2009) (Chapter 6). Then he can explore the posture intelligently to his own elastic limit.

The key clue to this, or any other posture, is in the ease and flow of the breath and the subtle ability to transmit the breathing motion through the whole pose and body, rhythmically. That is through the expansion, release, squeeze, release cycle mentioned earlier. When this is not

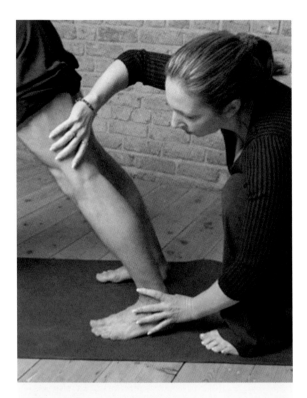

Figure 12.7

Once a principle ballet dancer, Alexander is more than capable of 'stretching' his body in Dog Pose, heels to the ground. However, to optimise elasticity, every joint is seen for its role in the tensional balance of the whole. This includes the relationship of the back to the front and the continuity throughout their longitudinal organisation, from fingertips to feet and coccyx to crown. (Model: Alexander Filmer-Lorch. Reproduced with kind permission from Charlie Carter Photography).

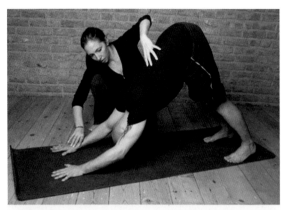

Figure 12.8

Subtle adjustment gives feedback to tension the pose in suitable balance at each of the joints, breathing in to the potential length as it unfolds, without forcing stretch. (Model: Alexander Filmer-Lorch. Reproduced with kind permission from Charlie Carter Photography).

compromised there is no need for extraneous, unnecessary tightness, floppiness or strain: only a suitable containment of the whole, to move or hold a pose.

A yoga style more focused on holding the pose for 1–2 minutes can also be perfectly facilitated. By growing and breathing the body into stillness, we can stretch more instinctively, exploring the fundamental yogic principles of the 'steady and the sweet' (*sthiram* and *sukham*). This takes us beyond technique to the inner experience where yoga really lives and is capable of flourishing, for each unique individual.

For the more dynamic practice, it encourages containment and spring-loaded tension or potential: the stored energy capacity for the next posture in a flowing sequence (Chapter 10). Thus it primes the tissues for effortless and contained transition between asanas at the variable speeds. We nourish our loading history by accumulating balance, poise and adaptability, from speed to stillness and beyond.

Summary

Yoga practice is an exploration of balance and integration on many levels. By exploring the breath in the postures, sequences and different styles of practice the stretch-release-squeeze-release-in-motion principle is naturally complemented. Our form rests in the neutral potential that we call release, although it is biotensegrally orchestrated and always poised in tensional integrity for potential movement. As a force transmission system with innate elastic properties, dependant upon how we use the body and respect this unifying feature, the fascial matrix and yoga express and enhance each other in all their variety and possibility.

References

Avison, J. (2015) *YOGA: Fascia, Form & Functional Movement*. Handspring Publishing, Edinburgh.

Bertolucci, L.F. (2011) Pandiculation: nature's way of maintaining the functional integrity of the myofascial system? *J Bodyw Mov Ther*. 15(3):268–80.

Broad, W.J. (2012) *The Science of Yoga*. Simon & Schuster, New York.

Flemons, T. (2006) *The Geometry of Anatomy*. www.intensiondesigns.com [Accessed Oct 2014]

Henson, J.J., Yates, T., Biddle, S.J.H., Edwardson, C.L., Khunti, K. Wilmot, E. G. Gray, L. J., Gorely, T., Nimmo, M.A. & Davies, M.J. (2013) Associations of objectively measured sedentary behaviour and physical activity with markers of cardiometabolic health. *Diabetolgia* 56(5): 1012–1020.

Ingber, D.E. (2006) The Architecture of Life. *Scientific American*, January 1998. http://time.arts.ucla.edu/Talks/Barcelona/Arch_Life.htm [Accessed Oct 2014].

Langevin, H.M. (2006) Connective tissue: a body-wide signaling network? *Med Hypotheses* 66(6): 1074–1077.

Levin, S.M. (2012) Comments on Fascia Talkshow, Episode 7, Biotensegrity (Avison) www.bodyworkcpd.co.uk (19.09.12 webinar). See Further Information

Levin, S. (2013) Comments on Biotensegrity and Elasticity (email). See Further Information

Levin, S.M. (1995) The importance of soft tissues for structural support of the body. *Spine*. 9:357–363.

Levin, S.M. (1990) The primordial structure. In: Banathy BH, Banathy BB (Eds) *Proceedings of the 34th annual meeting of The International Society for the Systems Sciences*. Portland, vol. II, pp. 716–720. This article will explore the icosahedron as the primordial biologic structure, from viruses to vertebrates, including their systems and sub-systems. www.biotensegrity.com

Levin, S. (2006) Tensegrity, the New Biomechanics. In: Hutson, M. & Ellis, R. (Eds), *Textbook of Musculoskeletal Medicine*. Oxford University Press, Oxford. Updated http://www.biotensegrity.com/tensegrity_new_biomechanics.php.

Martin, D.C. & Levin, S.M. (2012) Biotensegrity: The mechanics of fascia. In: Schleip, R., Findlay T.W., Chaitow, L. & Huijing, P.A. (Eds) *Fascia: The Tensional Network of the Human Body*. Elsevier, Edinburgh, Chapter 3.5. See Further Information & Levin, S. M.

Myers, T.W. (2009) The Superficial Back Line. *Anatomy Trains*. Elsevier, Edinburgh, Chapter 3.

Richards, D. (2012) University of Toronto, Assistant Professor Medical Director, David L. MacIntosh Sport Medicine Clinic: Doug Richards on Stretching: The Truth: Nov 2, 2012.

Schleip, R. (2003) Fascial plasticity – a new neurobiological explanation; Part 1. *J Bodyw Mov Ther*. 7(1), 11–19.

Schleip, R. (2011) Principles of Fascia Fitness. www.terrarosa.com.au, Issue 7.

See Further Information for additional reference to Schleip R.

Further Information

Bears at grouse mountain

Grouse Mountain in Vancouver, http://www.grousemountain.com/wildlife-refuge. There is a 'BearCam' facility and it is possible to watch Coola and Grinder in hibernation. Researchers and Rangers in the park run a blog and films about the bears (and other wildlife at the reserve) and their hibernating habits.

Carter, C., photography

Courts, K. www.yoga-nut.co.uk

Filmer-Lorch, A. (2012) *Inside Meditation*. Troubador Publishing, Leicester, UK.

Guimberteau, J.C. see Handspring Publishing, www.handspringpublishing.com and http://www.guimberteau-jc-md.com/en/

Hamilton, B. see www.tensegrity.com for tensegrity models.

Ingber, D.E. (1993) Cellular tensegrity; defining new rules of biological design that govern the cytoskeleton. *J Cell Sci*. 104 (3)m 613–627.

Jager, H. & Klinger, W. (2012) Fascia is alive. In: Schleip, R., Findlay T.W., Chaitow, L. & Huijing, P.A. (Eds) *Fascia: The Tensional Network of the Human Body*. Elsevier, Edinburgh, Chapter 4.2.

Levin, S. see www.biotensegrity.com for a variety of articles and papers and instructional video material

McDermott, S. see *Wildlife Conservation Photography* www.wildearthilluminations.com Images of animal behaviour and movement in their natural habitat.

Schmidli, S. see www.samirayoga.co.uk

Snelson, K. see http://kennethsnelson.net/articles/TheArtOfTensegrityArticle.pdf

Woolley, D. see www.davidwoolleyphotography.com and www.limitlesspictures.com

CHAPTER 13

Fascia oriented Pilates training

Elizabeth Larkam

The movement system created by Joseph Hubertus Pilates (1880–1967) served the bedridden after World War I broke out in 1914, when he taught in a camp for enemy aliens in Lancaster, England. Joseph Pilates took springs from beds and rigged up his earliest rehabilitation equipment for the internees (Pilates Method Alliance, 2013). Now Pilates programmes, informed by principles of fascia oriented training, (Müller & Schleip, 2011) (Chapter 11) improve standing balance, seated balance and proximal control of gait for polytrauma patients returning from Iraq and Afghanistan with amputations (Moore, 2009), trauma, traumatic stress, brain injury, and vestibular dysfunction (Larkam, 2013). Soldiers from Denmark, Israel and the United States demonstrate their fascia oriented Pilates programmes, informed by the organisation of the myofascial meridians (Myers, 2013) (Chapter 6) (Pilates Method Alliance DVD, 2013).

The principles of fascia oriented training correlate with Pilates movement principles

The principles of fascia oriented training (Müller & Schleip, 2011) (Chapter 11) can be correlated with the eight movement principles of the Pilates method. Table 13.1 matches the principles of fascia oriented training with an expanded list of Pilates movement principles (St. John, 2013).

Selected mat and reformer exercises provide examples of the related principles. (Note: Each mat and reformer exercise is pictured and described in detail in the *Pilates Instructor Training Manuals* listed in the Bibliography.) This chapter examines the effectiveness and the limitations of the original Pilates method to fulfill the principles of fascia oriented training.

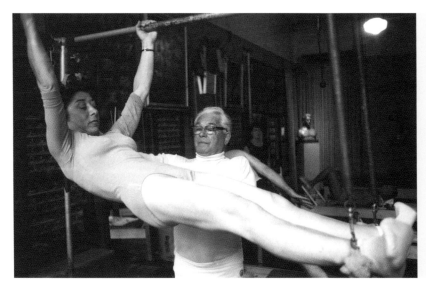

Figure 13.1

Joseph H. Pilates instructing a client in Hanging Pull Up on his Trapeze Table at Joe's Gymnasium, the 8th Avenue Studio, New York, New York, October 1961. The Universal Reformer is visible in the background. (Copyright I.C. Rapoport)

It also suggests how the original Pilates method of unique movement sequences and equipment created a foundation from which contemporary expressions of Pilates can be customised to train fascia. The chapter provides one example of how the classical mat exercise Leg Pull Front provides a foundation for the contemporary Pilates Reformer exercise, Jumping in Quadruped, that fulfills the principles of fascia oriented training. The Pilates movement principles are explained in *The Pilates Method Alliance Pilates Certification Exam Study Guide* (PMA, 2013) which states: 'The body is organised to move by **centring. Balanced muscle development** allows efficient

Table 13.1

Fascia oriented training principles and Pilates principles are similar. Selected Pilates Mat and Reformer exercises put each principle into practice.

Fascia oriented training principles	Pilates principles	Pilates mat exercise	Reformer exercise
1. Preparatory Counter-movement	Rhythm	Single Straight Leg Stretch	Jumping on Jumpboard
2. Flowing Movement Sequences The Ninja Principle	Flow	Roll Up	Standing Side Splits
3a. Dynamic Stretching	Rhythm	The Saw	Knee Stretch Knees Off/ Jackrabbit
3b. Tempo Variation fast and slow dynamic stretching	Rhythm	Fast – Single Leg Kick Slow – Roll Over	Fast –Stomach Massage with Round Back Slow –Side Stretch /Mermaid
3c. Whole-Body Movements simultaneously involving large areas of the fascial network	Whole body movement	Side Bend Twist	Long Stretch
3d. Multidirectional Movements with slight changes in angle	Balanced muscle development	Corkscrew	Feet in Straps
3e. Proximal Initiation	Centring	Teaser	Short Box Advanced Abdominals
4a. Proprioceptive Refinement	Concentration Control	Leg Pull Up (face ceiling)	Control Back (face ceiling)
4b. Kinesthetic Acuity	Precision	Double Leg Circles	Front Splits –Hands Up
5a. Tissue Hydration	Relaxation	Seated Spine Stretch Forward	Short Spine Massage
5b. Tissue Renewal	Breathing	Seated Spine Twist	Cleopatra
6. Sustainability for collagen remodeling	There is no matching Pilates principle.	Mat practice 20 minutes 2x/week for between six months and two years	Reformer practice 20 minutes 2x/week for between six months and two years

movement and proper joint mechanics. Constant mental **concentration** is required to fully develop the body. **Precision**, meaning exact, defined, specific, intentional movement is necessary for correct form. Only a few repetitions of each exercise are appropriate so that each repetition can be performed with the greatest **control**, using only the necessary muscles and effort necessary for each movement. **Breathing** promotes natural movement and **rhythm** and stimulates muscles to greater activity. Performance of the Pilates exercises is distinguished by always using the **whole body**.'

History of the Pilates method

The Pilates method has been in continuous use in the United States since 1926 when Joseph Pilates and his wife Clara immigrated to New York City from Germany. In 2010 there were 8,653,000 Pilates participants in the United States (Sporting Goods Manufacturers Association, 2010) and countless millions engaged in the practice of Pilates worldwide. For more than 40 years, J.H. Pilates created and documented a comprehensive movement system that reflected his own physical training and the physical culture of the times. In his youth, he practiced various physical regimens to overcome childhood ailments of rickets, asthma and rheumatic fever. The movement system Joseph Pilates created was influenced by his practice of bodybuilding, gymnastics, skiing, diving, martial arts and boxing. Joseph Pilates did not have any clinical or medical credentials (PMA, 2013). He was self-taught through movement experience, observation and reading. His ideas regarding spinal alignment (Pilates, 1934) were markedly different from the generally accepted view that optimal spine organisation requires a cervical and lumbar lordosis and a thoracic kyphosis. In fact, Joseph Pilates designed his entire movement system to straighten spinal curves, reflecting his belief that 'the normal spine should be straight to successfully function according to the laws of nature in general and the law of gravity, in particular… Proper carriage of the spine is the only natural preventive against abdominal obesity, shortness of breath, asthma, high and low blood pressure and various forms of heart disease. It is safe to say that none of the ailments here enumer-

ated can be cured until the curvatures of the spine have been corrected' (Pilates, 1934).

Mat exercises provide the foundation of the Pilates method

Thirty-four mat exercises form the foundation of the movement system that Joseph Pilates called 'Contrology'. Joseph Pilates states his philosophy in *Return to Life*, his book published in 1945: 'Faithfully perform your Contrology exercises only four times a week for just three months… you will find your body development approaching the ideal, accompanied by renewed mental vigor and spiritual enhancement.' (Pilates, 1945). Careful study of the mat exercises indicates that, although specific Pilates mat exercises may satisfy the fascia oriented training guideline 3d Multidirectional Movements with slight changes in angle, (Table 13.1), the majority of exercises will not, given their single plane orientation. Of the mat exercises pictured in *Return to Life Through Contrology*, 15 are organised in flexion in the sagittal plane. Only eight exercises emphasise extension in the sagittal plane. Spinal rotation of the spine is represented by only one exercise. Lateral flexion of the spine is represented by two exercises. Three exercises combine flexion and rotation. Joseph Pilates intended the remaining five exercises to be performed in a posterior pelvic tilt and lumbar flexion in order to flatten the lumbar lordosis. However, they may be practiced in a neutral pelvis and a neutral lumbar spine. The Catapult Mechanism of elastic recoil of fascial tissues 'can be achieved by muscular activation (e.g. against resistance) in a lengthened position while requiring small or medium amounts of muscle force only.' (Müller & Schleip, 2011) (Chapter 10). Given that 29 of the mat exercises are open kinetic chain for the lower extremity, these mat exercises are not optimal for developing elastic recoil in full weight bearing. Only four exercises are closed kinetic chain for both upper and lower extremities. Joseph Pilates performed many of the mat exercises with rather vigorous elastic bounces in the end ranges of available motion (Pilates, 1932–45) so even his open kinetic chain exercises can be used to develop elastic recoil (Chapter 11).

Joseph Pilates was a prolific inventor of exercise apparatus

Throughout his four decades of work in Joe's Gymnasium, Joseph Pilates continued to develop his movement system, inventing over 14 exercise apparatus that provide assistance, resistance and complexity to the organisation required by the mat exercises. The equipment frames provide a number of places to which springs or cords may be attached, creating movement environments that support a variety of vectors, making it possible to satisfy all the principles of fascia oriented training listed in Table 13.1. Joseph Pilates created a unique movement repertoire for each of his inventions.

Contemporary evolution of the Pilates method serves client and patient diversity

Nearly 90 years have passed since Joseph Pilates began working in a New York City boxer's training gym, teaching a diverse clientele. The proliferation of applications of Pilates techniques has resulted in an expansion of protocols for a wide range of diagnoses, conditions, and performance goals. Research on the properties and function of fascia, as well as the creation of Fascial Fitness (Chapter 11), influences interest in how to train fascia in Pilates.

Table 13.2

Use this Pilates Mat Fascia Training Guide to plan your mat classes and individual practice for thorough fascial training. Each exercise cultivates at least one of the fascia oriented principles and activates one primary and several secondary myofascial meridians.

	The myofascial meridians						
Fascia oriented training principles	Deep Front Line	Superficial Front Line	Lateral Line	Spiral Line	Superficial Back Line	Arm Lines	Functional Lines
Preparatory Counter-movement	Scissors	Single Leg Kick	Side Kick	Spine Twist	Swan Dive	Boomerang	Criss Cross
Flowing Movement Sequences	Jackknife	Neck Pull	Side Bend Twist	Corkscrew	Double Leg Kick	Push-ups	Hip Circles
Dynamic Stretching	Shoulder Bridge	Bicycle	Kneeling Side Kicks	Leg Circles with trunk rotation	Scissors	Swimming	The Saw
Tempo Variation	Rolling Like a Ball	Seal	Corkscrew	Hip Circles	Swimming	Swan Dive	Swimming
Whole-Body Movements	Double Leg Stretch	Roll Up	Mermaid Side Bends	Side Bend Twist	Roll Over	Push Ups	Swan Dive
Multidirectional Movements	Hip Circles	Kneeling Side Leg circles with knee bent	Kneeling Side Leg Circles	Single	Roll Over	Push Ups	Corkscrew
Proximal Initiation	The Hundred	Single Leg Stretch	Side Kicks	Criss Cross	Shoulder Bridge	Leg Pull Up	Criss Cross
Proprioceptive Refinement Kinesthetic Acuity	Open Leg Rocker	Rolling Like a Ball	Kneeling Side Leg Circles	Corkscrew	Leg Pull Up	Boomerang	Leg Pull Down
Tissue Hydration Tissue Renewal	Spine Stretch Forward	Double Leg Kick	Mermaid Side Bends	The Saw	Single Leg Kick	Mermaid Side Bends	The Saw
Sustainability for collagen remodeling	Practice a 20 minute mat programme twice a week for between six months and two years. Each week vary your exercise selection in order to maximise the benefits of fascia oriented training.						

Table 13.3

Use this Pilates Reformer Fascia Training Guide to plan your reformer classes and individual practice for thorough fascial training. Each exercise cultivates at least one of the fascia oriented principles and activates one primary and several secondary myofascial meridians.

The myofascial meridians							
Fascia oriented training principles	**Deep Front Line**	**Superficial Front Line**	**Lateral Line**	**Spiral Line**	**Superficial Back Line**	**Arm Lines**	**Functional Lines**
Preparatory Counter-movement	Jumping on Footplate	Quadruped Jumping with foot on jump board	Seated arm jumps with hand on footbar	Twist	Long Box Double Leg Kick	Quadruped Arm Jumps with hands on footbar	Snake
Flowing Movement Sequences	Jackknife	Long Spine Massage	Mermaid Short Box	Side Stretch Mermaid with rotation	Long Box Swan	Breast Stroke	Semicircle
Dynamic Stretching	Down Stretch	Thigh Stretch	Side Splits	Short Spine Massage with one foot in opposite strap	Tendon Stretch	Rowing Back I Round Back	Corkscrew
Tempo Variation	Short Box Advanced Abdominals	Coordination	Sidelying single leg jumps with foot on jumpboard	Seated arm jumps with trunk rotation, side toward footbar	Long Box Grasshopper	Rowing Back II –Flat Back	Single Leg Jackrabbit
Whole-Body Movements	Long Box Horseback	Back Splits Facing Straps	Star Side Support	Twist	Long Box Rocking	Long Back Stretch Slide	Conrol Front
Multidirectional Movements	Semicircle	Reverse Abdominals Oblique Variations	Cleopatra	Short box obliqe	Long Box Breaststroke with thoracic rotation	Kneeling Arm Circles	Kneeling Side Arms
Proximal Initiation	Bridging Pelvic Lift	Long Box Teaser	Tendon Stretch Single Leg Slide		Arabesque and Single Leg Elephant	Long Box Rocking	
Proprioceptive Refinement Kinesthetic Acuity	Long Box Teaser	Front Splits Hands up	Star / Side Support	Corkscrew	Control Back	Control Front (face carriage)	Control Front (face carriage)
Tissue Hydration and Renewal						Cleopatra	
Sustainability for collagen remodeling	Practice a 20-minute reformer programme twice a week for between six months and two years. Each week vary your exercise selection in order to maximise the benefits of fascia oriented training						

Fascial Fitness inspires development of Pilates teaching techniques

Although the Pilates movement principles can be considered a subset of the principles of fascia oriented training (Chapter 11), the design of fascia training programmes in the contemporary Pilates environment requires new consideration of all elements of Pilates programme design. Research on fascia suggests new criteria for exercise sequencing, new choices of movement tempo and rhythm and different language for verbal cueing, as well as clarification of the quality and direction of touch for tactile cues.

The practice of training fascia in Pilates has been inspired by the publication of Thomas W. Myers' book *Anatomy Trains - Myofascial Meridians for Manual and Movement Therapists*

(Chapter 6). Pilates teachers seeking to augment their movement education with interdisciplinary study applied the 11 myofascial meridians described by Myers to the Pilates mat and apparatus repertoire and began the paradigm shift from 'isolated muscle theory' to the 'longitudinal anatomy' (Myers, 2013). Figure 13.2 shows the 11 myofascial meridians drawn on Pilates mat and apparatus exercises, illustrating the effectiveness of this movement system for fascia oriented training. Table 13.5 provides the key to Figure 13.2, naming each myofascial meridian according to the model detailed by Myers in *Anatomy Trains*.

In 2010 Phillip Beach published *Muscles and Meridians* in which he proposed the Contractile Field model of movement. 'Seeing movement as whole organism fields of contractility that have evolved along functional pathways offers us fresh approaches to assessment and treatment of the moving body…Core patterns of contractility, allied to field-like behavior, suggest new ways to understand human movement' (Beach, 2010). The Contractile Field Theory has not yet exerted a significant influence on fascia oriented training in Pilates. This may be due, in part, to the complexity of his theories and the fact that *Muscles and Meridians* is less richly illustrated than *Anatomy Trains*. The publication in 2012 of *Fascia: The Tensional Network of The Human Body* (Schleip, Findley, Chaitow and Huijing) (Chapter 1), has inspired Pilates teachers to deepen their interdisciplinary study of the properties and function of fascia and apply these findings of research to movement education in the contemporary Pilates environment. Chapter 1.4, Deep fascia of the shoulder and arm and 1.5, Deep fascia of the lower limbs, by Carla Stecco and Antonio Stecco, may inform accuracy of movement sequencing and direction of tactile cues. 'While the bony insertions of the muscles actuate their mechanical actions, their fascial insertions could play a role in proprioception,

Table 13.4

Use this Fascia Training Guide for Pilates Chair, Trapeze Table, Step Barrel and Ladder Barrel to plan your studio client sessions and personal practice. Each principle of fascia oriented training is put in motion by at least one exercise from each piece of Pilates equipment.

Fascia oriented training	Wunda or combo chair	Trapeze Table/ Cadillac	Step barrel/ spine corrector	Ladder barrel
Preparatory Counter-movement	Swan on Seat	Rolling In and Out	Grasshopper	Lay Backs Scissors
Flowing Movement Sequences	Cat Kneeling	Roll Down	Side Stretch Sit Ups	Climb a Tree
Dynamic Stretching	Hamstring Stretch 1	Footwork Bend and Stretch	Bicycle	Standing Stretches
Tempo Variation	Step Downs	Leg Springs Magician Dolphin	Rolling In and Out	Leg Lifts Grasshopper
Whole-Body Movements	Pull Up Hamstring 3	Bridging	Overhead Stretch/Roll over	Swan Dive
Multidirectional Movements	Around the World	Circle Saw	Corkscrew	Leg Circles and Helicopter
Proximal Initiation	Handstand	Teaser Sprung from below	Lip Abdominal Series	Horse Back
Proprioceptive Refinement and Kinesthetic Acuity	Scapula Mobilization	Standing Arms Facing Away	Swimming	Short Box Abdominal
Tissue Hydration and Renewal	Side Body Twist Side lying Oblique	Side Bends	Side Sit Ups	Side Sit Ups
Sustainability for Collagen Remodeling	Practice a 20-minute programme twice a week for between six months and two years. Each week vary your exercise selection in order to maximise the benefits of fascia oriented training.			

contributing to the perception of movement' (Schleip et al., 2012). The Pilates movement principles of Precision, Control, Centring, Flow and Whole Body Movement all correlate with the fascia oriented training principle of Proprioceptive Refinement and Kinesthetic Acuity. Chapter 2.2 on Proprioception by Jaap van der Wal may guide Pilates teachers who seek clarity on the perception of movement. 'To understand the mechanical and functional circumstances of the fascial role in connecting and in conveying stresses and in proprioception, it is therefore more important to know the architecture of the connective and muscle tissue than the regular anatomical order or topography' (Schleip et al., 2012).

Reframe Pilates concepts with new understanding of the structure and function of fascia

'Fascia is the missing element in the movement/ stability equation. Understanding fascial plasticity and responsiveness is an important key to lasting and substantive therapeutic change' (Earls & Myers, 2010). In harmony with the fascia oriented training guideline of finding body movements that engage the longest possible myofascial chains (Müller & Schleip, 2011) and the Pilates movement principle of whole body movement, Earls and Myers remind us that, as of our second week of development, the fascial network is a unified whole and remains a single, unifying and communicating network from birth until death (Earls & Myers, 2010). Fascia oriented training shaped by research on the properties and function of fascia challenges the Pilates practice of muscle training and offers an invitation to reframe the inner unit of core control with an understanding of the Deep Front Line myofascial meridian (Myers, 2013) (Chapter 6).

The concept of lumbopelvic stability and the Pilates principle of balanced muscle development can be informed by an understanding of tensegrity, derived from 'tension' and 'integrity'. Myers and Earls suggest that we see the body as a single tensional webwork in which the bony struts 'float'

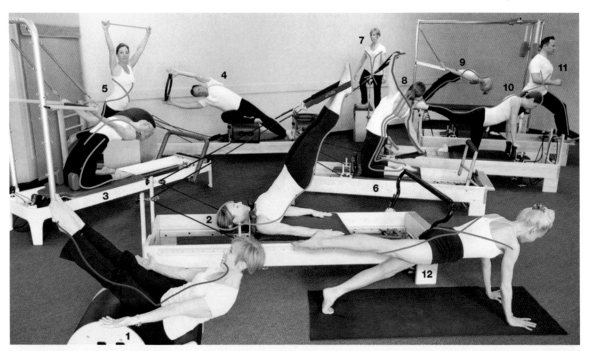

Figure 13.2

Myofascial meridians drawn on Pilates mat and apparatus exercises illustrate the effectiveness of this movement system for fascia oriented training. Table 13.2 names each myofascial meridian, each exercise, and the equipment based on the original designs of J. H. Pilates. (Copyright 2013, Elizabeth Larkam)

Table 13.5

Each model in Figure 13.2 performs a Pilates exercise that activates several myofascial meridians. The primary myofascial meridian is identified here together with the exercise name and equipment evolved from the inventions of J. H Pilates.

Myofascial Meridian drawn on Pilates mat and apparatus exercise	Pilates Exercise	Pilates Equipment
1. The Deep Front Line	Teaser Reverse	Clara Step Barrel
2. The Superficial Back Line	Long Spine Massage – advanced version	Reformer with Long Straps
3. The Superficial Front Line	Thigh Stretch with spine extension and left rotation	Reformer with Tower Push through bar
4. The Lateral Line	Mermaid/Dive for a Pearl	Leg Springs Magician Dolphin
5. The Spiral Line front section	Swan Dive Rotations	Ladder Barrel and Dowel in hands
6. The Spiral Line back section	Thigh Stretch – advanced version. Spine extension and right rotation	Reformer with Short Straps
7. The Front Functional Line	Side Lunge with Weight Shift – advanced version	Combo Chair and Rotator Disc under right foot
8. The Arm Lines Left – Deep Front Arm Line Right – Superficial Back Arm Line	Kneeling Arm Work and Thigh Stretch – advanced version. Spine extension and right rotation	Reformer with Short Straps
9. The Deep Front Line	Bridging	Trapeze Table with Push through bar
10. The Superficial Back Line	Jumping on Footplate in Quadruped	Reformer with Footplate (Footplate/Jumpboard is hidden behind model #6)
11. The Spiral Line front section	Standing/Side Splits with diagonal orientation	Reformer with Standing platform
12. The Back Functional Line	Leg Pull Front	Mat

(Earls & Myers, 2010) (Chapter 6). The internal balance of tension and compression enables the body to have internal integrity, to hold its shape no matter what its spatial orientation. Any deformation will create strain that is evenly distributed throughout the body. Any injury rapidly becomes a strain distribution patterned into the whole body and requires a whole-body assessment and whole-body treatment. Pilates teachers are challenged to see the whole body in terms of tensegrity, in order to develop coherent movement progamme designs that address the seamless neuro-myofascial web and develop motor control in support of functional movement.

Fascia oriented training has the principle of Proximal Initiation (Chapter 11). This matches with the Pilates principle of Centring. Joseph Pilates used the term 'powerhouse' to refer to the girdle of strength between the top of the pelvis and the bottom of the rib cage responsible for Centring or Proximal Initiation. Contemporary Pilates teacher education, influenced by

Diane Lee (2011), explains that the inner unit of core control is the key to efficient, graceful, balanced movement (St. John, 2013). The transversus abdominus, pelvic floor, multifidi and diaphragm all work together to stabilise the pelvis and lumbar spine.

Although lumbopelvic stability is related to core and abdominal strength, it includes all of the muscles that attach to the pelvis and spine through the action of the four outer units of core control: the anterior oblique sling system, the posterior oblique sling system, the deep longitudinal system and the lateral system (Chapter 7). All the outer units of core control play some role in virtually every Pilates exercise and in functional movement (St. John, 2013).

Augment fascia oriented Pilates training with fascial release for structural balance

Fascia oriented Pilates training may be integrated with manual therapy or fascial release for structural balance (Chapter 19). When one practitioner has acquired both skill sets, the client will be fortunate to receive fascia oriented training for motor control and movement education together with fascia release for structural balancing. If the practitioner has only one skill set, the client may seek two practitioners who can provide complementary sessions. Precise, whole body movement is necessary for training the fascia but may not be sufficient to facilitate efficient movement. The body as a tensegrity system responds to trauma, contracting and retracting around all axes (Earls & Myers, 2012). When fascial release for structural balance opens the body in one dimension, it seems to respond in all dimensions.

Design tactile cues to reinforce fascia oriented Pilates training

The tactile cues modeled by Joseph Pilates in his films (Pilates, 1932–1945) indicate a strong touch, sometimes forcefully pushing the client into the intended position. Fascia oriented training encourages a perceptual refinement of shear, gliding and tensioning motions in superficial fascial membranes (Müller & Schleip, 2011) (Chapter 1). This is inspired by the finding that the superficial fascia layers are more densely populated with mechanoreceptive nerve endings than the tissue situated more internally (Stecco et al., 2014) (Chapter 4). Although this perceptual refinement is recommended in terms of movement, it seems reasonable to apply this discovery to shaping tactile cues for fascia oriented Pilates training. By applying precise vectors at the depth of the superficial fascia layer, conveying myofascial continuity to a bony landmark or organ, a clear direction in space can be given. For example, in Figure 13.2, in exercise no. 12, the desired thoracic kyphosis has been lost. Accurate spinal organisation may be reinforced by placing the pads of the four fingers of the teacher's hand on the posterior spinous processes of the thoracic vertebrae between the scapulae. Instruct the client to bring the sternum up, in the direction of the vertebrae, bringing the spinous processes convex toward the ceiling. This cue activates the myofascial meridians of the arms, integrating them with all the myofascial meridians providing trunk support.

Another example of a tactile cue harmonious with fascia oriented training, involves exercise no. 10 in Figure 13.2. Support of the thoracolumbar junction has been lost, resulting in compression in the area of T11, T12, and L1. The palm surface of the instructor's fingers are placed on the anterior lateral surfaces of the lower ribs, guiding the ribs towards the back of the thorax, asking the client to draw the lower ribs in and up toward the ceiling. Tactile cues are to be used judiciously, to inform or encourage rather than to force or overwhelm. In fascia oriented Pilates training, the client is the active agent who has the responsibility of shaping the movement rather than the role of a passive recipient of instructor actions.

Fascia oriented Pilates training is a young field undergoing rapid development

The intentional practice of fascia oriented Pilates training has only been in development since 2001. The principles of fascia oriented training can inform all elements of Pilates programme design, including utilisation of all planes of motion, movement sequencing, tempo, duration, frequency, selection of resistance, verbal cues, touch cues and movement choices appropriate for clients with hypermobility (Chapter 8), fascial adhesions due to age, surgery, trauma (Chapter 5) or traumatic brain injury.

The work of the international community of Pilates teachers, who are evolving the field of fascia oriented Pilates training, occurs in Pilates studios throughout the world. In these movement laboratories, Pilates teachers engage in interdisciplinary enquiry and collaborate with clients to facilitate functional, elegant movement in activities of daily living, athletics and performance.

Practical Application

Transform a classical Pilates mat exercise, that addresses muscular function, into a Pilates reformer sequence that stimulates fascial tissues, satisfying the principles of fascia oriented training. In Figure 13.2, exercise 12, a Leg Pull Front is demonstrated. This classical mat exercise requires integration of all the Myofascial Meridians (Myers, 2013) (Chapter 6). However, Leg Pull Front does not satisfy the Fascia oriented Training Principles (Table 13.1) (Chapter 11). This demanding mat exercise provides limited opportunities for Preparatory Counter-movement, Flowing Movement Sequences, Tempo Variation and Multidirectional Movements, with slight changes in angle that lead to Tissue Hydration and Renewal. Leg Pull Front does not involve elastic recoil (Chapter 10). Contrast Leg Pull Front with the contemporary Pilates Reformer exercise shown in Photograph Figure 13.2, exercise 10. Jumping on the Footplate in Quadruped requires integrated action of all the Myofascial Meridians utilised in Leg Pull Front. (The Footplate, or Jump Board, is hidden by the person doing exercise 6.) One blue spring connects the reformer carriage to the frame. In addition to fulfilling the myofascial meridian requirements of fascia oriented training, exercise 10 satisfies a number of fascia-oriented principles. The dancer's demi plié or knee bend prepares for the ankle plantar flexion and knee extension required for each jump. This is Preparatory Counter-Movement (Chapter 11). Landing from each jump involves deceleration through the entire lower kinetic chain together with enhanced tensioning of the long fascial chains that connect the feet with the pelvic girdle, spine, thorax, shoulder girdle, arms and hands. This creates a flowing movement sequence, or the Ninja Principle. The jumps may be quick and small or slow and large. This is Tempo Variation. The jumping leg may be oriented in neutral hip rotation, external rotation or internal rotation. This fulfills Multidirectional Movements with slight changes in angle. The elastic recoil property of Reformer Jumping in quadruped makes additional demands on proprioceptive refinement and kinesthetic acuity, resulting in tissue hydration and tissue renewal.

References

Beach, P. (2010) *Muscles and Meridians.* Churchill Livingstone Elsevier.

Earls, J. & Myers, T. (2010) *Fascial Release for Structural Balance.* Chichester, Lotus Publishing.

Larkam, E. (2013) *Heroes in Motion.* DVD 9 minutes 31 seconds. Available through: Pilates Method Alliance <www.pilatesmethodalliance.org/i4a/pages/index.cfm?pageid=3401>
<https://www.youtube.com/watch?v=YdsTMB61dBo>

Lee, D. (2011) *The Pelvic Girdle.* 4th ed. Churchill Livingstone Elsevier.

Lessen, D. (2013) *The PMA Pilates Certification Exam Study Guide.* 3rd ed. Pilates Method Alliance Inc. Miami, Florida.

Moore, J. (2009) MPT,OCS, ATC, CSCS *Physical Therapist.* Lower Extremity Amputation: Early Management Considerations. Naval Medical Center San Diego Military Amputees Advanced Skills Training (MAAST) Workshop July 28–30. Comprehensive Combat and Complex Casualty Care Naval Medical Center, San Diego.

Muller, M.G. & Schleip, R. (2011) Fascial Fitness: Fascia oriented training for bodywork and movement therapies. *IASI Yearbook* 2011: 68–76.

Myers, T.W. (2013) *Anatomy Trains Myofascial Meridians for Manual and Movement Therapists.* 3rd ed. Churchill Livingstone Elsevier.

Myers. T. (2011) *Fascial Fitness: Training in the Neuromyofascial Web*. Available through: IDEA <http://www.ideafit.com/fitness-library/fascial-fitness>

Pilates, J.H. (1932–1945) *Joe and Clara Historic Video*. DVD 70 minutes. Available through Mary Bowen < www.pilates-marybowen.com/videos/video.html>

Pilates, J.H. & Miller W.R. (1945) *Return to Life Through Contrology*. Reprinted 2003. Presentation Dynamics Inc.

Pilates, J.H. (1934) *Your Health*. Reprinted 1998. Presentation Dynamics Inc.

Schleip, R., Findley, T.W., Chaitow, L. & Huijing, P.A. (2012) *Fascia: The Tensional Network of the Human Body*. Churchill Livingstone Elsevier.

Sporting Goods Manufacturers Association. (2010) *Single Sport Report – 2010 Pilates*. < sgmaresearch@sgma.com> < www.sgma.com>

St. John, N. (2013) *Pilates Instructor Training Manual Reformer 1*. Balanced Body University.

Stecco, L. & Stecco, C. (2014) *Fascial Manipulation for Internal Dysfunction*. Piccin Nuova Libraria S.p.A.

Further reading

Blom, M-J. (2012) Pilates and Fascia: The art of 'working in'. *Fascia: The Tensional Network of The Human Body*. 7 (22): 451–456. Churchill Livingstone Elsevier.

These five contemporary Pilates classes reflect the influence of fascia oriented training and the myofascial meridians discussed in the chapter. Viewers have a 15 day free trial on the Pilates Anytime website.

Earls, J. (2014) Born to Walk: *Myofascial Efficiency and the Body in Movement*. Lotus Publishing.

Larkam, E. (2012) *#1014: Reformer Workout Level 2 90 minutes*. http://www.pilatesanytime.com/class-view/1014/video/Elizabeth-Larkam-Pilates-Pilates-Class-by-Elizabeth-Larkam

Larkam, E. (2012) *#889: Reformer Workout Level 2/3 75 minutes*. http://www.pilatesanytime.com/class-view889/video/Elizabeth-Larkam-Pilates-Pilates-Class-by-Elizabeth-Larkam

Larkam, E. (2012) *#866: Wunda Chair Workout Level 2/3 60 minutes*. http://www.pilatesanytime.com/class-view/866/video/Elizabeth-Larkam-Pilates-Pilates-Class-by-Elizabeth-Larkam

Larkam, E. (2012) *#863: Mat Workout Level 2 50 minutes*. http://www.pilatesanytime.com/class-view/863/video/Elizabeth-Larkam-Pilates-Pilates-Class-by-Elizabeth-Larkam

Larkam, E. (2012) *#829: Pilates Arc Workout Level 2 60 minutes*. http://www.pilatesanytime.com/class-view829/video/Elizabeth-Larkam-Pilates-Pilates-Class-by-Elizabeth-Larkam

St. John, N. (2013) *Pilates Instructor Training Manual Mat 1*. 2nd ed Balanced Body University.

St. John, N. (2013) *Pilates Instructor Training Manual Mat 2*. 2nd ed Balanced Body University.

St. John, N. (2013) *Pilates Instructor Training Manual Reformer 2*. 2nd ed Balanced Body University.

St. John, N. (2013) *Pilates Instructor Training Manual Reformer 3*. 2nd ed Balanced Body University.

St. John, N. (2013) *Pilates Instructor Training Manual Pilates Chair*. 2nd ed Balanced Body University.

St. John, N. (2013) *Pilates Instructor Training Manual Trapeze Table*. 2nd ed Balanced Body University.

St. John, N. (2013) *Pilates Instructor Training Manual Barrels*. 2nd ed Balanced Body University.

Turvey, M.T. & Fonseca, S.T. (2014) The Medium of Haptic Perception: A Tensegrity Hypothesis. *Journal of Motor Behavior* Vol. 46, No. 3, 2014: 143–187.

CHAPTER 14

Training fascia in GYROTONIC® methodology

Stefan Dennenmoser

A short Gyrotonic history

The developer of the GYROTONIC EXPANSION SYSTEM®, Juliu Horvath, was a professional dancer with the Romanian State Ballet before relocating to the US where he continued his career with the NYC opera ballet and the Houston Ballet. Severe back problems and injury to his Achilles tendon, led him to develop his concept of complex undulating and elastic movements called Gyrokinesis®, also known as *yoga for dancers*. This was done entirely without the aid of equipment. As this proved to be too difficult for many people, Horvath came up with a family of training apparatuses to support three-dimensional, round movements. This system became well known under the name Gyrotonic (*gyros* = circle, *tonic* = tonify). The idea first spread within the dance community, and subsequently to fitness, physiotherapy and bodywork and was

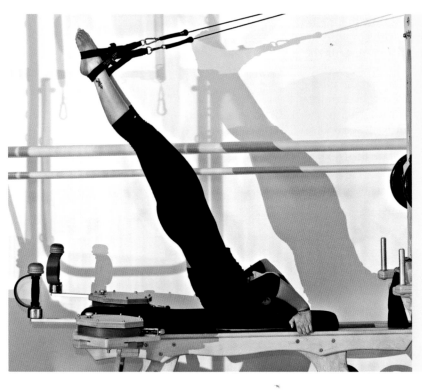

Figure 14.1
Release of bodyweight with legs supported by the apparatus

(photo: Gyrotonic-Master Trainer Fabiana Bernardes, Atelier do Movimento.
www.gyrotonic-sjcampos.com.br)

GYROTONIC and GYROTONIC EXPANSION SYSTEM are registered trademarks of Gyrotonic Sales Corp and are used with permission

enthusiastically received by young and old alike. The focus of Gyrotonic training is not increased muscular power but the improved coordination, elasticity and flexibility of the entire body as a system of movement. In addition, stimulating effects on the lymphatic system, the cardiovascular system, the autonomic nervous system and the energetic system have also been attributed to Gyrotonic training. 'Gyrotonic training increases the functional capacity of the entire organism in a harmonious way' (Horvath, 2002). Although the connective tissue was not explicitly mentioned here, today the fascial system would be included.

The unusual construction of Gyrotonic equipment can be attributed to the nonlinear, three-dimensional approach to movement. The original basic apparatus is known as the 'Pulley Tower Combination Unit'. It consists of two rotatable plates which are primarily moved with the hands, requiring a round and three-dimensional movement. The involved movement is not isolated. Instead it is carried out with the inclusion of the entire body wherein the spine functions as a stable yet flexible centre point for the movement. A second aspect of the construction of the equipment is the controlled release of the body via dynamic hanging from the extremities. This is the reason why training with the Gyrotonic equipment is sometimes described as 'swimming in space'.

Gyrotonic principles and the correspondence with fascial training

There is a clear synergy between the movement principles of Gyrotonic training and the structural training of the fascia, for example, Fascial Fitness (Chapter 11). Of great benefit is the adjustable level of effort, meaning that new movement patterns can still be ergonomically practiced. With a high level of concentration and coordinated exertion, specific movement habits may be optimised and made more economical without excessively stressing the structure. In such training, a befitting breathing pattern (Chapter 12) accompanies every movement so that the training contributes to intermuscular coordination.

It is noteworthy that nearly every training session begins with an *awakening of the senses*, a type of self-massage that includes rubbing and/or tapping all the areas of the body that can be reached. From a fascial perspective, this stimulates the superficial and deeper layers, in order to prepare the body for the forthcoming training (Chapter 4).

Principle 1: Stabilisation through contrast – reaching and lengthening

Classically, it was a given that movements occur by contraction, i.e. a pulling action of the muscles. In strength training, the active muscle, or agonist,

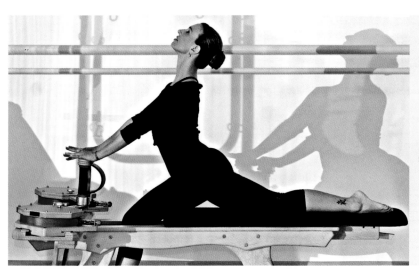

Figure 14.2

Pandiculated lengthening in multiple directions with legs, torso and arms in an advanced variation of the arch/curl exercise.

(photo: Gyrotonic-Master Trainer Fabiana Bernardes, Atelier do Movimento, www.gyrotonic-sjcampos.com.br)

is trained while the opposing musculature, or antagonist, must simply allow the movement. This leads to the resulting habitual shortness that is primarily seen in power athletes. (Here, we see problems involving muscular imbalance, the range of motion of joints and the joints themselves, as well as postural issues.) In contrast, if a cat, for example, is observed, the principle of lengthening, the reaching stretch that is the basis of Gyrotonic 'movements' and a key component of Fascial Fitness (Chapter 11), is entirely evident. Horvath goes further by recommending lengthening in opposing directions to better stabilise the body. Instead of defining a *fixed point,* as a stable segment and a *mobile point,* there is a pandiculating movement of expansion in at least two dimensions (Chapters 9 and 12). A sprawling, reaching and inner lengthening, which matches

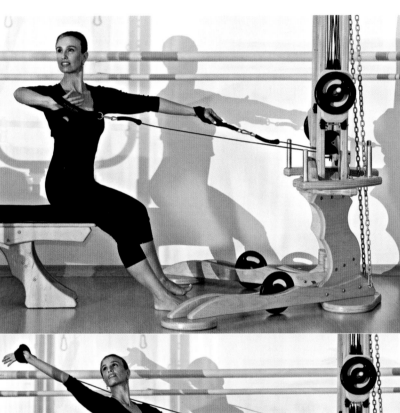

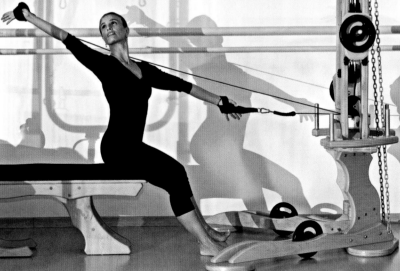

Figures 14.3 & 14.4

Central stability combined with dynamic movements of the whole body

(photo: Gyrotonic-Master Trainer Fabiana Bernardes, Atelier do Movimento, www.gyrotonic-sjcampos.com.br)

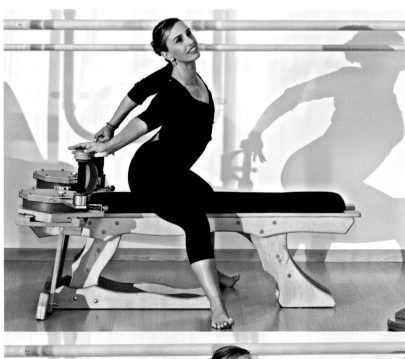

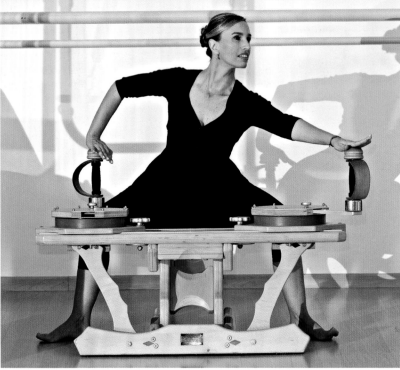

Figures 14.5 & 14.6
Narrowing the pelvis connects the body in a dynamic and elastic way

(photo: Gyrotonic-Master Trainer Fabiana Bernardes, Atelier do Movimento, www.gyrotonic-sjcampos.com.br)

the multivector varying stretches of the fascial structure.

In addition to the releasing effect on connective tissue adhesions, movement training also addresses the shortening that arises from one-sided strain leading to balance in movement. In movement practice, the client is challenged to generate a connection free of slack between the paired extremities as the arms lengthen upwards and the legs lengthen downwards. The same principle applies throughout the body. For example, sitting on an apparatus, the hands push or pull on rotating handholds in the same sense that the feet move as they are anchored to the floor. The spine is moved in the opposite direction. The result is a movement known as 'arch/curl' which is described biomechanically as an alternating and continuous flexion and extension of the torso.

Principle 2: Expanding and retracting – tracing inner/natural movements

The principle of expansion and retraction is closely related to the principle of lengthening. These inversely related forces occur simultaneously as well as in successive sequence. While, on the one hand, the extremities follow a reaching and expansion, a contraction of the body centre via the core musculature should still be present. This allows movements of the extremities arising from a stable centre. From a fascial perspective, there is a coupling of the myofascial tracks (Chapter 6) to a pre-tensioned centre of force in the torso as is primarily occurring with arm and leg work.

Alternatively, opposing forces, that happen successively, involve a dynamic change that follows the rhythm of the movement resulting in a continuous changing of the vectors of force. Horvath seized on an idea that is emphasised in fascial movement disciplines: the wavelike change in the dynamic and the direction of natural movements, a sign of internal movement impulses and a creative game with minimal variations (Conrad, 2007). Within the sequence of exercises, this change in prescribed movement cycles takes place. Moreover, it uses the elastic quality of the connective tissue (Chapter 10). In more advanced movements and sequences, with a high 'unwinding' factor, the creative elements move more into the foreground. The sequence of exercises, as well as the exercises themselves, still always allow for a harmonious change in opposing directions of movement.

Principle 3: Scooping around (creating space in) the joints – power stretches

In Gyrotonic, creating *space in the joint* is key. In fascial training, this is seen in the connection with capsular (pre)tensioning around the joint. It is the difference between a mechanical hinge movement, when lifting the arm, and a theatrically flowing gesture, that does more than only moving the bones. Instead, it defines the space through which the arm moves. The task involved in this so-called scooping, is to imagine that the specific body part is not part of the joint but instead moves around the joint, i.e. as if something was in the way that hindered the direct bending of the joint. Essentially, it is, again, a lengthening around the axis of the joint without a shortening on the inside of the joint. During such a movement, there should, therefore, be no compressive loading in the involved joint. This idea of scooping is realised by means of emphasising the pre-tensioning of the myofascial structure in the movement (Chapter 11).

Van der Wal described a 20–30% loss of power in linear muscle force in order to guarantee the clean and economical guiding of a joint (van der Wal, 2009). This is lost in the capsule-ligament structure. Through the conscious emphasis of this pre-tensioning around the joint, the mechanics of the joint, during the exercise as well as with everyday movements, can be markedly improved. Therapeutically, this effect is applicable where one seeks to relieve joint strain, for example in early osteoarthritis. As a result, the Gyrotonic movements take on and initiate a dance quality, a gesture that comes to resemble whole body movement.

Principle 4: Narrowing the pelvis – elastic recoil

In relation to the torso, which is always a participant in Gyrotonic movements, is the idea of a transfer of pre-tensioning that is focused on the pelvis. This is called *narrowing the pelvis* and aims to constantly make a mental connection between the two hip joints under tension. Through this held tension, the spine should be somewhat lengthened and at the same time stabilised, and the connection to the lower extremities should also be improved. This is an idea that is consistent with the tensegrity model (Ingber, 1998) (Chapter 6) with a resulting therapeutically important release of the spinal joints. The initiation of the movement is also projected into the abdominal and pelvic region, which has a positive effect on the flow of the movement. This *elastic recoil (Chapter 10)* seems to produce a suitable pre-tensioning in the central hip/pelvis area for the activation of a movement. For example, a golfer's swing that involves the elasticity of the whole body, allows the golfer to perfectly execute the swinging movement.

These tension distributing structures, running through the muscles and fascia of the pelvis, together with the three sheets of lumbar fascia and the related musculature (quadratus lumborum, transverse abdominals), which are involved in various movements like forward bending and walking (Vleeming, 2007) (Chapter 17), are responsible, in healthy people, for the optimisation of work done by the musculature in everyday movements.

Principle 5: Stimulation of the body – tactile feedback/body organisation

Within the structure of the fascia there are six times as many afferent nerve sensors as in the musculature (Stecco et al., 2008). This means that the body receives an overwhelming part of its kinetic feedback directly from the fascial system (Chapter 4). The wealth of information available requires more awareness than is available, so the body classifies it as unimportant. Through the unfamiliar body positions, guiding and releasing involved in training with Gyrotonic equipment, the movement centres are confronted with new information that comes into the conscious awareness and, in this way, contributes to improved coordination of movement. Additionally, proprioceptive awareness, as well as the input from the trainer are called on in order to eliminate

movements that are not economical and, instead, instil healthy movements. For this reason, Gyrotonic work is always carried out under the guidance of an instructor as this guided repetition of 'smooth' movements provides the perfect possibility for working on an individual's coordination and flexibility.

Principle 6: Vision guides the movement – using the body's reflexes

The posture and the level of tension in the body are always adjusted with regard to the position in which the head and the eyes are held (righting reflex). This arises from our earliest development of movement. Often a clear excess of tension can be found in the neck that hinders the coordinated movement of head and spine. When this coordination no longer happens automatically, the awareness of the person doing the exercises must be brought online and the head position, neck vertebrae and spinal curves brought into balance with one another. In this way, the myofascial meridians are maintained as a body-wide continuum that is free of blockages. Without control of the direction of the gaze, training the spine would yield disruption or disturbance. For this reason, in Gyrotonic training the proper direction to look is often part of the description of the movement.

Principle 7: Intention as the driving force – improving the quality/economy of movements

In addition to the external 'objective' information, the client has an internal idea of movement that is decisive in the realisation of that movement. In process-oriented disciplines, awareness of this missing intention is highlighted. By correcting this inner concept, there is also improvement in the movement.

One idea in Gyrotonic methodology is, to the extent possible, to start a movement from the centre of the body. A second is the equal distribution of the specific spinal movements over the length of the spine. Both increase internal awareness (Chapter 4) and pre-tensioning in the body and, in conjunction, visibly improve the quality of the movement (See arch/curl example).

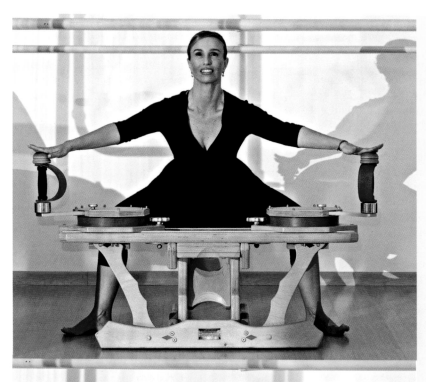

Figures 14.7 & 14. 8
Arch/curl exercise in symmetrical and asymmetrical variations

(photo: Gyrotonic-Master Trainer Fabiana Bernardes, Atelier do Movimento, www.gyrotonic-sjcampos.com.br)

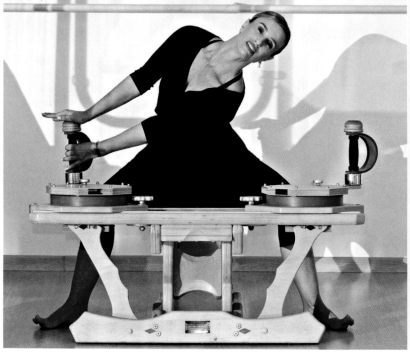

Principle 8: Corresponding breathing-patterns – creating a shear-motion within the tissue

For every exercise on a Gyrotonic apparatus, there is a corresponding breathing pattern. Like the movement, this needs to be trained and learned. Through its expanding and retracting character, inhaling and exhaling support the movement being worked (Chapter 12). It includes a mobilising movement via the involvement of the connective tissue and fascia. Commonly, an extension is accompanied by an inhalation and a movement into flexion with an exhalation so that in reaching, first and foremost, the ribs, the thoracic spine and the structures of the lung are mobilised in extension. In flexion, with the involvement of the transverse abdominal musculature, the structures of the lumbar spine and retroperitoneal space are mobilised and rounded. In this sense, heightened focus on the breath encourages movement of the extracellular connective tissue fluid and the hydration of the extracellular matrix is improved (Chapter 1).

Practical Examples

Arch/curl (basic exercise)

The most well-known Gyrotonic movement, and also often the first practiced, is the 'arch/curl'. This movement is normally done in sitting and includes the use of rotating plates. It starts with an extension of the spine as the torso is pushed forward onto the hands, which hold the grips. The movement is supported with a light activation of the legs, in order to encourage length in the torso. Pre-tensioning of the fascial connections and the joint capsules, through a targeted muscle contraction, the pelvis and the torso, should be included in this so that the 'reaching' movement of the spine is kept safe and the client does not fall into an uncontrolled lordotic posture. In addition, the so-called *5th line*, a conceptual middle line through the inside of the body, is not allowed to shorten and instead remains at the same length. Moreover the client focuses on their breathing and, specifically, the inhalation during the extension movement. In this position, looking forward and up, both hands guide the two grips of the rotational plates to the end-points of the movement of their

rotation. At the same time, the extension through the torso and spine should be maintained. This may be difficult for beginners to accomplish. The reflexes involved and the opposing lengthening makes absolute sense of the myofascial meridians (Chapter 6). This way, the hands and feet are more supportive and included in the stretch. There are even recommendations for the position of the fingers and toes. Nonetheless, the forces should be in balance to such an extent that the movements could theoretically be done without equipment.

After reaching the turnaround point of the rotating plate, all of the directions of force and movement are reversed: the feet push into the floor in order to move the spine toward flexion forward, the back is rounded and the exhalation phase is begun. Like a four-legged animal, hands and feet are again active to provide support and length away from the body. The torso also lengthens away from the extremities. The 5th line should nonetheless remain 'long'. Again – although the movement looks easy and natural – this may be hard to achieve without extensive practice.

At the end of the curl movement, if the back has wandered far back between the hands and the person doing the exercise is clearly sitting behind their sitting bones, there is again a change in the direction of force as the client 'uprights' themselves from the feet up and begins the sequence from the start. Throughout the arch/curl, the narrowing of the sides of the pelvis and the related pre-tensioning should be maintained. The breathing pattern used supports the incorporation of the 'so-called' deep musculature.

The arch/curl can be clearly viewed as a movement that is relevant for the fascia due to the elastic movement at the turnaround point (Chapter 11). It is the pre-tensioning of the torso that gives the client the possibility to swing back and forth, between extension and flexion. If this movement quality is practiced, the breath and the connection to hands and feet make sense. The pelvis, as the centre of the movement, gives the undulation of the body the ease it needs to resolve existing immobility and tension.

Arch/curl can be carried out with rotation in either direction of the plates but, as described, this only takes place in the sagittal plane. To move beyond this plane, and put greater demand on the spine, there are a number of variations that combine the basic movements with a sideways bending and rotation of the spine.

Due to the varied and complex movements done on the Gyrotonic devices, the training always takes place under one-on-one guidance with an instructor. The greater aim is to improve the quality of movement and eliminate stored movement patterns. The apparatus offers a certain level of guidance and support, but still leaving the client a lot of freedom in working out the movements.

Limitations of and problems with Gyrotonic methodology

Most fascial qualities can be trained with the help of Gyrotonic exercises: elasticity, interconnect-edness, flexibility, stabilisation and lengthening into the movement (Chapter 11). This list is not exhaustive and a certain level of competence in movement is assumed. That is not to say that those without experience cannot train on a Gyrotonic device. However, the familiar grace of the movements only appears with sufficient flexibility and coordination. Those who lack motor skills sometimes seem 'lost' when engaged in a discipline that was developed by a dancer.

Some movement patterns are not considered thoroughly and are accepted as 'normal'. This could include external rotation in the legs, a 'straight back' or overly depressed shoulders. Although the majority of clients benefit from these outcomes, in terms of advice, in the therapeutic field there exists a prevailing need for explanation and discussion.

References

Bertolucci, L.F. (2011) Pandiculation: Nature's way of maintaining the functional integrity of the myofascial system? *J Bodyw Mov Ther.* 15(3): 268–280.

Calais-Germaine, B. (2005) *Anatomy of Breathing.* Seattle: Editions DesIris.

Conrad, E. (2007) *Life on Land.* Berkeley: North Atlantic Books.

Findley, T.W. & Schleip, R. (2007) *Fascia research: basic science and implications for conventional and complementary healthcare.* Munich: Elsevier Urban & Fischer.

Horvath, J. (2002) *GYROTONIC® presents GYROTONIC EXPANSION SYSTEM®,* New York: GYROTONIC® Sales Corporation.

Ingber, D. (1998) The architecture of life. *Scientific American Magazine.* January.

Müller, D.G. & Schleip, R. (2012) Fascial Fitness: Suggestions for a fascia-oriented training approach in sports and movement therapies. *In: Fascia, the tensional network of the human body.* Edinburgh: Churchill Livingstone.

Stecco, C., Porzionato, A., Lancerotto, L. et al. (2008) Histological Study of the deep fascia of the limbs. *J Bodyw Mov Ther.* 12(3): 225–230.

Van der Wal, J. (2009) The architecture of the connective tissue in the musculoskeletal system: An often overlooked functional parameter as to proprioception in the locomotor apparatus. In: Hujing, P.A., et al., (Eds.) *Fascia research II: Basic science and implications for conventional and complementary health care.* Elsevier GmbH, Munich, Germany.

Vleeming, A. (2007) *Movement, Stability and Lumbopelvic Pain.* Edinburgh: Churchill Livingstone.

Further reading

Benjamin, M. (2009) The fascia of the limbs and back – a review. *Journal of Anatomy.* 214(1): 1–18.

Fukashiro, S., Hay, D.C. & Nagano, A. (2006) Biomechanical behavior of muscle-tendon complex during dynamic human movements. *J Appl Biomech.* 22(2): 131–47.

Fukunaga, T., Kawakami, Y., Kubo, K. et al. (2002) Muscle and tendon interaction during human movements. *Exerc Sport Sci Rev.* 30(3): 106–110.

Maas, H. & Sandercock, T.G. (2010) Force transmission between synergistic skeletal muscles through connective tissue linkages. *J Biomed Biotechnol.* Article ID 575672.

Müller, D.G. & Schleip R. (2011) Fascial Fitness: Fascia oriented training for bodywork and movement therapies. [Online] Sydney: *Terra Rosa e-magazine.* Issue no. 7. Available from: http://www.scribd.com/fullscreen/52170144&usg=ALkJrhhvc3ughAKnmhBGk-6B1r-0Olcg2Pw [accessed 1 April 2013]

Muscolino, J.E. (2012) Body mechanics. *Massage Therapy Journal.* [Online] Available from: http://www.learnmuscles.com/MTJ_SP12_BodyMechanics%20copy.pdf [accessed 1 April 2013]

Myers, T.W. (1997) The Anatomy Trains. *J Bodyw Mov Ther.* 1(2): 91–101.

Stecco, C., Porzionato, A., Lancerotto, L. et al. (2008) Histological Study of the deep fascia of the limbs. *J Bodyw Mov Ther.* 12(3): 225–230.

Zorn, A. & Hodeck, K. (2012) Walk With Elastic Fascia – Use Springs in Your Step! In: Dalton, E. *Dynamic Body.* Freedom From Pain Institute.

CHAPTER 15

How to train fascia in dance

Liane Simmel

Introduction

Dancers, especially ballet dancers, are easily spotted on the street as they seem to move differently from other people. Not only do they tend to walk with turned out legs but their bodies also seem to show a 'connectivity', that allows for lightness, elasticity and elegant movement quality.

Dance is taught and learned through the dancer's own body experience. The body knowledge of generations of dancers and dance teachers is passed on in the studios, adapted by each individual dancer and tested practically over a wide variety of different body 'types'. Dance offers a great source of body expertise and movement knowledge, gained through physical experience, however this knowledge has yet to be proven scientifically.

Since the 1980s there has been an increasing interest in dance from a medical perspective. In its early years, the new medical field of dance medicine focused mainly on the dancer's health, their working conditions, typical dance injuries and injury prevention (Allen & Wyon, 2008) (Hincapié et al., 2008) (Jacobs et al., 2012) (Laws et al., 2005) (Leanderson et al., 2011) (Malkogeorgos et al., 2011) (Simmel, 2005). Analogous to the development in sports medicine, where the focus is moving away from the management of sport injuries to a broader definition of a medicine of exercise (Brukner & Khan, 2011), dance medicine is widening its horizons towards the dancer's body expertise, motor learning abilities and the general training methods in dance (Ewalt, 2010) (Twitchett et al., 2011) (Wyon, 2010). It is the expanded knowledge in medical research, sports medicine and exercise science that allows for a deeper scientific understanding of many of the traditional training methods in dance.

The dancer's high degree of flexibility (Hamilton et al., 1992), exceptional balance (Bläsing et al., 2012) (Crotts et al., 1996) and remarkable coordination of whole-body movements (Bronner, 2012) are combined to their suppleness and elegance. Dancers seem to be an ideal model for a well-trained fascial system. This leads to the question: How does dance training support fascial fitness?

Many dancers describe their dance training as an outstanding training for body connectivity. As a dancer, in transition to her second profession, states: 'Searching in all varieties of sports, I could not find any other athletic training which provides the same feeling of a whole-body training as the dance training does. After a ballet class, my body feels trained from head to toe'. The recently expanded research in the fascial field might help to find a scientific explanation for this reported body experience. Meanwhile, looking at dance training from a fascial training perspective supports today's training recommendations and adds further ideas which might increase the effectiveness of fascial fitness training (Chapter 11).

Dance training

In contrast to many sports, where the attention is focused on achieving measurable external goals, dance places its general emphasis not only on the outer shape and the outcome of the movement but also on the perception and awareness of the sensations within the dancer's body (Hanrahan, 2007) (Koutedakis & Jamurtas, 2004).

It is the ability to perceive, classify and react to one's individual inner body perspective that creates a sophisticated dancer. Dance seems to be a special combination between strong athletic performance ability and high body perception and awareness.

When speaking of dance and dance training, one has to keep in mind the enormous variety of different dance techniques. From classical ballet, modern and contemporary dance to street and break dance, tap or afro; almost any dance style can be seen on stage and might be part of a dancing choreography. This great diversity in dance styles places high demands on the dancer's body. Obviously, there is not one specific training method that can provide everything dancers need for their fitness (Angioi et al., 2009) (Wyon et al., 2004). However, even today for many dancers the classical ballet technique seems to be the basis of their dance career as well as their daily training routine. Even dance companies, who mainly perform contemporary dance or dance theatre, tend to offer daily ballet classes to their dancers. Enriched with somatic principles and contemporary dance elements, these classes seem to offer helpful training methods, most of which developed practically by trial and error, but still have not been investigated scientifically.

With the integration of somatic movement education in dance, listening to the body and responding to perceived sensations, by consciously questioning movement habits and altering movement patterns (Eddy, 2009), became an important tool in teaching and learning dance. Dance and somatic approach influenced each other mutually with the dancer's experience supporting somatic investigation and the somatic approach being applied to the dance technique (Bartenieff & Lewis, 1980). By addressing the inner body perspective, dance stimulates both the proprioception and interoception of the body. The highest density of proprioceptive and interoceptive receptors are found within the fascial tissue (Schleip et al., 2012) (Chapter 1), so the fascial net plays an important role in the perception of inner sensations. Thus, training body awareness seems to be intensively associated with the fascial body network.

Fascial Fitness

'Form follows function'. This statement by the American sculptor Horatio Greenough, which addressed the organic principles in architecture (McCarter, 2010), is quoted in many bodywork methodologies to refer to the impressive adaptability of body tissues. How the body is used and the way the individual tissue is put under strain influences its formation and architecture. It is this principle that forms the basis for many training methods in dance. Targeted dance exercises allow the body's tissues to adapt to the increasing strain by building up correspondingly.

Research has shown that fascial tissue is particularly adaptable to regular 'strain'. When put under increasing physiological stress, it reacts to the loading patterns by remodeling the architecture of its collagenous fibre network, resulting in a change in length, strength, elasticity and an increasing ability to withstand shearing forces (Müller & Schleip, 2012) (Chapter 11). In contrast, ageing processes and lack of movement lead to a more haphazard and multidirectional arrangement of the collagenous fibres, diminishing the elasticity of the fascial net (Järvinen et al., 2002) (Chapter 1). Thus the local architecture of the fasciae reflects the individual history of previous strain and movement demands.

To achieve adaptation effects in human fascial fibres, the strain applied needs to exceed the degree of normal daily life activities (Arampatzis, 2009). This recommends a specific fascial training that stimulates the fibroblasts to build up an elastic and springy fibre architecture (Chapter 2). Movements that load the fascial tissues over multiple extension ranges while using their elastic springiness seem to be especially efficient. As many dance exercises require a great range of motion and a variety of movement angles, dance offers a large repertoire of exercises to maintain and train the strength, elasticity and shearing ability of the fascial tissue.

Dance offers both training and challenge to the fascial network. Different from most sports, dance sequences are, in general, practiced on both right and left sides, as well as backwards and forwards. Through these multidirectional whole-body movements, dance allows for a great variety of motion, which calls for a high shearing ability of the fascial system. Additionally, by putting a special focus on the alignment and placement of the body, dance supports the shaping of the fascial network. With targeted flexibility training being an integral part of most dance classes, dance seems to increase general myofascial mobility. Counter movements, dynamic muscle loading and fascial rebound are part of many dance steps. This challenges the elastic storage capacity of the fascial tissue (Chapter 10). Furthermore, by focusing on inner body awareness while performing exercises, dance can trigger new proprioceptive sensations.

Dance facilitates Fascial Fitness through:

- Multidirectional whole body movements
- Alignment and placement of the body
- Targeted flexibility training
- Counter movements, dynamic muscle loading and fascial rebound
- New proprioceptive sensations.

Fascial focus in dance training

Although findings from fascial research are only beginning to be included specifically, many dance elements, dance exercises and dance corrections address the fascial connective tissue in their practical application and are congruent with the suggestions made for Fascial Fitness training (Müller & Schleip, 2012) (Chapter 11). The following will give further insight into dance-implemented fascial training and, in addition, will offer some supplementary dance related ideas for general Fascial Fitness training.

Fascial release

As research has shown, lack of movement quickly fosters the development of additional cross-links in fascial tissue (Järvinen et al., 2002). It seems a natural conclusion that whole-body mobility is an

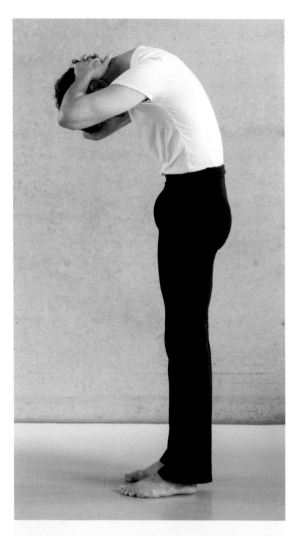

Figure 15.1
Release of the dorsal fascia

important prerequisite for the elasticity and shearing ability of the fascial net. In our daily movement habits, we are far away from using the full range of motion our joints would permit. Instead, we stick to accustomed movement patterns which further and further limit our range of motion and reduce mobility. This is where the targeted mobilisation exercises of dance come to the fore. In the following, the dorsal fascial net is used as an example for the application of a specific fascial release exercise.

Exercise: Release of the dorsal fascia

This exercise gradually releases the dorsal fasciae starting from the cervical area down to the heels. Standing upright, feet parallel and hip-width apart, with the hands lying crossed on the back of the head. Slowly roll down, starting from the top of the head. When an initial stretch can be felt at the back of the spine, stop the 'rolling-down' and gently increase the pressure on the head, resisting by performing an isometric contraction of the back muscles. Hold the contraction for eight seconds, then release the tension and slowly continue rolling-down, stopping at any newly felt stretch. Slowly proceed in this manner until reaching the deepest possible stretching position (Figure 15.1).

Exercise: Release of the plantar fascia

This exercise focuses on releasing the plantar fascia of the feet while preloading the dorsal fasciae. Standing in the yoga downward-facing-dog position, feet parallel and hip-width apart. Feel the connection between the soles of the feet and the hands flat on the floor, focusing on the stretch of the dorsal fascia. Shift the weight onto the hands and walk slowly step-by-step towards the hands

using the elasticity of the sole of the foot to deepen the stretch on the dorsal fascia (Figure 15.2).

Stretching variety

The fibres of the fascial 'system' are primarily shaped by tensional strain rather than by compression (Schleip & Müller, 2013) (Chapter 11). This fact, and the decrease in range of motion that usually accompanies ageing, reducing the shearing ability between distinct fascial layers, leads to a strong recommendation for regular stretching in order to remodel, train and maintain the fascial tissue. Using variations of different stretching styles seems to be more effective than sticking to one method only. Thus alternating between slow passive stretches at different angles and dynamic and bouncing stretches has been recommended (Chaitow, 2003). Research suggests that fast dynamic stretching is even more effective for fascial training when combined with a preparatory counter movement (Fukashiro et al., 2006) (Chapter 11).

Dance uses a wide variety of stretching and flexibility methods throughout its training. Passive stretching methods are common to increase general flexibility. The typical multidirectional

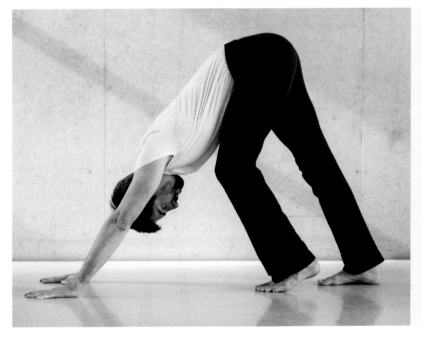

Figure 15.2
Release of the plantar fascia

movements, with slight changes in angle, while deepening the stretch offer an effective training for the fascial system. Active and dynamic stretching is naturally integrated into most dance steps. Each high extension of the legs and each kick elongates the fascial tissue and puts tensional strain on the fascial fibres. The dynamic swinging used in leg swings (Chapter 11), whether while lying on the floor or standing, stimulates the serial arranged tendinous and aponeurotic tissue fibres. What makes all these stretches in dance highly effective, are the long myofascial chains that are involved when focusing on the elongation of the body and enlarging the movement. Stretching seems to be more effective when the myofascial chain that is engaged in the body movement is longer (Myers, 1997) (Chapter 6).

Exercise: Dynamic stretching of the back of the leg

For a more comprehensive stimulation of fascial tissue, this exercise uses a dynamic muscular loading pattern in which the muscle is briefly activated while in its lengthened position. For this purpose Müller and Schleip (2012) propose soft elastic bounces at the end ranges of available motion (Chapter 11). Standing upright, feet parallel and hip-width apart, with the balls of the feet standing on a stair. Be aware of the connection between heel and head letting the head easily 'float' on the cervical spine, and slowly lower the heel. At the end of the available movement, perform soft elastic bounces, lowering the heel even further. Finish the exercise with a short isometric engagement of the calf muscles while still in the deepest stretching position (Figure 15.3).

Preloading – counter movements

The elasticity of the fascial tissue is the key to its high capacity to store kinetic energy. Using the dynamic catapult effect of the fascial fibres allows for an energetic and elastic movement, not only when jumping and running but also in daily activities, i.e. walking (Sawicki et al., 2009) (Chapter 17). The higher the demands on velocity and momentum, the more the elasticity of the fascial system comes into account. In a healthy fascial system, to actively preload the fascial tissue before the

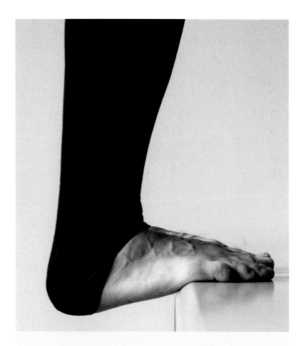

Figure 15.3
Dynamic stretching of the back of the leg

action starts facilitates the dynamic impulse. This can be made use of by starting a movement with a slight counter movement in the opposite direction, thus preloading the fascial fibres. While performing the actual movement, the stored energy will dynamically release in a passive recoil action thereby using the catapult effect of the fascial tissue (Chapter 10).

Preparatory counter movements are common in dance. Many dance exercises implement the energy loading momentum as preparation for a dance step. Using a deep demi-plié (bending the knees without lifting the heels off the floor) before jumping or in preparation for a pirouette, loads the fascial tissue and allows for a dynamic passive recoil of the elastic system to start the actual movement. The principles of fall, rebound and recovery, as used in many contemporary dance techniques (Diehl & Lampert, 2011), seem an ideal training for the preloading and recoil capacity of the fascial tissue. Breathing in before bending backwards, increases the elastic tension of the fascial body suit and thus elongates the spine, diminishing the pressure on the discs as well as the intervertebral joints.

Exercise: Leg swings

The focus of this exercise is on the preloading of the posterior fascial chain. Lying supine, both knees bent, feet parallel and aligned with the sit bones. The right knee drops to the left side. The momentum of the movement allows the lower right leg to swing along the floor to the left, thereby also rotating the pelvis to the left. The entire right posterior fascial chain from the shoulder to the foot becomes preloaded, supporting the right leg, at the end of its loading capacity, to swing back along the floor to the starting position. The left side takes over the momentum, starting to swing to the right, preloading the left posterior fascial chain. Repetitive alternation between right and left swing preloads the fascial chains and facilitates the passive recoil action at the end of the preloading capacity (Figure 15.4).

Cyclic training

When putting fascial tissue under strain, fluid is pressed out of the stressed zone, similar to a sponge being squeezed. When releasing the strain, this area will refill with fluid, coming from the surrounding tissue, the lymphatic network and the vascular system (Schleip et al., 2012). Proper timing of the duration of the individual loading and unloading phases is important to facilitate optimal rehydration, as the short pause gives the tissues the chance to absorb nourishing fluid thereby boosting the fascial metabolism. A cyclic training that alternates periods of intense strain with targeted breaks is therefore a recommended component of Fascial Fitness training.

In general, rhythm plays an important role in dance, by using music as an external "pacemaker", by focusing on the individual's breathing pattern or by engaging with the inner rhythm of the movement itself. Rhythmically loading and

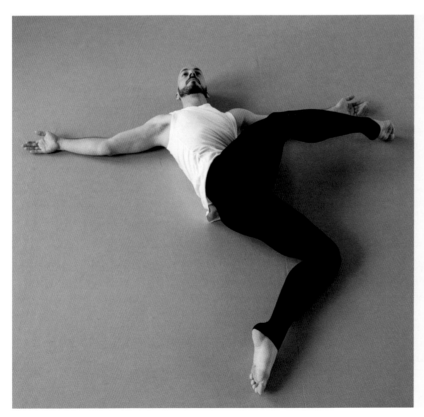

Figure 15.4
Leg swings

unloading the fascial tissue comes naturally in dance, alternating between stretching and releasing, between elongating and contracting (Chapter 10). Thus many dance exercises implement a cyclic fascial training and hence support fascial health.

Fascial awareness

Good coordination and awareness of one's whole-body connectivity are essential keystones for dance. Allowing movements to fluently continue through the body, focusing on maintaining the alignment and elongating the body lines, brings focused attention to the fascial network. Dance, especially contemporary dance, implements a large repertoire of fascial awareness exercises, which focus on the body's inner communication network and the stretching of the connecting tissue.

Exercise: Rocking the dorsal fasciae on the floor

Focus on the dorsal fascia to facilitate its mobility. Lying supine, both legs parallel with the feet in dorsal flexion, anchoring the heels into the floor. Rhythmically point and flex the feet allowing the momentum to continue up to the head, gently flexing and extending in the upper cervical joint. Feel the connectivity from the toes up to the head and register the impulse of the feet as it induces the motion of the head.

Exercise: Awareness of whole body connectivity

Elongate and mobilise the lateral fascial chain: lying supine, legs stretched, arms opened out to the side with palms facing towards the ceiling. Start with the impulse of the right foot slowly pulling the right leg across to the left side, allowing the pelvis and spine to follow. Feel the resistance by firmly keeping the right arm and shoulder on the floor. To keep the stretch dynamic, alternate the pulling impulse between right leg and right arm. Roll back to the starting position taking time to compare both sides of the body, then continue the exercise on the left side (Figure 15.5).

Supplementary fascial training through dance

As well as offering a large selection of exercises for Fascial Fitness training, dance also offers helpful supplementary ideas to support and increase general fascial training. Although these practices have been inspired by physical feedback and are not yet proven scientifically, they have been applied practically by generations of dancers and have helped dancers to gain 'whole body connectivity' for

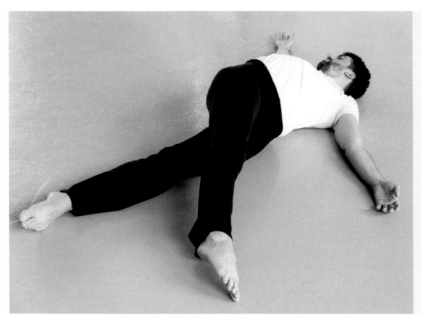

Figure 15.5
Awareness of whole body connectivity

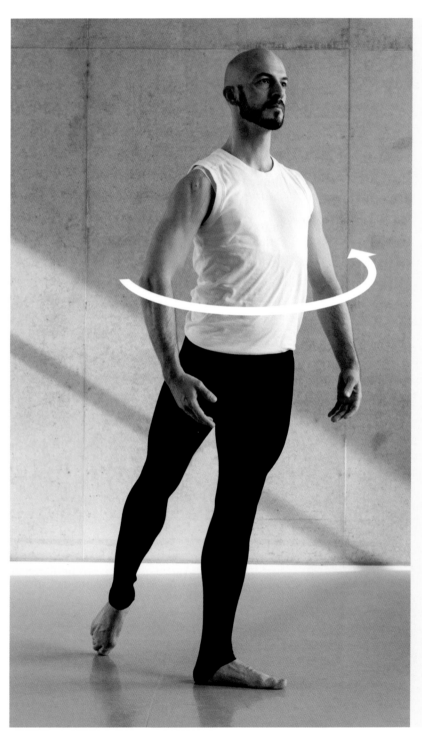

Figure 15.6

In order to achieve an economic equilibrium the dancer performs a small rotation of the spine to the left when lifting the right leg to the back.

which they are renowned. By performing most of the exercises equally on both sides, dance provides a general balancing out of the body. Regarding fascial training, there are four movement principles, which are fundamental to almost every dance training and which, in application to the specific Fascial Fitness training, could increase its effectiveness.

> Increase fascial fitness training by the use of dance-specific movement principles:
> - Awareness of oppositions
> - Elongation
> - Counter movements
> - Momentum and rebound.

The awareness of oppositions is a key for body connectivity. As a preparation for the exercise, the dancer is focusing on the specific body parts affected by the movement to follow, their connection and their separation. This allows for the feeling of space and elongation yet connection between the opponents. For example, when bending the upper body to the right side, the left foot firmly keeps its contact to the floor. The two opponents, head and left foot, stay connected, thus allowing elongation and stretching of the fascial tissue on the left of the body.

When lifting one leg off the floor or using the arms for expressive dance movements, dancers tend to focus on the elongation of their extremities. With the image of widening the movement into space, filling out the surrounding area, the dancers increase their bodily borders. From the perspective of fascial training, this elongation of the extremities allows for further loading and pre-stretching of the fascial tissue.

Keeping one's balance is crucial in dance. To achieve a natural equilibrium, regardless of the performed dance movement, the dancer makes use of small counter movements that allow for stability and counter strain. For example, to achieve economic equilibrium a small rotation of the spine to the left may be used when lifting the right leg to the back (Figure 15.6). Fascially speaking this small counter movement allows loading of the corresponding fascial tissue.

Jumping, rolling on the floor or lifting, all of these dance movements demand the perfect timing of the impulse, momentum and rebound: the optimal timing in releasing the preloaded fascia. A cat-like jump with a noiseless landing requires a high level of elasticity within the fascial tissue, using the body like a spring, preloading its fibres in preparation for the movement. Applying this momentum and rebound to daily life activities, for example, by using the elastic rebound while walking fast or climbing stairs, allows for an implemented Fascial Fitness training (Chapter 11).

Although these dance movement principles still require further research regarding their effect on the fascial tissue, applying them into Fascial Fitness training might add helpful aspects and increase its effectiveness.

Dance uses a wide variety of fascial training techniques and principles, which are nowadays recommended and supported by an increasing body of evidence. In its practical application, dance provides ideas for further research in fascial fitness training. However, with its highly complex movement patterns and its whole-body integration, dance remains scientifically challenging. Yet further studies on the dancer's body expertise might help to deepen the understanding of fascial structures and their 'trainability'.

References

Allen, N. & Wyon, M. (2008) Dance Medicine: Artist or Athlete? *Sportex Medicine* 35: 6–9.

Angioi, M., Metsios, G.S., Metsios, G., Koutedakis, Y. & Wyon, M.A. (2009) Fitness in contemporary dance: a systematic review. *Int J Sports Med* 30(7): 475–484.

Arampatzis, A. (2009) Plasticity of human tendon's mechanical properties: effects on sport performance. *ISBS – Conference Proceedings Archive* 1(1).

Bartenieff, I. & Lewis, D. (1980) *Body Movement: Coping with the Environment*. Routledge.

Bläsing, B., Calvo-Merino, B., Cross, E.S., Jola, C., Honisch, J. & Stevens, C.J. (2012) Neurocognitive control in dance perception and performance. *Acta Psychol* 139(2): 300–308.

Bronner, S. (2012) Differences in segmental coordination and postural control in a multi-joint cancer movement: Développé arabesque. *J Dance Med Sci* 16(1): 26–35.

Brukner, P. & Khan, K. (2011) *Brukner & Khan's Clinical Sports Medicine*. Australia: McGraw-Hill Book Company.

Chaitow, L. (Ed). (2003) 'The stretching debate' Commentaries by: J. Beam, DeLany, J. Haynes, W., Lardner, R., Liebenson, C., Martin, S., Rowland, P., Schleip, R., Sharkey, J., & Vaughn, B. Response by: Herbert, R. & Gabriel, M. *J Bodyw Mov Ther*. 7(2): 80–98.

Crotts, D., Thompson, B., Nahom, M., Ryan, S. & Newton, R.A. (1996) Balance abilities of professional dancers on select balance tests. *J Orthop Sports Phys Ther*. 23(1): 12–17.

Diehl, I. & Lampert, F. (Eds). (2011) *Dance Techniques. 2010:* Tanzplan Germany (1. Aufl.). Leipzig: Seemann Henschel.

Eddy, M. (2009) A brief history of somatics practices and dance: historical development of the field of somatic education and its relationship in dance. *Journal of Dance and Somatic Practices* 1(1): 5–27.

Ewalt, K.L. (2010) Athletic Training in Dance Medicine and Science. *J Dance Med Sci*. 14(3): 79–81.

Fukashiro, S., Hay, D. & Nagano, A. (2006) Biomechanical behavior of muscle-tendon compl. *J Appl Biomech* 22(2): 131–47.

Hamilton, W., Hamilton, L., Marshall, P. & Molnar, M. (1992) A profile of the musculoskeletal characteristics of elite professional ballet dancers. *Am J Sports Med* 20(3): 267–273.

Hanrahan, S.J. (2007) Dancers perceptions of psychological skills. *Rev Psicol Deporte* 5(2).

Hincapié, C.A., Morton, E.J. & Cassidy, J.D. (2008) Musculoskeletal Injuries and Pain in Dancers: A Systematic Review. *Arch Phys Med Rehabili*. 89 (9): 1819–1829.

Jacobs, C.L., Hincapié, C.A. & Cassidy, J.D. (2012) Musculoskeletal Injuries and Pain in Dancers. *J Dance Med Sci*. 16 (2): 74–84.

Järvinen, T.A.H., Józsa, L., Kannus, P., Järvinen, T.L.N. & Järvinen, M. (2002) Organization and distribution of intramuscular connective tissue in normal and immobilized skeletal muscles. An immunohistochemical, polarization and scanning electron microscopic study. *J Muscle Res Cell Motil*. 23(3): 245–254.

Koutedakis, Y. & Jamurtas, A. (2004) The Dancer as a Performing Athlete: Physiological Considerations. *Sports Med* 34(10): 651–661.

Laws, H., Apps, J., Bramley, I. & Parker, D. (2005) *Fit to Dance 2: Report of the Second National Inquiry Into Dancers' Health and Injury in the UK*. Regina Saskatchewan, Canada: Newgate Press.

Leanderson, C., Leanderson, J., Wykman, A., Strender, L.-E., Johansson, S.-E. & Sundquist, K. (2011) Musculoskeletal injuries in young ballet dancers. *Knee Surg Sport Tr A*. 19(9): 1531–1535.

Malkogeorgos, A., Mavrovouniotis, F., Zaggelidis, G. & Ciucurel, C. (2011) Common dance related musculoskeletal injuries. *Journal of Physical Education & Sport* 11(3): 259–266.

McCarter, R. (2010) *Frank Lloyd Wright*. (6th edition). London: Reaktion Books.

Müller, D.G. & Schleip, R. (2012) Fascial Fitness. In *Fascia: The Tensional Network of the Human Body. The Science and clinical application in manual and movement therapy* (S. 465–75). Elsevier.

Myers, T.W. (1997) The Anatomy Trains. *J Bodyw Mov Ther*. 1(2): 91–101.

Sawicki, G., Lewis, C. & Ferris, D. (2009) It pays to have a spring in your step. *Exerc Sport Sci Rev*. 37(3): 130–138.

Schleip, R., Duerselen, L., Vleeming, A., Naylor, I.L., Lehmann-Horn, F., Zorn, A., Jaeger, H. & Klingler, W. (2012) Strain hardening of fascia: static stretching of dense fibrous connective tissues can induce a temporary stiffness increase accompanied by enhanced matrix hydration. *J Bodyw Mov Ther*. 16(1): 94–100.

Schleip, R., Findley, T.W., Chaitow, L., (Eds), P.A.H., Myers, A.T., Willard, F.H. et al. (2012) *Fascia: The Tensional Network of the Human Body: The Science and Clinical Applications in Manual and Movement Therapy*. Churchill Livingstone Elsevier.

Schleip, R. & Müller, D.G. (2013) Training principles for fascial connective tissues: Scientific foundation and suggested practical applications. *J Bodyw Mov Ther*. 17(1): 103–115.

Simmel, L. (2005) *Dance Medicine - The dancer's workplace. An introduction for performing artists*. Berlin: Unfallkasse.

Twitchett, E.A., Angioi, M., Koutedakis, Y. & Wyon, M. (2011) Do increases in selected fitness parameters affect the aesthetic aspects of classical ballet performance? *Med Probl Perform Ar. 2*. 6(1): 35–38.

Wyon, M.A. (2010) Preparing to Perform Periodization and Dance. *J Dance Med Sci*. 14(2): 67–72.

Wyon, M., Abt, G., Redding, E., Head, A. & Sharp, N.C.C. (2004) Oxygen uptake during modern dance class, reheasal, and performance. *J Strength Cond Res*. 18(3): 646–649.

Further reading

Clippinger, K. (2007). *Dance Anatomy and Kinesiology*. Champaign: Human Kinetics.

Franklin, E. (2012) *Dynamic Alignment Through Imagery*. Champaign: Human Kinetics.

Solomon, R., Solomon, J. & Minton, S. (2005) *Preventing Dance Injuries. An interdisciplinary perspective*. Champaign: Human Kinetics.

Todd, M. (2008) *The Thinking Body*. Gouldsboro: Gestalt Journal Press.

Welsh, T. (2009) *Conditioning for Dancers*. Gainesville: University Press of Florida.

CHAPTER 16

The secret of fascia in the martial arts

Sol Petersen

We live in two worlds, one on either side of our skin. The very survival of the Ninja or the hunting wild cat is dependent on their alertness and presence in both worlds. Body-Mindfulness is what I call this embodied awareness and aliveness. Its full expression is found in martial arts mastery. Body-Mindfulness is a calm, open state of present-time awareness of inner and outer body experiences, including sensory stimulations such as pressure, touch, stretch, temperature, pain, tingling, physical movement and position in space, visual, auditory and olfactory impressions. An integral aspect of Body-Mindfulness is fascial awareness: the capacity to sense our body-wide network of myofascial tissue in stillness and in movement. We can develop this skill and build the elastic potential of the connective tissue system (Chapter 1) in fine, coordinated, controlled martial training such as tai ji, karate and kung fu forms, then actualise this controlled power in explosive high speed movements.

The quest for ultimate power and awareness in self-defence and attack is an ancient one. Two thousand years ago the masters, who trained tendon power, knew something intuitively that science has only recently validated. Shaolin training and tai ji masters both recognised the vital importance of conditioning and strengthening the fascia and connective tissues to build and protect the body's Qi energy (life force).

Since research has shown that it is the organ of stability and the seat of our proprioception, the fascia has finally received the attention it deserves. In fact, most musculo-skeletal injuries involve inappropriate loading of the connective tissues and fascia, not the muscles. Therefore, the fascia must be considered an important factor in peak performance and training. The pioneers in the

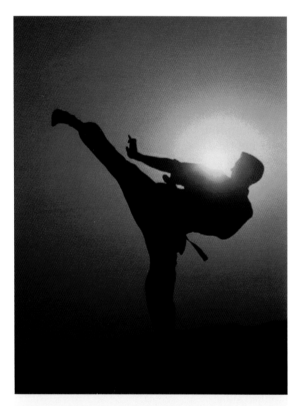

Figure 16.1

Shaolin KungFu training develops fascial strength

SiFu Pierre Yves Roqueferre

new fascia research define fascia more broadly than traditionally. They recognise fascia as the soft tissue component of the connective tissue system permeating the entire human body as one interconnected tensional network. It includes tendons, ligaments, joint and organ capsules, membranes, dense sheets and softer collagenous layers

(Chapter 1). In the new Fascial Fitness approach there is an emphasis on developing elasticity, of acknowledging the stress-responsive nature and tensional integrity of fascial tissue, of specifically conditioning and hydrating the fascia for appropriate stress-loading, as well as appreciating its recently discovered proprioceptive qualities (Chapter 11).

This chapter explores some of the implications of the current research and how Fascial Fitness, attained through physical training and Body-Mindfulness, is one of the secrets for success in martial arts mastery.

The Mindful heart and spirit

Our capacity for training in martial arts pivots around our heart, spirit, motivation, and understanding our place in the universe. If this were not the case, why would we train with the passion required to achieve the highest excellence? The Qi expressed in martial arts practice follows the deepest intention of our heart and mind, and according to Chia, our fascial planes. 'The fascia are extremely important in Iron Shirt Chi Kung; as the most pervasive tissue they are believed to be the means whereby Qi is distributed along acupuncture meridians.' (Chia, 1988).

There are unusual instances in life where, for example, a woman who would not usually be seen as very strong, has accessed the strength to lift a car and save her child. Her shock, fear and desire enable her to transcend her usual capacity. Her muscles clearly were not strong enough to lift the car. How did she do it? Perhaps like the kangaroo, which also does not have strong enough muscles to jump very far but can spring great distances with tendon and fascia power (Chapter 10), her fearless mind and tendon power took her beyond her usual physical limits.

Lee Parore, naturopath and author of Power Posture, trains top New Zealand athletes. Former trainer for world heavyweight boxer, David Tua, he sees awareness as primary. 'Technology is the key to high performance training but we are often looking at the wrong technology. The key isn't machine training or muscle bulk. It is awareness and then self-awareness. It is a fire inside us.' (Parore, 2013).

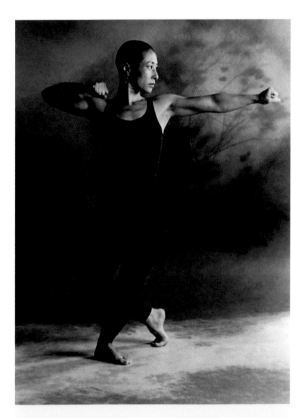

Figure 16.2

The Qi follows the intention of the heart and mind

Harumi Tribble, dancer and choreographer

Fascial awareness, an integral aspect of Body-Mindfulness

Robert Schleip considers the connective tissues as the global connecting network, a listening system for the whole body: 'Science now recognises this richly innervated body-wide fascial web as the seat of our interoception and proprioception, our very embodiment.' (Schleip, 2013). In fact, the fascia is more richly innervated than our muscles. So when we say our muscles are sore it may be that we are feeling our fascia or our fascia is feeling our muscles (Chapter 1).

Cirque du Soleil acrobat, Marie Laure, combines a high degree of Body-Mindfulness as well as enormous core strength and endurance in her performances with her partner. One might assume this would translate into rigidity in her fascial or muscle tissue. On the contrary, as a therapist with the physiotherapy team during their New Zealand tour, I experienced her myofascial tissue to be surprisingly supple and her physique hardly bulked. This is in line with a comment by Stuart McGill, author of *Ultimate Back Fitness and Performance*, 'The hallmark of a great athlete is the ability to contract and relax a muscle quickly and to train the rate of relaxation' (McGill, 2004). This skill is essential to achieve speed in kicking and punching.

Fascial awareness enables the martial arts practitioner to relax the muscles and fascia and be fully present in their internal and external worlds. This enables martial artists to use their bodies to sense nuances in the balance of the other's body and manipulate or deflect the other's expended energy to their own advantage.

Huang Sheng Shyan was famous for his powerful issuing of the Tai Ji-jin or elastic force. His training method involves precise attention to the internal changes of muscles, tendons and fascia. Patrick Kelly, Tai Ji teacher and author, speaks about this awareness where internal relaxation means every muscle in the body elongates and actively stretches under the pressure, rather than contracts and shortens (or holds unchanged) in a tense resistance. 'We can say that the basis of the secret is just this: Tai Ji-jin is motivated by the yi (mind intention) energised by the Qi, issued from the root and transmitted through the body in a wave of stretching muscles' (Kelly, 2007). Intense physical training, without self-awareness, will not produce the highest results. If we do not develop our inner and outer sensing, we will not achieve awareness of the space around us (our opponent) or in the sword we hold. Quite simply, our fascia is a vital sensory organ and fascial awareness is an important key in martial training.

Building fascial resilience and fascial armouring

Iron Shirt is an ancient Kung Fu method that profoundly understands the stress-responsive nature of the bones and fascia. Wolff's law states that bone, in a healthy person or animal, will adapt to the loads under which it is placed. If loading increases, the bone will remodel itself over time to become stronger. Iron Shirt strengthens muscles, tendons, fascial sheaths and bones, by sub-

jecting them directly and gradually to increasing stress. The important detail here is 'gradually'. Internal energy visualisation combined with breath and body conditioning are used to cultivate the Qi power. 'The Qi that is generated is then stored in the fascial layers where it works like a cushion to protect the organs' (Chia, 1986).

This concept of Qi between tissue layers helps to explain an experience I had with a Singaporean Tai Ji master. It is 1981. I am waiting at a table to ask if I can study with him. He walks out, smiles, reaches across, pinching the skin of my forearm between his thumb and forefinger, rolling it back and forth in different places for about ten seconds. 'Yes', he says, 'I can see you have been practising Tai Ji for a while. Good practice creates elasticity between the tissue layers.'

Lau Chin-Wah was a senior student of Master Huang. I studied with him in Kuching, East Malaysia. Our practice centred on refining the form, Pushing Hands and White Crane Quick Fist. Sometimes Chin-Wah would just throw his arm, as if it was an enormous wet rag or rope, against a stone wall, apparently not hurting himself at all. He said the secret was to totally relax the muscles and fascia of the arm and also to condition and harden the bones to become like steel, by training with a partner, hitting bony forearms and shins against each other. This is extremely painful initially but becomes easier and may transform the marrow and substance of the bones and soft tissues (Chia, 1988). Chin-Wah spoke of the Qi inside gathering to meet the force of an attack. He said that when he was centered, aligned in his structure and his body and energy field were one, his fascia, bones and soft tissues became like impenetrable armour enabling him to have a heavy roof tile broken over his head as if it were nothing. Our fascial system is clearly capable of adapting and strengthening itself in response to progressive loading.

Fascial fitness keys for martial arts training

The capacity to relax: The source of speed

In boxing drills, fighters need to become experts at letting go of all muscle tension. A system that is genuinely relaxed does not need to overcome tension to ignite itself for immediate response.

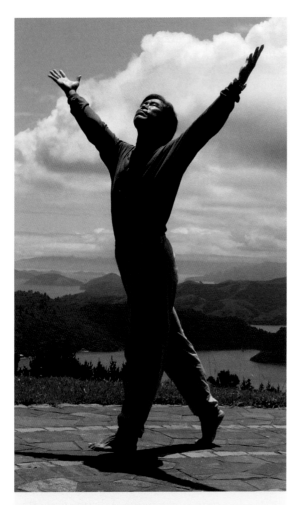

Figure 16.3
Demonstrates energising the Qi in long anterior myofascial chains

Master Li Jun Feng

'You don't want muscle bulk for true speed and strength in boxing but resilient fascia like Spiderman' (Parore, 2013). In Tai Ji Pushing Hands, the players must be willing to be pushed over, to learn to use elastic fascia force instead of relying on muscular strength to combat force. Master Huang was simultaneously totally relaxed yet totally stable. To push him was to feel drawn into empty space and then be sent flying.

Bruce Lee, the famous Kung Fu master, was not a big man. At only 1.7 m (5' 8') and 68 kg (150 lbs),

he often defeated opponents who were both larger and much heavier. One day, he demonstrated his one-inch punch to a sceptical, burly man who was astonished as he flew back 5 meters into the swimming pool. When asked how he had done it Lee said, 'To generate great power you must first totally relax and gather your strength, and then concentrate your mind and all your strength on hitting your target' (Hyams, 1982).

Your fascial resilience affects your field of physical potential

Neuroscientists call the space around the body peripersonal space (Rizzolatti et al., 1997). Recently, brain mapping techniques have confirmed what Tai Ji Master Mak Ying Po once said to me, 'You must extend your feeling sense out around your body. When you move the sword through space, feel the length of it, the tip, as if it was part of your body' (Mak Ying Po, 1976). Similarly, in *The Body Has a Mind of Its Own* the Blakeslees say, 'Your self does not end where your flesh ends, but suffuses and blends with the world, including other beings. Thus when you ride a horse with confidence and skill, your body maps and the horse's body maps are blended in shared space' (Blakeslee & Blakeslee, 2007). The acrobatic kick-boxer and the Kung Fu master both rely on the combination of intense movement training and their refined body awareness. This enables them to respond without hesitation to the slightest change in their field of physical potential. As Master Huang said, 'If you are thinking, it's too late' (Huang, 1980).

Tensegrity strength: Stabilising the myofascial system

Those studying the fascial matrix have compared the body to a tensegrity structure, a structure of tensional integrity. Unlike a pile of bricks, our bones do not touch each other but are spaced by cartilage or soft tissues and the skeletal relationships are maintained by the tension and span of the global myofascial system: in some ways like a tent. It is interesting that barefoot runners may endure less shin splints than runners in protective shoes (Warburton, 2001). Barefoot runners strike the ground more gently with more of the forefoot than runners in conventional shoes. Viewed in a tensegrity way, this reduces the stress transmitted to the shin bones and joints and spreads it throughout the entire fascial and skeletal framework where it is stored as elastic energy (Chapter 10). Balance exercises, such as slack line, wobble board, Swiss ball, rock climbing, etc., challenge and train our fascia and internal strength to develop spontaneous tensegral adaptability.

I observed Cirque du Soleil acrobats maintaining their core stabilisation through 'animal-like' stretches and play, consistent practice of their art and specific exercises to strengthen the flexors, extensors, lateral torso and hip muscles for movement in all three functional planes. This core stabilisation and core stiffening is essential for hyper-mobile acrobats to avoid injury. The capacity for a resilient, tensegral whole body stabilisation is paramount for martial artists.

The no inch punch: The preparatory counter movement at its most subtle

In boxing and Wing Chun punching training, we see the value in spring loading, pre-tensioning as a preparation to unleash the explosive punch. In actual fighting, however, it is vital that this underlying preparatory counter movement is not telegraphed to our opponent. It may be that, in fighting situations, martial artists use a second style, a briefly sustained pre-stretching and pre-loading of their fascial tensegrity web, while the muscles prevent the release of recoil-power until the precise moment for the perfect delivery (Chapter 11).

Alan Roberts, Aikido teacher said, 'In Aikido, Cheng Hsin and Jiu Jitsu, there is definitely an avoidance of communicating preparatory counter movements as they forewarn an opponent's intention. Much of the purpose of the internal training is to develop the ability to strike with immediacy and power. This is even more of a concern in the sword arts, where efficiency, speed, accuracy and the unexpected are highly prized' (Roberts, 2013).

Huang was known throughout the Chinese martial arts world for his capacity to effortlessly throw opponents many metres. Not only was he not extending his hands and arms but, paradoxically, they almost appeared to be withdrawing as the person flew back, as if from an electric shock. In

Tai Ji, the deep stance, focused breath and cultivation of Qi in the lower Dan Tien, as the weight is shifted, is a systematic spring-loading and preparatory counter movement stored for the issuing force to be delivered.

Peter Ralston, author of *The Principles of Effortless Power*, when asked about Bruce Lee's one-inch punch placed his hand on the person's chest saying, 'You don't need an inch,' and knocked him 6 meters across the room, with little visible movement.

Actively stretching the fascia for true elasticity

Our body is designed for active loading. 'We are hard-wired to move, for survival, pleasure, creative self-expression and optimal function. The body has an inherent vocabulary of coordinated movements that develop naturally and concurrently with brain development. I refer to these as primary movements and postures. In cultures where people squat, sit cross-legged on the floor as a matter of course and walk barefoot at least sometimes, they cultivate their internal strength and fascial flexibility, which last into old age. On the other hand, many Westerners, even in their teens and certainly as they get older, struggle to squat flat-footed and sit upright on the floor. This loss of primary postures, movements and healthy fascial functioning is more and more evident in our chair-based society' (Petersen, 2009).

Our movement repertoire is locked into our breathing pattern. Each breath is a physical and energetic impulse into the myofascial system (Chapter 11). In martial arts, abdominal and reverse abdominal breathing is an integral part of the training. The quest for full and powerful range of motion of the arm, spinal and leg myofascial chains in kicks, punches, blocks and evasive movements amplifies the fascial stretch and flexibility in both the core of the body, the powerhouse of our internal strength, and the engine of our entire breathing mechanism.

Many find stretching an invaluable part of martial arts training. The classic holding of long passive stretches is not something we see much in the animal kingdom. Animals naturally and spontaneously roll, actively stretch and rub their soft tissues and joints against the ground or trees, which neutralises built up stress, nourishes and rehydrates their myofascial system (Bertolucci, 2011). If we are well embodied, our stretching will be more of a natural occurrence, with less need for a special regime (Chapter 9).

Many trainers now suggest not stretching immediately before exercise but to warm up and mobilise the joints and tissues instead. Experience suggests fast, dynamic stretching, which occurs in many kicks and punches, is beneficial for the fascia when performed correctly: soft tissues should be warm and abrupt movements avoided. Rhythmic controlled bouncing at the end range may also be effective (Chapter 10).

'Fascia research is highlighting the fusion of passive and active tissue. Thus, when combining the fascial systems of the body, the objective in my view is to tune the passive and active tissues and their interaction. This enables optimal strength, speed, and power through a system that reduces injurious stress concentrations. This is a higher concept than simply stretching. Tuning tissue enhances performance, for example, when jumping. If the hamstrings are overstretched, only the active component of the muscle can create force. But great jumpers often have tighter hamstrings where they can time the muscle recoil with the elastic recoil of fascia and connective tissue, creating a higher resultant force. Thus more stretching is not the answer. Enough mobility is needed for the task but no more. The muscle creates force and so does tuned fascia. Consequently we have a better result' (McGill, 2013).

Train the fascia through forms and Kata for total warrior fighting strength

'To prepare for mixed martial arts or real fight situations, it is important to realise, that functional strength can only be developed through exercises that not only work major muscle groups but also improve the condition and flexibility of the fascial planes,' says 8th degree black belt Grand Master, Lance Strong. 'Kata or Forms training has a huge effect on developing fascial strength and your ability to apply that strength in many different directions, while still maintaining your body's centre and balance. Virtually no form of exercise, other than kata, tai ji or yoga, and some cross-training exercises, develop this ability' (Strong, 2013).

Conditioning the fascial body

It takes time to build fascial resilience: 'It takes two to three years to build an aikido body that is elastic and strong enough for the training practice. Most injuries occur in the tendons and ligaments and are caused by over-training too early or trying to practice techniques more roughly than is appropriate' (Roberts, 2013).

The Shaolin monks knew that, for positive results and to avoid injury, they could only do the intense bone conditioning every second or third day. We now know that collagen has a slow renewal cycle with a half-life of approximately one year, so after two months fascial training we may have little to show but much more after six or twelve months (Chapter 1). In martial arts fascial training, a long-term progress orientation is encouraged alongside loading, and particularly eccentric loading, rather than repetition. With free weights or kettlebells (Chapter 23), medium weights are used to train the fascia and heavier weights for the muscles.

To achieve the best results, fascial training is limited to two or three times a week. On the other hand, daily exercise can have great value for our brain, muscles and cardiovascular system. Short intense boot camp trainings should be avoided as this often propagates compartment syndromes and fascial inflammation.

'If tolerated by the joints, training should include a component that demands 100% neural drive to the muscles. This is usually accomplished by training at speed. The actual static load need not be that great. Good form in all exercise promotes sparing of the joints but ensures optimal tensioning all along the musculoskeletal linkage' (McGill, 2013). McGill gives the example of a slow grinding bench press versus standing and falling into a push-up position, where the hands are on a low box, then immediately exploding back up to the standing position. The box height is adjusted so that this is barely possible. The neural drive is exceptional as is the tuning of the fascia, passive tissue and active muscle system.

To maximise the tensegral power of the myofascial system, we should cultivate structural awareness and learn how physical alignment can be a foundation for both the ultimate relaxation and the ultimate expression of power. Effortless power is a consequence of setting up the right conditions through conscious training and this includes training the fascial body.

Healthy fascia for a healthy body

The fascial web, rather than the muscles alone, provides a framework for storage and release of kinetic energy (Chapter 10). It governs the spring-loaded joint mechanisms for the leg, arm, spinal chains and the entire system. Without good nutrition and hydration the fascia will let you down.

'The foundation for top performance has to be health, so before serious training with an athlete I test the liver, heart, blood and get the nutrition right so the Qi can move through the body' (Parore, 2013). The body's acid/alkaline balance, hormonal influences, lymph and blood flow all have a strong affect on the fascia and this affects our fitness. We rehydrate fascia with an inclusion of appropriate resting times for tissue and viscoelastic recovery. An active life and light nutrition support the fascia and muscles better than a sedentary life style. On a heavy red meat diet with saturated fats and refined sugar products we may cultivate stress hormones and chronic inflammation.

Fascial restrictions and scarring can affect and inhibit a martial arts practice (Chapter 2). For self-care maintenance and injury healing, foam rollers, massage balls and self-massage can be helpful. Some therapists use stone massage tools or powerful herbal liniments to reduce fascial scarring. New interventions such as injecting medical ozone and vitamin cocktails may assist in fascial recovery. Adhesions can also be released with integrative myofascial approaches such as osteopathy, acupuncture, integral aquatic therapy and structural integration.

Fascial awareness and embodiment: Training for Life

The path of the ultimate warrior, in traditional martial arts teachings, is not just the path of the fighter. It is a path of service, love and protection for our community. It demands us to access the deeper qualities of the warrior: focus, energy, perseverance and dedication to a cause bigger than ourselves. This heart, this spirit, is the essence of the internal power of the martial arts. It is foundational for reaching peak performance, recovering from an injury or building resilience to deal with the inherent challenges of life. Buddha said, 'Mindfulness is the sole path to freedom' (Goldstein, 1976). So perhaps, we shouldn't be surprised that Mindfulness is a source for unlimited potential in the movement arts and that it has been at the cutting edge of psychotherapeutic methods for the last decade. Contemporary Western culture and the media tend to draw us away from our deeper body awareness. A committed martial arts practice is a daily returning to ourselves. True masters in the martial arts are rare beings who have achieved the ultimate physical expression and the deepest Body-Mindfulness, with the consequent fascial awareness and peace of mind. This is built step-by-step during a lifetime of training as they integrate their art into every dimension of their life and well-being. As Master Huang said, 'Eat, sleep and practice Tai Ji.' (Huang, 1980).

Be assured Body-Mindfulness need not be a serious task. To expand your fascial repertoire is to become elastically playful. It involves bringing a new creative attitude, not only to your martial arts practice but also to simple everyday activities like standing on one leg to brush your teeth, always sitting on the floor to watch television, studying stretching with a local cat and regular practice of the flat-footed squat. It is never too late to begin your fascial training. Stella is an 88-year-old student in my Tai Ji class. When she began at the age of 80, she struggled to climb the stairs to the practice room and to accomplish even basic movements. At 88, her practice has lightness and flow. Her balance has improved impressively. She carries her success in every step.

In conclusion, giving attention to your fascial body is practically important and, combined with Mindfulness, these will be the best tools to manage your training. The fruits of bringing Body-Mindfulness into a martial arts practice and your life are a new 'aliveness', an enthusiastic resilient energy and a generous self-care attitude. Tools we all need for a long and healthy life.

References

Bertolucci, L. (2011) Pandiculation: nature's way of maintaining the functional integrity of the myofascial system? *JBMT*. Jul.

Blakeslee, S. & Blakeslee, M. (2007) *The Body Has a Mind of its Own*. New York: Random House.

Chek, P. (2004) *How to Eat, Move and Be Healthy!* San Diego, CA: A C.H.E.K Institute Publication.

Cheng Man-ch'ing, Robert W. Smith, R. (1967) *T'ai-Chi: The 'Supreme Ultimate' Exercise for Health, Sport and Self-Defense*. Rutland, Vermont: Charles E. Tuttle Co.

Chia, M. (1988) *Bone Marrow Nei Kung*. Thailand: Universal Tao Publications, 32.

Chia, M. (2002) *Tan Tien Chi Kung: Empty Force, Perineum Power and the Second Brain*. Rochester, Vermont: Destiny Books.

Chia, M. (2007) *Iron Shirt Chi Kung I*. Thailand: Universal Tao Publications.

Dalton, E. et al. (2011) *Dynamic Body: Exploring Form, Expanding Function*. Freedom From Pain Institute.

Goldstein, J. (1976) *The Experience of Insight*. Boulder, Colorado, USA: Shambala Press.

Hibbs, A.E. et al. (2008) Optimizing performance by improving core stability and core strength. *Sports Med*. 38, (12.) 995–1008.

Huang Sheng Shyan, (1980) Personal interview.

Hyams, J. (1982) *Zen in the Martial Arts*. New York: Bantam.

Kelly, P. (2007) *Infinite Dao*. New Zealand: Taiji Books.

Kelly, P. (2005) *Spiritual Reality*. New Zealand: Taiji Books.

Master T.T. Liang, (1977) *T'ai Chi Ch'uan For Health and Self-Defense: Philosophy and Practice*. United States, New York: Random House.

Master Gong Chan, Master Li Jun Feng, (1998) *Sheng Zhen Wuji Yuan Gong: A Return to Wholeness*. 2nd ed. Makati, Philippines: International Sheng Zhen Society.

McDougall, C. (2010) *Born To Run: The hidden tribe, the ultra-runners, and the greatest race the world has never seen*. London: Profile Books Ltd.

McGill, S. (2004) *Ultimate Back Fitness and Performance*. Waterloo. Ontario, Canada: Wabuno Publishers.

McGill, S. (2013) Personal interview.

McHose, C. & Frank, K. (2006) *How Life Moves: Explorations In Meaning And Body Awareness*. Berkely, Carlifornia: North Atlantic Books.

Myers, T. (2009) *Anatomy Trains: Myofascial Meridians for Manual and Movement Therapists*. 2nd ed. Churchill Livingstone Elsevier.

Myers, T. (2011) *Fascial Fitness: Training in the Neuromyofascial Web*. United States: IDEA Health & Fitness Inc.

Ni, Hua Ching, (1983) *8000 Years of Wisdom: Conversations With Taoist Master Ni, Hua Ching*. Malibu, California: *The Shrine The Eternal Breath of Tao and Los Angeles* (Book 1), CA: College of Tao & Traditional Chinese Healing.

Parore, L. (2002) *Power Posture: The Foundation of Strength*. Vancouver, British Columbia: Apple Publishing Company Ltd.

Parore, L. (2013) Personal interview.

Petersen, S. (2006) *How Do I Listen? Applying Body- Psychotherapy Skills in Manual and Movement Therapy*. Missoula, Montana: The International Association of Structural Integration (IASI).

Petersen, S. (2009) *Cultivation Body-Mindfulness: The heart of Structural Integration*. Missoula, Montana: The International Association of Structural Integration (IASI).

Ralston, P. (1989) *Cheng Hsin: The Principles of Effortless Power*. Bekerly, California: North Atlantic Books.

Random, M. (1977) *The Martial Arts*. Paris, France: Fernand Nathan Editeur.

Roberts, A. (2013) Personal interview.

Rolf, I.P. (1977) Rolfing: The Integration of Human Structures. New York: Fitzhenry & Whiteside Limited.

Schleip, R. & Müller, D.G. (2012) Training principles for fascial connective tissues: Scientific foundation and suggested practical applications. *J Bodyw Mov Ther*.

Stecco, L. & Stecco, C. (2008) *Fascial Manipulation*. Padua: Piccin Publisher.

Strong, L. Personal interview.

Further reading

Desikachar, T.K.V. (1995) *The Heart of Yoga: Developing A Personal Practice*. Rochester, Vermont: Inner Traditions International.

Feldenkrais, M. (1981) *The Elusive Obvious*. Capitola, CA: Meta Publications.

Joiner, T.R. (1999) *The Warrior As Healer: A Martial Arts Herbal For Power, Fitness, And Focus*. Rochester, Vermont: Healing Arts Press.

Lao Tsu (translated by Gia-Fu Feng & Jane English, J.), (1972) *Tao Te Ching*. United States, New York: Random House.

Levine, P.A. (1997) *Waking the Tiger: Healing Trauma*. Berkely, California: North Atlantic Books.

Mann, F. (1972) *Acupuncture: The Ancient Chinese Art of Healing*. 2nd ed. London: William Heinemann Medical Books Ltd.

Moore, R. & Gillette, D. (1990) *King Warrior Magician Lover*. New York, NY: HarperCollins Publishers.

Rizzolatti, Fadiga, L., Fogassi, L. & Gallese V. (1997). The Space Around Us, Science magazine.

Sieh, R. (1992) *T'ai Chi Ch'uan*. Berkeley, California: North Atlantic Books.

Warburton, M. (2001) Barefoot running. *Sport Science*. Dec; 5(3).

CHAPTER 17

Elastic walking

Adjo Zorn

Years ago I used to think of walking as a chore, much like doing the dishes. Until recently, walking was one of the main physical activities necessary for survival. So I thought that in this day and age we could count ourselves lucky that this was no longer the case. But then I happened upon a curious conjunction of apparently unrelated and disquieting facts that led me to examine the science of walking. Those facts were as follows:

- The cause of back pain is completely unclear in eight out of ten cases (Deyo & Weinstein et al., 2001) (Kendrick et al., 2001).

- There is a large and strong anatomic structure in the lower-back region, the elastic lumbodorsal fascia, which is consistently ignored by the multi-million dollar back-pain research industry (Tesarz et al., 2011). Until very recently, there was little indication as to whether or not this fascia could cause back pain (Taguchi et al., 2009) (Tesarz et al., 2011).

- Although this structure acts as the tendon of the latissimus-dorsi muscle, and thus directly connects the arms and legs, it too has generally been ignored by biomechanics researchers studying human movement.

- Gait analysis, the term for the science of walking, analyses different walking patterns only as pertains to certain clinical cases, such as in the use of prosthesis, certain forms of paralysis or Parkinson's disease. Gait analysis has paid little attention to the walking patterns of healthy people, which are as unique as their handwriting.

- It is almost a tenet of gait analysis that walking, as opposed to running, is an inelastic, muscle-driven pendulum movement (Alexander, 1991) (Sawicki et al., 2009).

I began to wonder whether some people walk 'incorrectly' and develop back pain, while others walk 'correctly' and don't experience any. In addition, I began to wonder whether those who walk 'incorrectly' actually fail to use their 'big' fascia, while those who walk 'correctly' use the fascia and thus maintain its elasticity (Jackson, 1998) (Burton et al., 2004).

With my background in mechanical engineering, I came to realise that the lumbodorsal fascia is excellently located. Given its elastic properties (Chapter 10) (Maganaris, 2002), it should actually function as an effective engine for walking. Being a Rolfer, I have the opportunity to observe many lower backs on the treadmill. Unfortunately, in most cases I can hardly detect any internal movement in the *lumbodorsal area*. This was very different in certain parts of Africa. In remote villages in Zambia and Ghana, people displayed quite a lot of movement in the area of the *lumbodorsal fascia*. There, the daily struggle for survival requires a great deal of walking for adults and children alike. In Europe, on the other hand, natural walking has become practically superfluous at work, and has fallen out of fashion as a leisure activity. We drive cars, ride the subway, go to the gym, cycle or jog. But hardly anyone simply goes for a walk.

This is where I would like to make a contribution towards a new understanding of walking. Not only is walking, besides running, probably our most natural way of moving, the one that most closely corresponds to our body structure, but it can also be a dynamic form of meditation, that is to say, walking can easily combine movement and contemplation. Now, while it is true that almost anyone can lumber around or shuffle their feet, I believe that walking 'correctly' is actually a great challenge.

My hypothesis is that to walk 'correctly', you need to walk 'elastically'. For this reason I have, in recent years, sought to understand natural walking from two different angles. On the one hand, I have used the exact mathematical principles of Newtonian mechanics to calculate a computer-based model of walking as an elastic operation (Zorn & Hodeck, 2011). On the other hand, I have gathered empirical experience from showing my Rolfing clients how to walk elastically. Both approaches

have made it clear that elastic walking entails very precise coordination, that is to say, it requires the right amount of force to be applied at precisely the right time, much like the force that is needed to keep a child's swing in motion (Chapter 10).

In terms of the laws of physics, movement on an even surface does not require energy. If it were not for friction, a body that was set in motion at one point in time would continue rolling or sliding indefinitely. The same goes for a bouncing ball

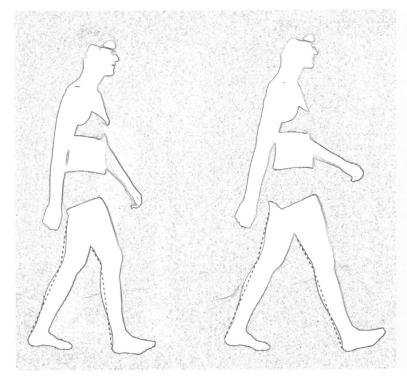

Figure 17.1

Two different ways of using the knee in the stance leg

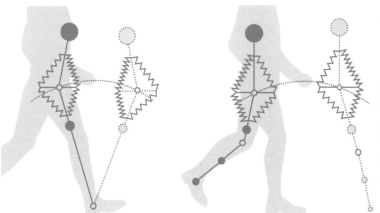

Figure 17. 2

The elastic springs of the hip pull the stance leg up, act as a brake as it drops down, maintain the balance of the upper body, accelerate the swing leg and brake its movement again. (The circles symbolise the body's centres of mass.)

or a jumping kangaroo, both using elastic springs in which, for a short moment, energy is stored and then re-used. My hypothesis is that this very principle may apply to a walking person. However, just as the air pressure in a bouncing ball has to be just right, the fascial springs of a jumping kangaroo and a walking person need to have the appropriate amount of tension (Chapters 1 and 10).

A muscle is mainly comprised of one part, containing the contracting fascicle, and another, containing the tendon. The right tension can be achieved at very low energy cost if the muscle fascicles contract in a way that they maintain a *constant* length while the connected tendon (and further fasciae) can change their length, stretch and recoil (Fukunaga et al., 2001). In other words, the elastic tendon does all the work, at almost zero energy cost while the fascicles just maintain a kind of initial tension, at very low energy cost. Please note that this process should not to be confused with a muscle acting isometrically as a whole, where the fascicles and the tendon *together* maintain a constant length (Chapter 10).

In what follows I set out some advice to help readers to explore elastic walking. Of course, learning movement out of a book is a questionable endeavor. Therefore, I ask that you view this as an experimental proposition. (For a theoretical discussion hereof, see Zorn, 2011.)

1. Walking with straight legs

Humans are the only animals whose stance leg can be straight like a column while walking (Sockol et al., 2007). The rotation of this 'column' around the ankle is what produces the typical up-and-down motion of the torso in human walking, a motion that is also unique in the animal kingdom. Admittedly, nowadays many people tend to walk with slightly bent knees, thus preventing any elastic stretching, a problem that is only exacerbated by the current trend that favours standing with bent, supposedly 'relaxed' knees (Figs. 17.1 and 17.4).

If the back leg is properly extended in the final stance phase, then the psoas, rectus femoris and the triceps surae muscles, along with their fasciae are stretched and loaded. When the stance leg starts to become the swinging leg, these muscles recoil and unload, thus accelerating the lower leg forward like a slingshot (Ishikawa et al., 2005) (Schleip, 2013). In

the final stage of the swing, the swinging leg, *if* it reaches complete extension, comes to a halt due to the stretching of the gluteus maximus muscle and its fasciae, especially the lumbodorsal fascia and the iliotibial tract (Fig. 17.2). Incidentally, this explains the oblique and almost horizontal direction of the gluteus maximus fibres, something that makes little sense for a hip extensor in the standing posture (Fig. 17.3).

After the heel strike, this same stretch pulls the weight of the torso upwards onto the new, rotating stance leg. After the mid-stance position has been reached, the downward fall of the torso stretches the psoas, the rectus femoris and the triceps surae regions once again (Fig. 17.2).

In terms of physics, the potential energy of the weight of the falling body is transformed into the energy of a stretched spring: the psoas and gastrocnemius gently catch the body weight. The elastic energy is then converted into the kinetic energy of an accelerating flywheel: the psoas and gastrocnemius propel the lower leg upwards and forwards. Subsequently, the kinetic energy is transferred into elastic energy again: the glutmax and the iliotibial tract cause the swinging lower leg to brake. Finally, the elastic energy is transformed back into potential energy: the gluteus maximus and the iliotibial tract lift the body weight upwards, via the hip. All of this only works if the knee of both the stance leg and the swing leg, in its final phase, is straight (Zorn & Hodeck 2011).

2. Take long steps

The stretches described above are only possible if you take long steps (Fig. 17.4). Make your stride as long as you can and observe how your pelvis then rotates in the horizontal plane, stretching the fasciae in your lower back (Figures 17.2 and 17.3). Don't forget to keep up a brisk pace!

3. The centre of the heel

Most often, people carry their weight on the outer edge of their feet. Unfortunately, some trainers and therapists even recommend this. In my opinion, to achieve dynamic-elastic walking, you really only need to use two points of the foot (see CH and BT, Figure 17.5) and, in between those points, the elastic anti-shock arch with the plantar fascia on the medial side of the foot (Ward et al., 2003)

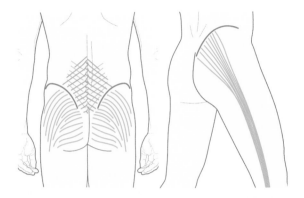

Figure 17.3

The smooth fibre extending from the lower leg to the lower back.

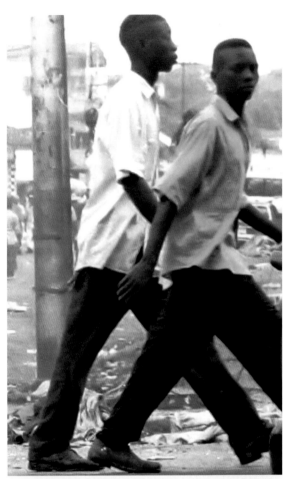

Figure 17.4

Walking in Ghana: long steps, straight knees, upper bodies forward.

(Roux et al., 2009) (Inman et al., 1981, p16). The foot then rolls up exactly at those two points CH (leg forward) and BT (leg back). In order for the heel to touch down precisely *in the middle* (at point CH), a 'centre-of-heel' awareness is needed (Figs. 17.5 and 17.6). You need to feel this point while walking (see also Chapter 15).

It may be the case that the outer edge of the foot is only important for balancing on one leg, like the training wheels a child uses when learning to ride a bike.

4. Pressure with the ball of the foot

At point BT, and only at that point, there is a sesamoid bone that can function like a ball of a ball bearing. When your stance leg gets close to its furthest back position, try pushing down and towards the back, with your *knee straight*, on to the main joint of the big toe, as if you wanted to make the earth roll away. What you would actually do is give yourself a push forward but the first description works better in terms of imagining what you have to do. This way, you roll off exactly on the sesamoid bone and stretch the triceps surae region. Interestingly, the stretch of the gastrocnemius muscle, with its sling shape around the condyles, then helps to prevent over-stretching of the knee.

5. Carry your pelvis

As a general principle of human posture, bones are not usually balanced on top of each other around a central axis. Rather, they form hook-shaped units that are suspended in tension through muscles and fasciae (Chapter 1). If you fell asleep standing up, for instance, your head would drop forward and then your knees would buckle because the neck and calf muscles would lose tension. An alert human poise requires steady tautness in the body. In terms

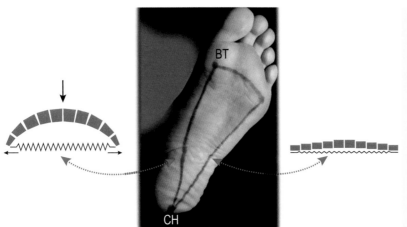

Figure 17.5

The elastic anti-shock structure is located on the medial
side of the foot.

of evolution, this can be traced back to the fact that it was probably more beneficial for early humans to react quickly in case of an attack by a predator than it was for them to be able to stand around in a cool, energy-saving pose. Nowadays, people can afford to be lazy and outsmart this dynamic tensional principle by lounging in their ligaments. For instance, some people sink into locked knees instead of standing in a posture of active balance. Less obviously, the pelvis too needs to be actively balanced with certain tautness (Rolf, 1989) and 'the passive part of the lumbodorsal fascia requires the reduction of lordosis in order to become tightened.' (Gracovetsky et al., 1987) (Adams et al., 2007) (Chapters 13 and 14). Instead, many people let the front of the pelvis drop down, lock the lumbar vertebrae, buckle the vertebral column, and disable the lumbar fascia (Adams, 2001) (Smith et al., 2008). Unfortunately, there are many alternative movement or posture teachers who continue to promote this posture by telling their students: 'relax your belly!' Similarly, some physiotherapists regard the rectus abdominis muscle as being 'superficial' and therefore automatically assume that it is generally over-activated. In my opinion, the rectus abdominis muscle is often too inactive (Porterfield & Derosa, 1998), sometimes along the oblique abdominal muscles, not only among those with a 'relaxed' belly but also among bodybuilders with impressive but rigid six-packs. In fact, this large muscle should *pull up* the pubic bone with agility and, thereby,

adjust the balance of the pelvis and fine-tune its position with respect to the quickly changing forces during movement (Fig. 17.7, Arrow A).

Furthermore, this muscle should form an elastically tensioned abdominal wall (McGill, 2001) that functions as a partner to the diaphragm for breathing. This should not to be confused with sucking in the belly. 'The importance [of the rectus abdominis] in erect posture is universally recognised... True strength is not hardening; it is resilience, adaptability, stability. It is characterised by elasticity' (Rolf, 1989). Currently, some readers probably feel that the role of the rectus abdominis muscle is overvalued and that I miss proper mention of the transversus abdominis muscle. Please keep in mind that the main focus here is not on stability but on elasticity.

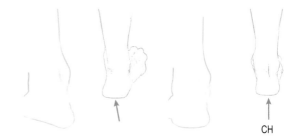

Figure 17.6

Effective use of the elastic structure of the sole requires the correct placement of the heel.

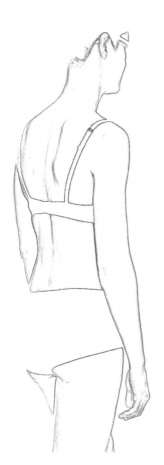

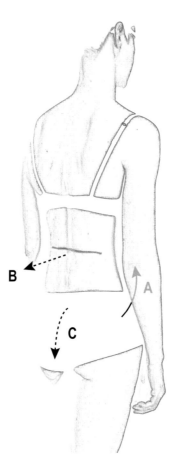

B

A

C

Figure 17.7

Balancing the pelvis and stabilising the lower spine for
people who otherwise let the
pelvis drop in front.

Arrow A: Carrying the pelvis
at the pubic bone.

Arrow B: 'Waistline back!' (Ida
Rolf). Making sure the vertebral column does not buckle.

Arrow C: Dropping the sacrum. Stretching the lumbodorsal fascia.

If your usual walking style includes short steps, a dropped pelvis, and a hollow back, then your hip flexors have most likely not developed the range of motion necessary to carry your pelvis as described above. Reconditioning the hip flexors through stretching by undertaking elastic walking will probably take effort, determination, and patience but will eventually pay off.

6. A sideline: Elastic breathing

This is not actually a part of walking but it is essential in terms of having an elastically tensioned abdominal wall. Diaphragmatic breathing has a great impact on the autonomic nervous system and on stress-related conditions. Elastic breathing is not possible when the belly protrudes forward flaccidly, due to a lack of rectus abdominis tone as described above, or when the belly is sucked in, through a shortening of the upper transversus abdominis muscle. Equally unhelpful for elastic breathing is a six-pack, if all that it does is look good but is actually rigid. In elastic breathing, you feel the stretching of the tensioned abdominal wall every time you breathe in. In the give-and-take of breathing, the rectus abdominis muscle and the diaphragm behave like strong, rhythmic dance partners cradling the internal organs in their movement (Chapter 12).

7. The pinnacle: Letting the sacrum drop

This is possibly the most difficult part of my whole proposition. If the long muscles and fasciae in front fail to do their job of stabilising the spinal column, some short muscles in the back then get involved as a kind of emergency back up

(Bergmark, 1989) (Reeves et al., 2007). This creates a paradoxical situation. These muscles become overactive and, sooner or later, overloaded in a region which is already too short: the over-lordotic lower back.

People in this situation may easily be able to relax the lumbar muscles if they bend forward to tie their shoelaces but they may not be able to relax these muscles at all when doing a physical activity. This situation is not uncommon among

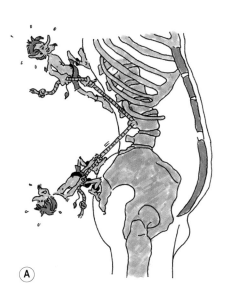
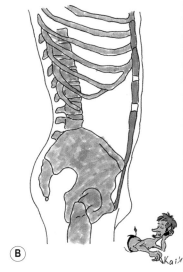

Figure 17.8

If the front muscles allow the spine column to buckle, some of the muscles in the back have to work very hard.

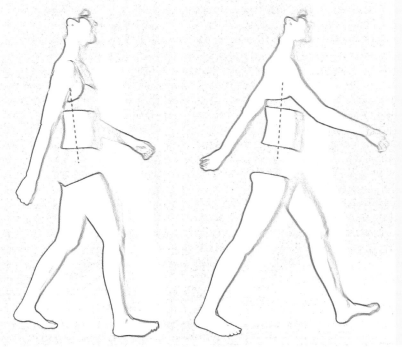

Figure 17.9

To walk energetically, the upper body needs to bend forward slightly.

professional athletes and dancers with lower back pain. What people in that situation need is the ability to relax their back muscles, i.e., to let the sacrum bone drop down while performing a forceful physical move (Figure 17.7, arrow C). The ability to carry out such subtle, fine movement is also absolutely necessary in terms of being able to balance the pelvis and to walk using the elastic fasciae in the back. It is, of course, impossible to teach this 'intellectually' but, according to my knowledge, the techniques of Tai Ji Quan come closest to such training (see also Chapter 15).

If the elastic fasciae in the lower back are able to stretch and recoil in walking, a wave-like motion swings through the spine and the lumbar vertebrae. Thus, all fascial structures in the lower spine stretch appropriately and have little reason to develop pain.

8. Move your upper body

Although traditional gait analysis regards the upper body as a mere 'passive passenger' (Perry, 1992), I think that the elastic fasciae of the lower back are there to be used in walking. For this to happen, the fasciae need to have a healthy level of tension, instead of being crumpled. For dynamic elastic walking, the lower back needs to be elongated in a certain way. This means the upper body should have a slight forward tilt. This forward tilt will likely feel quite odd at first, as if you might fall forward, and often causes people to look downwards. Look towards the horizon instead (Fig. 17.9).

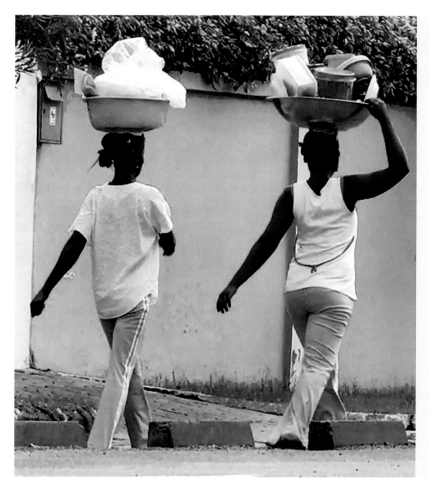

Figure 17.10

Walking in Ghana: using the arms.

9. The arms are important too

While you are walking, let your arms swing backwards much further and more vigorously than usual. If the arms swing far enough and the legs make the long strides, described above, then the pelvis and the upper body will show torsion movements and merrily stretch their fasciae. Furthermore, the heel of the forward foot is then able to touch the ground as softly as a cat's paw (Chapter 16) (Fig. 17.10).

11. Walk more often

Leave your car or bike where it's parked and walk more often. Walk to a station further down the street. Take a longer walking route when you leave work.

Park your car on the other side of the park and walk home. Get yourself good wet and cold weather gear. Walk briskly so that your circulation rate increases slightly and treat yourself to a little more oxygen. Get your children used to walking too! If people complain to you about back pain, then ask them: How often do you walk? *How* do you walk? Don't be surprised if you catch yourself smiling for no reason while walking elastically. After all, you might come to discover the joy of walking, as I eventually did.

Acknowledgement
I owe a great debt of gratitude to Kai Hodeck, PhD, fellow physicist and Rolfing practitioner. The critical acuity of his generous feedback helped dismantle my favourite hypotheses and generally improve this chapter.

References

Adams, M.A. & Dolan, P. (2007) How to use the spine, pelvis, and legs effectively in lifting. In Vleeming, A., Mooney, V. & Stoeckart, R. (eds.) *Movement, Stability and Lumbopelvic Pain*, vol. 2: 167–183, Edinburgh: Churchill Livingstone.

Adams, M.A. & Dolan, P. (2001) Spinal Dysfunction And Pain: Recent Advances In Basic Science, in Vleeming, A. (ed.) (2001) 4th Interdisciplinary World Congress on Low Back & Pelvic Pain: *Moving from Structure to Function*, Montreal, Canada, November 8–10.

Alexander, R.M. (1991) Energy-saving mechanisms in walking and running. *J. Exp. Biol.* 160: 55–69.

Bergmark, A. (1989) Stability of the lumbar spine. A study in mechanical engineering. *Acta Orthop Scand.* Suppl 230: 1–54.

Burton, K., Balague, F., Cardon, G., Eriksen, H.R., Henrotin, Y., Lahad, A., Leclerc, A., Mueller, G. & van der Beek, A.J. (2004) *European Guidelines for Prevention in Low Back Pain*. European Commission, COST Action B13, from www.backpaineurope.org.

Deyo, R.A. & Weinstein, J.N. (2001) Low back pain. *N Engl J Med.* 344(5): 363–370.

Fukunaga, T., Kubo, K., Kawakami, Y., Fukashiro, S., Kanehisa, H. & Maganaris, C.N. (2001) In vivo behaviour of human muscle tendon during walking. *Proc Biol Sci.* 268(1464): 229–233.

Gracovetsky, S., Zeman, V. & Carbone, A.R. (1987) Relationship between lordosis and the position of the centre of reaction of the spinal disc. *J Biomed Eng.* 9(3): 237–248.

Inman, V.T., Ralston, H.J. & Todd, F. (1981) *Human Walking*. Baltimore: Williams and Wilkins.

Ishikawa, M., Komi, P.V., Grey, M.J., Lepola, V. & Bruggemann, G.P. (2005) Muscle-tendon interaction and elastic energy usage in human walking. *J Appl Physiol.* 99(2): 603–608.

Jackson, R. (1998) 'Postural Dynamics: Functional Causes of Low Back Pain', in B.P. D'Orazio (ed.) *Low Back Pain Handbook*, 159–194. Butterworth-Heinemann.

Kendrick, D., Fielding, K., Bentley, E., Miller, P., Kerslake, R. & Pringle, M. (2001) The role of radiography in primary care patients with low back pain of at least 6 weeks duration: a randomised (unblinded) controlled trial. *Health Technol Assess.* 5(30): 1–69.

Langevin, H.M. & Sherman, K.J. (2006) Pathophysiological model for chronic low back pain integrating connective tissue and nervous system mechanisms. *Med Hypoth.* 68: 74–80.

Maganaris, C.N. & Paul, J.P. (2002) Tensile properties of the in vivo human gastrocnemius tendon. *J Biomech.* 35(12): 1639–1646.

McGill, S.M. (2001) Achieving Spine Stability: Blending Engineering and Clinical Approaches. in A. Vleeming (ed.) 4th Interdisciplinary World Congress on Low Back & Pelvic Pain: Moving from Structure to Function, Montreal, Canada. November 8–10: 203.

Perry, J. (1992) Gait Analysis: Normal and Pathological Function, SLACK Inc, Thorofare, NJ.

Porterfield, J. & Derosa, C. (1998) *Mechanical Low Backpain – Perspectives in Functional Anatomy*. Philadelphia: Saunders.

Reeves, P. N., Narendra, K.S. & Cholewicki, J. (2007) Spine stability: The six blind men and the elephant. *Clin. Biomech.* (Bristol, Avon) 22: 266–274.

Rolf, I.P. (1989) Rolfing: *Reestablishing the natural alignment and structural integration of the human body for vitality and well-being.* 1st edition. Rochester, Vt: Healing Arts Press.

Roux, M., Baly, L. & Gorce, P. (2009) Could the study of ground reaction forces be an indicator of the footwear stability during locomotion?. *Science Sports.* 24: 27–30.

Sawicki, G.S., Lewis, C.L. & Ferris, D.P. (2009) It pays to have a spring in your step. *Exerc Sport Sci Rev*. July; 37(3): 130.

Schleip, R. & Müller, D.G. (2013) Training principles for fascial connective tissues: Scientific foundation and suggested practical applications. *J Bodyw Mov Ther*. 17(1): 103–115.

Smith, A., O'Sullivan, P. & Straker, L. (2008) Classification of sagittal thoraco-lumbo-pelvic alignment of the adolescent spine in standing and its relationship to low back pain. *Spine*. 33(19): 2101–2107, from doi:10.1097/BRS. 0b013e31817ec3b0.

Sockol, M.D., Raichlen, D.A. & Pontzer, H. (2007) *Chimpanzee locomotor energetics and the origin of human bipedalism*. *PNAS* 104(30): 12265–12269.

Taguchi, T., Tesarz, J. & Mense, S. (2009) The Thoracolumbar Fascia as a Source of Low Back Pain. In P.A. Huijing, et al. (eds.) *Fascia Research II: Basic Science and Implications for Conventional and Complementary Health Care*. 251. Munich: Urban & Fischer.

Tesarz, J., Hoheisel, U., Wiedenhofer, B. & Mense, S. (2011) Sensory innervation of the thoracolumbar fascia in rats and humans. *Neuroscience*. 194: 302–308.

Ward, E.D., Smith, K.M., Cocheba, J.R., Patterson, P.E., Phillips, R.D., Ward, E.D., Smith, K.M., Cocheba, J.R., Patterson, P.E. & Phillips, R.D. (2003) In vivo forces in the plantar fascia during the stance phase of gait: sequential release of the plantar fascia. William J. Stickel Gold Award. *Journal of the American Podiatric Medical Association*. 93(6): 429–442.

Zorn, A., Schmitt, F.J., Hodeck, F.H., Schleip, R. & Klingler, W. (2007) The spring-like function of the lumbar fascia in human walking. In T.W. Findley and R. Schleip (eds.) *Fascia Research: Basic Science and Implications for Conventional and Complementary Health Care*. 188–189.

Zorn, A., Schleip, R. & Klingler, W. (2010) Walking with elastic fascia: Saving energy by maintaing balance. In A. Vleeming (ed.) *7th Interdiciplinary World Congress on Low Back & Pelvic Pain*, Los Angeles, Nov 9th– 12th. 340–341.

Zorn, A. & Hodeck, F. (2011) Walk With Elastic Fascia: Use the Springs in your Step! in E. Dalton (ed.) *Dynamic Body: Exploring Form, Expanding Function*, 1st edition. 96–123, Freedom From Pain Institute, Oklahoma City, OK.

CHAPTER 18

Functional training methods for the runner's fascia

Wilbour Kelsick

Running is big business. Participation has increased exponentially in the last three decades at both the amateur and the professional level. On average, runners cover approximately 70–80 miles (110–130 km) a week but, at times, can be thwarted with a variety of injuries. First I should mention that running is an elastic movement in the body's gait mechanism. An improved efficiency or energy saving motion can be achieved when close to ideal elastic bounce in the running gait is attained (Chapter 10). The beauty of functional fascial training is that it can not only prevent injuries but can also increase running efficiency. This chapter focuses on how functional fascial training can address the elastic components of the running and walking mechanism (Chapter 17).

Running injuries are related to poor running technique, minimal or poor elastic bounce, muscle weakness (for example, hip abductors), muscle imbalances in running structure (for example, pelvic trunk muscles), biomechanical faults (over-pronation of feet, valgus of the knee), micro-trauma from overuse and an inadequately trained elastic fascial net. All of the above can influence each other, creating a collage of epidemiological causes for running injuries. Studies show that the majority of running injuries can be summed up as micro-trauma to collagenous tissues (Elliott, 1990) (Stanish, 1984).

It has been well documented that over 70% of recreational runners will sustain an injury during a one-year period (Caspersen et al., 1984) (Rochcongar et al., 1995) (Ferber et al., 2009).). For instance, more than 80% of running injuries are below the knee suggesting some common mechanism might be the culprit. (Ferber et al., 2009). Evidence does not support any one segmental region but more a global involvement of musculoskeletal running structures. Excessive pronation as a causative factor in over use injuries is well documented (Clarke et al., 1983) (Messier et al., 1991). Also hip and pelvic mechanism weakness and imbalance, or poor stabilisation, are now believed to be one of the major links to lower body running injuries. For example, iliotibial band compression syndrome (ITBCS) and patella femoral syndrome (PFS) (Fredericson et al., 2000) (Horton & Hall, 1989) (Livingston, 1998) (Mizuno et al., 2001) (Witvrouw et al., 2000). The aforementioned studies indicate that the causes of majority of running injuries are related, or have some link to, inefficiency in the structural integrity of the running mechanism (the musculoskeletal system). It is, therefore, obvious that the prevention, pre-habilitation and rehabilitation of such injuries must address these causes in a practical manner. This leads to the proposed functional approach to train the runner's fascia from a global prospective.

However, at this point the following questions must be addressed:

- What do we mean by functional training?
- What is the purpose of strength training for runners?
- What do we mean by fascial training?
- What functional fascial training is specific to runners?

What do we mean by functional training?

The definition that is used in this context for Functional Training is training that is specific to the body movement that you are attempting to execute.

In more detail: functional training is the concept of using functional exercise (i.e. sports-specific exercises) which more closely reproduces the movement pattern of a sport (for example, running) and can be modulated to improve the sum of parts, all of the bio-mechanical movement pattern or physiological profile of the sport. For example, in running the biomechanical pattern would be stride distance or frequency and the physiological profile would be aerobic power for a distance runner. In functional training, the exercise must be global (i.e. using the whole body as much as possible) and not training isolated body regions.

Functional training could be any sport-specific activity that moves an injured, deconditioned athlete or physically dysfunctioning individual towards safe return to sport or activities as soon as feasible.

What is the purpose of strength training for runners?

Running performance is dependent not only on a combination of aerobic and anaerobic capabilities, which vary based on the distance of the event, but also on other factors related to lower and upper body power and strength (Hudgens et al., 1987).

It has been documented that force and power are strongly correlated with running performance for short distances (i.e. sprints, hurdles) (Meylan & Malatesta, 2008) (Mikkola et al., 2011) (Kale et al., 2009). For example, plyometric (Meylan & Malatesta, 2008) resistance (Mikkola et al., 2011) and explosive strength training (Buchheit et al., 2010) (Spurrs et al., 2003) has shown significant improvement in sprint training.

In contrast, middle and long distance running have few studies which correlate that force and power improve performance. However, a few well-designed studies have recently proven that explosive strength training can improve the running economy of middle and long distance runners to a significant degree. (Ferraut et al., 2010) (Kelly et al., 2009) (Mikkola et al., 2007).

Hence the evidence is now clearer that strength training can help improve trunk pelvic, hip and lower extremity strength both concentrically and eccentrically thus improving running efficiency and performance. (Author's observation, unpublished data.)

The mechanism for this improved performance in distance runners is thought to be related to improved muscle (Fletcher et al., 2010) (Dumke et al., 2010) and tendon stiffness (Dumke et al., 2010) and the elastic properties of the fascial net (Tapale et al., 2010)(Huijing & Langevin, 2009) (Schleip, 2003) (Chapter 10). Therefore, the evidence for adapting exercises that train the fascial tissue net, as well as muscles and tendons, is paramount in decreasing and preventing running injuries and improving running economy.

What do we mean by fascial training?

In the past, training for athletes focused mainly on conventional cardiovascular fitness, muscular strength and power and neuromuscular coordination. The classical biomechanical tradition of considering the body as functioning in separate segments, with attached levers, is no longer feasible in the light of new research on fascial function in the whole body (Desmouliere et al., 2005) (Huijing, 2007) (Kubo et al., 2006) (Schleip, 2003). **You cannot train body parts in isolation and expect to have efficient global functioning.**

Running, in its true form, is mostly an elastic event (Bosch & Klomp, 2001) (Legramandi et al, 2013). The mechanism of running involves storing of energy during the deceleration or breaking phase (during foot ground contact) and releasing energy during the push off phase (Legramandi et al., 2013). Using an elastic recoil technique (Chapter 10) will allow the runner to be more efficient, placing less stress on their musculoskeletal system and eventually decreasing their injury rate. **Training for runners must be elastically functional and global in its approach, inclusive of the entire body mechanism and not just the lower extremities.**

There is evidence to support that different fascial elements are affected by different loading styles and fascia has an important role in maintaining muscle function (Steven et al., 1981) (Ingber, 2008). Typical weight training loads the muscle in its normal range of motion, therefore strengthening fascial tissues arranged in series with active muscles fibres. This type of loading has minimal effect on the intramuscular fibres that are arranged in parallel to active muscle fibres and also extra-muscular fascia. (Huijing, 1999) (Latrides et al., 2003) (Fukashiro et al., 2006). This evidence reinforces that, during functional training of the runner's fascial net, exercises must have a dynamic varied loading pattern with rhythm to have an effect on the elastic components and resilience of the body's fascial net.

The concepts of functional training for the runner arise from these insights. The functional training programme, designed in this context, will address the running mechanism from a global perspective with exercises geared to train the runner's elastic fascial component as well as the muscle, ligaments and tendons. The functional fascial exercise protocol for the runner is carried out with a certain amount of rhythm and an explosive component.

In maintaining form, or activated structural integrity, the body is able to set up its own internal and external anchor to create the dynamic stability needed as one segment generates power and the other stabilises (Ingber, 2008). This creates the alternate movement pattern designed for running. This patterning is classified as the on/off switching mechanism required for alternate body segmental movement in walking and running (Chapter 17).

What functional fascia training is specific to runners?

It has been documented that the manner, slow or fast, in which connective tissue is loaded will determine whether the tissue will exhibit a more elastic type or more hypertrophy (i.e. volume) (Kubo et al., 2003) (Kjaer et al., 2009) (Chapter 5).

In nature, kangaroos and gazelles are excellent examples of elastic storage and the release of energy during their movement patterns (Kram & Dawson, 1998) (Chapter 10). The human fascial net seems to have similar elastic behaviour (i.e. kinetic energy storage and release) in our daily activities of walking, running or jumping (Sawicki et al., 2009) (Chino et al., 2008). This justifies the

approach of functional training for the runner's fascial net using explosive, rhythmic type exercise movement patterns. (Fukunaga et al., 2002) (Kawakami et al., 2002)

The functional fascia training concept

The fact that human fascia behaves elastically is now documented (Chino et al., 2008) (Kubo et al., 2006). It stores energy and returns it quickly, as seen in cyclic movements like walking and running (Chapter 17) (Kubo et al., 2006) (Chino et al., 2008) (Legramandi et al., 2013).

Running elastically uses less muscle power, i.e. less metabolic energy (glucose) requirement, and more of the elastic fascia feature of the tissue, thus storing and returning energy back during propulsion. Global functional training for runners' fascia is designed to train the elastic fascia net of the entire body (i.e. muscle, tendons, ligaments). The mode of exercise includes bounding or plyometric movements, preparatory countermovement, unilateral movement patterns, exercise which mimics the mechanism of running (for example, single leg hops, single leg squats, etc.). The exercise protocol avoids slow, jerky type movement patterns, repetitive constant angled movements, movement with mono tempo/rhythm, muscular dominant movement, segmental isolation type movement pattern and minimises constant loading thus encouraging variable loading of the runner's tissues. In addition, research suggests that the fascial system is better trained by using a variety of vectors/angles, loads and rhythm (Huijing, 2007) (Chapter 11).

We cannot delve into this topic without mentioning the importance that running posture and technique plays in enhancing running efficiency and performance. In a correct sprinter's, posture, for example, they are a considerable height off the ground in the flight phase with a well positioned body preparing for the landing phase (a very important body position to maximise horizontal distance travel through the air). As coach Mike Murray says about sprinting posture: 'Attitude is attitude.' Although it is not possible to discuss the concept of running technique in this context in this chapter, it should be noted that it is a crucial piece of the puzzle in preventing running injuries and improving performance.

Exercise protocol for training the runner's fascia

Sports conditioning programmes need to be optimally individualised and sports specific because the limits of peak performance are highly variable even within the same discipline of sport. As described above, the purpose of these exercises is geared to train and strengthen the elastic components of the runner's fascia, muscle and tendons. Energy is stored in the eccentric phase of motion and immediately released on the concentric phase. The exercises are preceded by an eccentric pre-stretch (counter movement) (Chapter 11) that loads the muscle and prepares it for the ensuing concentric contraction. This coupling of the eccentric - concentric muscle contraction is known as the stretch-shortening cycle, which physiologically involves the elastic properties of the tissues (fascia, muscle) and proprioceptive reflexes (Tippett & Voight, 1995) (Radcliffe & Farentinos, 1985). The fact that connective tissue has a high capacity of adaptability and resilience makes it ideal for this type of training where loading forces, shearing and strain are highly variable. Connective tissue has the ability to continuously remodel its fibrous network when specific functional strain or load is applied to it (Langevin et al., 2010) (Chen et al., 1997) (Chapter 5).

In designing any exercise strengthening programme, there are some basic exercise prescription guidelines which must be taken into consideration and a few important questions that need to be asked: Why are you doing the activity? What is the goal of the activity? Is it for fitness maintenance or for competition? Note that the basic principles of training will also apply here (i.e. principles of adaptation (acute and chronic), specificity, overload, and progressive over load, stress-rest, contraction, control, ceiling, maintenance, symmetry and overtraining) (Kraemer, 1994) (Fleck & Kraemer, 1997). In this context we cannot address all these principles but they are found in detail in physiological texts on training (Fleck & Kraemer, 1997).

First, the exercise prescription must consider the total demands of the programme and ensure that the volume of exercise is not excessive, which can negatively interfere with the optimal physiological adaptation and performance. To ensure an effective prescription the following should be considered: (Kraemer & Koziris, 1992) (Fleck & Kraemer, 1997) (Tippet & Voight, 1995).

- the concept of periodisation of the training programme and goals of training
- developing a well planned exercise recovery and rest protocol by using the principles of periodisation
- understanding the balance between strength/power (intensity) and aerobic and anaerobic (volume) training.

In addition, the key resistance training programme components should be considered when designing functional fascia type exercises (Fleck & Kraemer, 1997) (Kraemer, 1994). These components are:

1. **Needs analysis** – this addresses questions about fascial net, muscle groups or body segments to be trained, the energy/metabolic systems involved (aerobic, anaerobic), the type of muscle action (eccentric or isometric).

2. **Acute programme variables** – this deals with choice, order, number of sets, rest period between sets and amount of load (intensity).

3. **Chronic programme manipulation** – this addresses the principles of periodisation as a means of designing long term programmes.

4. **Administrative concerns** – this deals with equipment needs in the gym (free weights, machines assisted resistance-isokinetics, jump platforms, etc.).

Exercise posture

These exercises are geared more towards middle distance and recreational runners. Due to space constrains in this chapter only eight exercises have been documented.

All exercises are performed in a 'Closed Kinetic Chain' posture to increase joint compressive forces, improve joint congruency and muscular co-contraction/activation which will overall enhance the stability of the body segments targeted (Lefever, 2011). Proper foot placement is paramount. The ankle should be in a 'locked' position attained by dorsi-flexion. Then an 'active' plantar flexion action has to take place just prior to ground impact. This well-timed coordinated action of the foot creates the stiffness in the lower extremity chain required to create reactive strength (Winkler, 2010 unpublished). This action ensures a pre-stretch and engages the elastic components of calf structures. Engagement/activation of the neuromuscular components of the trunk, pelvis, pelvic floor and lower extremities is also necessary.

Exercise mode

All exercises are done explosively with quick repeated rhythm/tempo to enhance the elastic effect of the fascia, muscle and tendon tissues.

Pre-exercise preparation

This preparation should be about 15 minutes and consists of the following to enhance general body mobility, ankle and foot ground reactiveness:

- 3–5 min jogging
- Low amplitude ankle/foot bouncing with initial active dorsiflexion and plantar flexion when landing on ground
- Standing lower extremity swings from hips
- Walking lunges with quick tempo
- Sideway scissors runs – lower extremity crossovers
- Double ankle hops with dorsiflexion of foot landing on balls of the feet
- Hip mobility drills – flexion and extension hip swings.

Functional training exercises for the runner's fascia

(Collaboration with Coach Gary Winckler)

These exercises are designed to target and exploit the elastic components in the fascia net, muscle and tendon tissues. The exercise execution (mode) must be explosive, rhythmic and reactive. Attention to global body posture and technique execution is crucial to experience the full benefits.

1. Extended arm overhead with resistance: Rectus abdominus & anterior chain eccentric strengthening

Purpose

To build anterior trunk anchoring strength for abdominal and lateral wall muscles (transversus, internal and external obliques) which transmits forces from the back structures mainly thoraco-lumbar fascia (TLF). The rectus abdominus, abdominals, pelvis, hips all work eccentrically to improve balance, coordination and force transmission in single leg stance.

Position/posture

Stand upright engage trunk anterior and posterior musculature, pelvic floor and hip structures. Hands are overhead with extended elbows.

Start position

Stand facing away from anchor of elastic tubing or pulley weight cables, which is anchored at the height of extended forearm overhead. Alternately you can use an individual assistant (as an anchor) to hold the tubing.

Movement technique

- Flex one hip with flexed knee (e.g. like running stance) with your thigh in midline and your pelvis level.
- Check your alignment then begin to march or walk against the overhead resistance.
- Increase pace from a walk to a slow jog maintaining tension on the elastic strap at all times.

The key is to be as upright as possible and try not to over extend the spine/trunk but main good tension of the elastic strap as you move forward. You can also use cable pulley weights for this exercise.

Dosage

Set: 3–6
Reps: 10–20 steps
Rest: 1–2 minutes

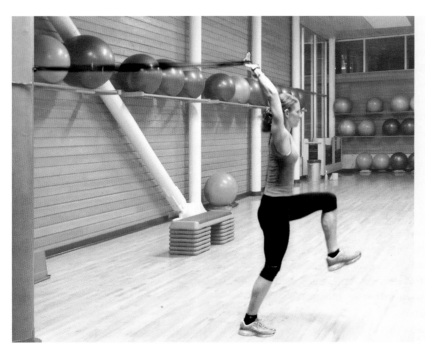

Figure 18.1
Over-head pull: Eccentric
resistance for anterior
abdominals/trunk

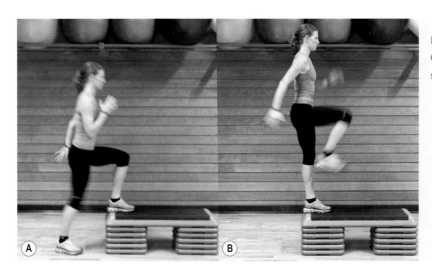

Figure 18.2 A & B
Quick step-ups and walking
step-ups

2. Quick step-ups

Purpose

To strengthen trunk, pelvis, hip, knee, ankle and foot. Improve coordination and balance in single leg stance.

Position/posture

Stand upright engage anterior and posterior trunk musculature, pelvic floor, hip structures.

Start position

Stand facing a step or box.

Movement technique

- Your front leg on the step/box (12-14") with your thigh in midline and your pelvis level-back leg on ground.
- Check your alignment then quickly push with the back leg lifting it off the ground and pushing your body straight upward.
- Step off with the leg, which was first on the box.
- Repeat alternating leg.
- The key is to push off with the back leg/leg on the ground not the front leg/leg on the box.

Dosage

Set: 3–6
Reps: 10–20
Rest: 1–2 minutes

3. Low amplitude double leg hop over mini hurdles

Purpose

Develops elastic strength, speed and explosive power of lower leg and pelvis, especially the gluteals, hamstrings, quadriceps and gastrocnemius-ankle complex. It enhances the elastic fascial components in the trunk, pelvis, hip, knee, ankle and foot.

Position/posture

Stand upright engage trunk anterior and posterior musculature, pelvic floor, hip structures. Step up two mini hurdles 6–12 inches high about one-stride length apart.

Start position

Stand upright about half a stride length in front of hurdles with shoulders slightly forward, head up. Elbows are at 90° and hands at sides with thumbs up.

Movement technique

- Begin by doing a countermovement downward and jump as high as possible flexing legs so the feet arrive under the buttocks. Bring the knees up medium high and forward for each jump to ensure maximum lift.
- To land, ensure the ankle is dorsiflexed. Jump forward again with the same cycle of leg and foot pattern.
- Execute as rapidly as possible always moving forward.
- The key is to gain moderate height and maximum distance without affecting repetition rate.

Dosage

Set: 3–6

Reps: 10–20

Rest: 1–2 minutes

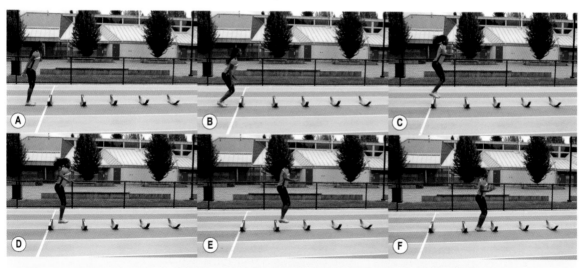

Figure 18.3 A–H
Double leg hops over mini hurdles

4. Double leg ankle jumps

Purpose

Develops elastic strength, speed and explosive power of lower leg and gastrocnemius-ankle complex. It enhances the elastic fascial components of the lower knee, ankle and foot.

Position/posture

Stand upright engage trunk anterior and posterior musculature, pelvic floor, hip structures.

Start position

Stand upright, both feet on the ground and hands by your side.

Movement technique

Push off the ground and immediately dorsiflex the ankle joint. The knee should be in extension. On landing ensure your foot is dorsiflexed and land on the balls of your feet. Repeat the sequence rapidly, maintaining an extended knee. Remain basically in the same spot.

Dosage

Sets: 4

Reps: 15–30

Rest: 2 minutes

5. Single leg ankle hops

Purpose

Develops elastic strength, speed and power of lower leg and gastrocnemius-ankle complex. It enhances the elastic fascial components of the lower knee, ankle and foot.

Position/posture

Stand upright engage trunk anterior and posterior musculature, pelvic floor, hip structures.

Start position

Stand upright both feet on the ground and hands by your side.

Movement technique

Push off the ground on one leg only leaping forward and immediately dorsiflexing the ankle joint. Try to land one stride length ahead on the ball of your feet. The knee should be in extension. On landing ensure your foot is dorsiflexed and land on the push off leg on the ball of your feet. Repeat the sequence rapidly, maintaining an extended knee and alternating legs.

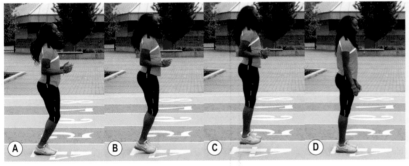

Figure 18.4 A–D
Double leg ankle jumps

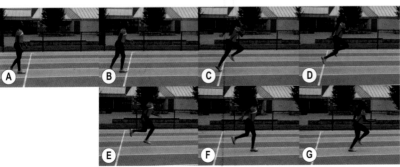

Figure 18.5 A–G
Single leg ankle hops

Dosage

Sets: 4
Reps: 15–30
Rest: 2 minutes

6. Split squat jump

Purpose

Develops elastic strength, speed and power of lower leg and pelvis especially the hip flexors, gluteals, hamstrings, quadriceps and gastrocnemius-ankle complex. It enhances the elastic strength of fascial components in trunk, pelvis, hip, knee, ankle and foot. The goal is to attain maximum height.

Position/posture

Stand upright and engage trunk anterior and posterior musculature, pelvic floor, hip structures as in the previous exercises.

Start position

Place feet shoulder-width apart, bend the front leg 45–90° at the hip and 45–90° at the knee.

Movement technique

Using counter movement technique – drop down into a half squat position and stop that movement and explode upward and forward as far as you can with a scissor like motion. Land with feet/ankle in dorsiflexion so that you land on balls of feet in a split squat position and immediately repeat the sequence initiating the pushing and jumping phase to propel the body forward. Cover about 30–40 metres.

Dosage

Sets: 4
Reps 15–30 (30–40m)
Rest: 2 minutes

7. Quick walking lunge

Purpose

Develops elastic strength, speed and power of the lower leg and pelvis especially the hip flexors, gluteals, hamstrings, quadriceps and gastrocnemius-ankle complex. It enhances the elastic strength of fascial components in trunk, pelvis, hip, knee, ankle and foot. The goal is to attain good rhythm.

Position/posture

Stand upright, engage trunk anterior and posterior musculature, pelvic floor, hip structures as in the previous exercises.

Start position

Place feet shoulder width apart, bend one leg to 90° at the hip and 90° at the knee attaining more or less a running stance.

Movement technique

Lunge foreword quickly with the unsupported leg. As soon as contact is made with the ground, recover the hind leg and use it to repeat the lunge. Land with feet/ankle in dorsiflexion so you land on the balls of the feet in a split squat position and immediately repeat the sequence initiating the pushing phase on the front leg to propel the body forward. Cover about 30–40 metres.

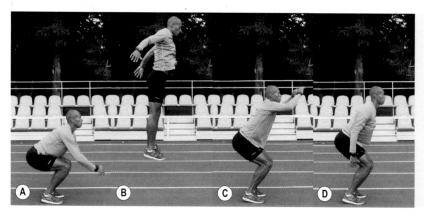

Figure 18.6 A–D
Split squat jump

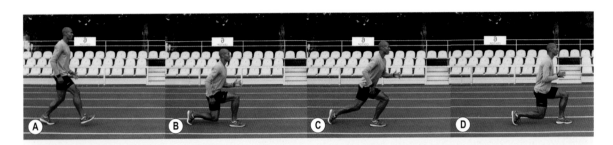

Figure 18.7 A–D

Quick walking lunge

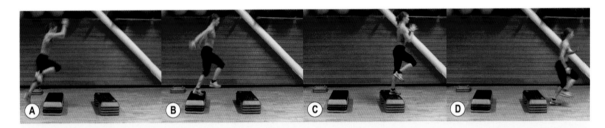

Figure 18.8 A–D

Alternate leg box Jumps

Dosage

Sets: 4

Reps: 15–30 (30–40m)

Rest: 2 minutes

8. Alternate leg box jumps

Purpose

Develops elastic strength, speed and explosive power of lower leg and pelvis especially the hip flexors, gluteals, hamstrings, quadriceps and gastrocnemius-ankle complex. It enhances the elastic fascial components in the trunk, pelvis, hip, knee, ankle and foot.

Position/posture

Stand upright, engage trunk anterior and posture musculature, pelvic floor and hip structures.

Start position

Stand upright on one leg, with one leg in front of the other, as if taking a step. Shoulders slightly forward and head up. Arms are at the sides.

Movement technique

Begin the exercise by pushing off with the back leg. Drive the knee up to the chest to achieve a maximum height and distance as possible before landing. Extend the driving foot outward quickly. Cycle the arm in contra-lateral motion in the air for balance. Repeat sequence using alternate leg on landing.

Dosage

Sets: 2–4

Reps: 8–12 (40 metres)

Rest: 2 minutes

References

Bosch, F. & Klomp, R. (2001) *Running-Biomechanics and exercise physiology in practice.* Churchill Livingstone.

Buchheit, M., Mendez-Villanueva, A., Delhomel, G., Brughelli, M. & Ahmaidi, S. (2010) Improving repeated sprint ability in young elite soccer players: Repeated shuttle sprints vs. explosive strength training. *J Strength Cond Res.* 24: 266–271.

Caspersen, C.J., Powell, K.F., Koplan, J.P., Shirley, R.W., Cambell, C.C. & Sikes, R.K. (1984) The incidence of injuries and hazards in recreational and fitness runners. *Med Sci Sports Exerc.* 16: 113–114.

Chen, C.S. et al. (1997) Geometric control of cell life and death. *Science.* 276(5317): 1425–1428.

Chino, K. et al. (2008) In vivo fascicle behaviour of synergistic muscles on concentric and eccentric plantar flexion in humans. *J Electromy Kines.* 18(1): 79–88.

Clarke, T.E., Frederick, E.C. & Hamill, C.L. (1983) The effects of shoe design parameters on rearfoot control in running. *Med Sci Sports Exerc.* 15: 376–381.

Desmouliere, A., Chapponier, C. & Gabbiani, G. (2005) Tissue repair, contraction, and the myofibroblast. *Wound Repair Regen.* 13(1): 7–12.

Dumke, C.l., Pfaffenroth, C.M., McBride, J.M. & McCauley, G.O. (2010) Relationship between muscle strength, power and stiffness and running economy in trained male runners. *Int. J Sports Physiol Perform.* 5: 249–261.

Elliott, B.C. (1990) Adolescent overuse sporting injuries: a biomechanical review. *Aust Sports Commission Program.* 23: 1–9.

Ferber, R., Davis, I.S., Noehren, B. & Hamill. J. In press Retrospective biomechanical investigation of iliotibial band syndrome in competitive female runners. *J Orthop Sports Phys Ther.*

Ferber, R., Hreljac, A. & Kendall, K. (2009) Suspected Mechanisms in the Cause of Overuse Running Injuries: A Clinical Review. *Sports & Health* May–June.

Ferrauti, A., Bergerman, M. & Fernandez-Fernandez, J. (2010) Effects of a concurrent strength and endurance training on running performance and running economy in recreational marathon runners. *J Strength Cond Res.* 24: 2770–2778.

Fleck, J., & Kraemer, W.J. (1997) Designing resistance training programs. *Library of Congress Cataloging-in-Publication Data.* 4: 88–106.

Fletcher, J.R., Esau, S.P. & MacIntosh, B.R. (2010) Changes in tendon stiffness and running economy in highly trained distance runners. *Eur J Appl Physiol.* 110: 1037–1046.

Fredericson, M., Cookingham, C.L., Chaudhari, A.M., Dowdell, B.C., Oestreicher, N. & Sahrmann, S.A. (2000) Hip abductor weakness in distance runners with iliotibial band syndrome. *Clin J Sport Med.* 10: 169–175.

Fukashiro, S., Hay, D.C. & Nagano, A. (2006) Biomechanical behavior of muscle-tendon complex during dynamic human movements. *J Appl Biomech.* 22(2): 131–147.

Fukunaga, T., Kawakami, Y., Kubo, K. & Kanehisa, H. (2002) Muscle and tendon interaction during human movements. *Exerc Sport Sci Rev.* 30(3): 106–110.

Horton, M.G. & Hall, T.L. (1989) Quadriceps femoris muscle angle: normal values and relationships with gender and selected skeletal measures. *Phys Ther.* 69: 897–901.

Hudgens, B., Scharafenberg, J., Travis Triplett, N., & McBride, J.M. (1987) Relationship Between Jumping Ability and Running Performance in Events of Varying Distance. *J Strength Cond Res.* 27(3): 563–567.

Huijing, P. (2007) Epimuscular myofascial force transmission between antagonistic and synergistic muscles can explain movement limitation in spastic paresis. *J Biomech.* 17(6): 708–724.

Huijing, P.A., & Langevin, H. (2009) Communicating about fascia: History, pitfalls and recommendations. In P.A. Huijing et al. (Eds.) *Fascia Research II: Basic Science and Implications for Conventional and Complementary Health Care.* Munich, Germany: Elsevier GmbH.

Huijing, P.A. (1999) Muscle as a collagen fiber reinforced composite: a review of force transmission in muscle and whole limb. *J Biomech.* 32(4): 329–345.

Ingber, D. (2008) Tensegrity and mechanotransduction. *J Bodyw Mov Ther.* 12(3): 198–200.

Kale, M., Alper, A., Coşkun, B. & Caner, A. (2009) Relationship among jumping performance and sprint parameters during maximum speed phase in sprinters. *J Strength Con Res.* 23: 2272–2279.

Kawakami, Y., Muraoka, T., Ito, S., Kanehisa, H. & Fukunaga, T. (2002) In vivo muscle fibre behaviour during countermovement exercise in humans reveals a significant role for tendon elasticity. *J Physiol.* 540(2): 635–646.

Kelly, C.M., Burnett, A.F. & Newton, M.J. (2010) The effects of strength training on three-kilometre performance in recreational women endurance runners. *J Strength Cond Res.* 23: 1633–1636.

Kjaer, M., Langberg, H., Heinemeier, K., Bayer, M.L., Hansen, M., Holm, L., Doessing, S., Konsgaard, M., Krogsgaard, M.R. & Magnusson, S.P. (2009) From mechanical loading to collagen synthesis, structural changes and function in human tendon. *Scand J Med Sci Sports.* 19(4): 500–510.

Kraemer, W.J. (1994) *The physiological basis for strength training in mid-life. In sports and exercise in midlife.* Ed. S.L. Gordon, 413–33. Park Ridge, IL: American Academy of Orthopaedic Surgeons.

Kraemer, W.J. & Koziris, L.P. (1992) Muscle strength training. Techniques and considerations. *Physical Therapy Practice* 2: 54–68.

Kram, R. & Dawson, T.J. (1998) Energetics and biomechanics of locomotion by red Kangaroos (Macropus rufus). *Comp Biochem Physiol B.* 120(1): 41–49.

Kubo, K. et al. (2006) Effects of series elasticity on the human knee extension torque-angle relationship in vivo. *Res Q Exercise Sport.* 77(4): 408–416.

Kubo, K., Kanehisa, H., Miyatani, M., Tachi, M. & Fukunaga, T. (2003). Effect of low-load resistance training on the tendon properties in middle-aged and elderly women. *Acta Physiol Scand.* 178(1): 25–32.

Langevin, H. et al. (2010) Fibroblast cytoskeletal remodeling contributes to connective tissue tension. *Journal of Cellular Physiology*. E-pub ahead of publication. Oct. 13, 2010.

Latrides, J. et al. (2003) Subcutaneous tissue mechanical behavior is linear and viscoelastic under uniaxial tension. *Connective Tissue Research*. 44(5): 208–217.

Lefever, S.L. (2011) *Therapeutic Exercise – Moving Toward Function*. Lippincott William & Wilkins. 14: 313–317.

Legramandi, M.A., Schepens, B. & Cavagna, G.A. (2013) Running humans attain optimal elastic bounce in their teens. *Sci. Rep.* 3. 1310; DOI:10.1038/srep01310.

Livingston, L.A. (1998) The quadriceps angle: a review of literature. *J Orthop Sports Phys Ther*. 28: 105–109.

Mackey, A.L., Heinmeier, K.M., Koskinen, S.O. & Kjaer, M. (2008) Dynamic adaptation of tendon and muscle connective tissue to mechanical loading. *Connect Tissue Res*. 49(3): 165–168.

McBride, J.M., Blow, D., Kirby, T.J., Haines, T.L., Dayne, A.M. & Triplett, NT. (2009) Relationship between maximal squats strength and five, ten and forty yard sprint time. *J Strength Cond Res*. 23: 1633–1636.

Messier, S.P. & Davis, S.E. & Curl, W.W. (1991) Etiologic factors associated with patellofemoral pain in runners. *Med Sci Sports Exerc*. 23: 1008–1015.

Meylan, C. & Malatesta, D. (2008) Effects of in-season plyometric training within soccer practice on explosive actions in young players. *J Strength Cond Res*. 23: 369–403.

Mikkola, J., Rusko, H., Nummela, A., Pollari, T. & Hakkinen, K. (2007) Concurrent endurance and explosive type strength training improves neuromuscular and anaerobic characteristics in young distance runners. *Int J Sports Med*. 28: 602–611.

Mikkola, J., Vesterinen, V., Taipale, R., Capostango, B., Hakkinen, K. & Nummela, A. (2011) Effect of resistance training regimens on treadmill running and neuromuscular performance in recreational endurance runners. *J Sports Sci*. 29: 359–1371.

Mizuno, Y., Kumagai, M. & Mattessich, S.M. (2001) Q-angle influences tibiofemoral and patellofemoral kinematics. *J Orthop Res*. 19: 834–840.

Myers, T. (2009) *Anatomy Trains: Myofascial Meridians for manual movement and Therapist*. New York: Churchill-Livingston.

Radcliffe, J. & Farentinos, R. (1985) Plyometrics: Explosive power training. Library of Congress Cataloguing-in-Publication Data. 5: 30–72.

Rochcongar, P., Pernes, J. & Carre, F. (1995) Occurrence of running injuries: a survey among 1153 runners. *Sci Sports*. 10: 15–19.

Sawicki, G.S., Lewis, C.L. & Ferris, D.P. (2009) It pays to have a spring in your step. *Exerc Sport Sci Rev*. 37(3): 130–138.

Schleip, R. (2003) Fascial plasticity – a new neurobiological explanation. *J Bodyw Mov Ther* 7(1) 11–19, 7(2): 104–116.

Schleip, R. & Klingler, W. (2007) Fascial strain hardening correlates with matrix hydration changes. In: Findley TW, Schleip R (eds.) *Fascia Research – Basic science and implications to conventional and complementary health care*. Munich: Elsevier GmbH. 51.

Smirniotou, A., Katsikas, C., Paradisis, G., Argeitaki, P., Zacharogiannis, E. & Tziortzis, S. (2008) Strength-power parameters as predictors of sprinting performance. *J Sports Me Phys Fitness* 48: 447–454.

Spurrs, R.W., Murphy, A.J. & Watsford, M.L. (2003) The effect of plyometric training on distance running performance. *Eur J Appl Physiol*. 89: 1–7.

Stanish, W.D. (1984) Overuse injuries in Athletes: a prospective. *Med Sci. Sports Exerc*. 16: 1–7.

Steven, R. et al. (1981) Role of Fascia in maintaining muscle tension and pressure. *Appl Physiol: Respirat Environ Exercise Physiol*. 51(2): 317–320.

Tapale, R.S., Mikkola, J., Nummela, A., Vesterinen, V., Capostango, B., Walker, S., Gitonga, D., Kraemer, W.J. & Hakkinen, K. (2010) Strength training in endurance runners. *Int J Sports Med*. 3: 468–476

Tippett, S. & Voight, M.L. (1995) Functional progressions for sports rehabilitation. Library of Congress Cataloging-in-Publication Data. 6: 74–75.

Witvrouw, E., Lysens, R., Bellemans, J., Peers, K. & Vanderstraeten, G. (2000) Open versus closed kinetic chain exercises for patellofemoral pain: a prospective, randomized study. *Am J Sports Med*. 28: 687–694.

Further reading

Bissas, A.l. & Havenetidis, K. (2008). The use of various strength-power tests as predictors of sprint running performance. *J Sports Med Phys Fitness* 48: 49–54.

Chaudhry, H., Schleip, R., Ji, Z., Bukiet, B., Maney, M. & Findley, T. (2008). Three-dimensional mathematical model for deformation of human fasciae in manual therapy. *J Am Osteopath Assoc*. 108(8): 379–90.

Cichanowski, H.R., Schmitt, J.S., Johnson, R.J & Niemuth, P.E. (2007) Hip strength in collegiate female athletes with patellofemoral pain. *Med Sci Sports Exerc*. 39: 1227–1232.

Duffey, M.J., Martin, D.F., Cannon, D.W., Craven, T. & Messier, S.P. (2000) Etiologic factors associated with anterior knee pain in distance runners. *Med Sci Sports Exerc*. 11: 1825–1832.

Dugan, S.A. & Bhat, K.P. (2005) Biomechanics and analysis in running gait. *Phys Med Rebabil Chin N Am*. 16: 603–623.

Fagan, V. & Delahunt, E. (2008) Patellofemoral pain syndrome: a review on the associated neuromuscular deficits and current treatment options [published online ahead of print July 14, 2008]. *Br J Sports Med PMID*: 18424487.

Ferber, R. & Kendall, K.D. (2007) Biomechanical approach to rehabilitation of lower extremity musculoskeletal injuries in runners. *J Athl Train*. 42: S114.

Hennessy, L. & Kilty, J. (2001) Relationship of the stretch-shortening cycle to sprint performance in trained female athlete. *J Strength Cond Res*. 15: 326–331.

Hunter, J.P., Marshall, R.N. & McNair, P.J. (2005) Relationship between ground reaction force impulse and kinematics of sprint-running acceleration. *J Appl Biomech.* 21: 31–43.

Grinnell, F. (2008) Fibroblast mechanics in three dimensional collagen matrices. *J Bodyw Mov Ther.* 12(3): 191–193.

Grinnell, F. & Petroll, W. (2010) Cell motility and mechanics in three-dimensional collagen matrices. *Annual Review of Cell and Developmental Biology.* 26: 335–361.

Hrysomallis, C. (2012) The effectiveness of resisted movement training on sprinting and jumping performance. *J Strength Cond Res.* 26: 299–306.

Hudgens, B., Scharafenberg. J., Travis Triplett, N. & McBride, J.M. (2013) Relationship Between Jumping Ability and Running Performance in Events of Varying Distance. *J Strength Cond Res.* 27(3): 563–567.

Ingber, D. (1998) The architecture of life. *Scientific American.* January. 48–57.

Kraemer, W.J. (1982) Weight training: What you don't know will hurt you. *Wyoming Journal of Health, Physical Education, Recreation and Dance.* 5: 8–11.

Koplan, J.P., Powell, K.E. & Sikes, R.K. (1982) The risk of exercise: an epidemiological study of the benefits and risks of running. *JAMA.* 248: 3118–3121.

Langevin, H. (2006) Connective tissue: A body-wide signaling network? *Medical Hypotheses.* 66(6): 1074–1077.

Macera, C.A., Pate, R.R. & Powell, K.E. (1989) Predicting lower-extremity injuries among habitual runners. Arch Intern Med. 149: 2565–2568.

Myers, T.W. (1997) The Anatomy Trains. *J Bodyw Mov Ther* 1(2): 91–101.

CHAPTER 19

Understanding mechano-adaptation of fascial tissues: Application to sports medicine

Raúl Martínez Rodríguez and Fernando Galán del Río

Introduction

Physical activity is associated with an improved quality of life. However, being physically active carries a risk factor of injury and re-injury (McBain et al., 2012). It is estimated there are approximately three million annual injuries in the United States directly related to organised sports. Of these, approximately 770,000 require physical treatment (Armsey & Hosey, 2004). In this context it is necessary to understand the influence of the fascial system on both the origin of muscular and tendinous injuries related to sport practice and on their associated treatment. This is mainly from the perspective of the connective tissue role, not only acting as a 'packing organ', but also as a mechanosensitive tissue capable of restructuring and redesigning itself under various stimuli derived from repetitive overuse (Schleip et al., 2012) (Chapter 1). Thus, high mechanical demands carve the soft tissue, thereby generating an overcompensation mechanism, on both contractile and non-contractile areas, and feature a collagen synthesis increase in muscular fascia, tendon, capsules and ligaments (Khan & Scott, 2009). As a consequence, the involvement of fascial tissue in human movement, as regards its capacity to absorb and transmit mechanical forces via different musculoskeletal structures, may be distorted and, hence, be at the origin of local and remote dysfunctions. From a therapeutic standpoint, skillful application of manual forces on the fascial system conditions and reverses collagen overproduction processes, thus improving tissue functionality and optimising rehabilitation mechanisms of musculoskeletal injuries.

This chapter also introduces fascial techniques as part of the rehabilitation protocols and treatment of arthrofibrosis, following bone and joint injuries after sport trauma.

Tissue adaptation of muscle fascia and tendon from overuse

Through a complex mechanism, known as mechanotransduction (Chapters 2 and 5), mechanical forces distributed and transmitted over the tridimensional and continuous connective tissue network, act at cellular level and eventually induce morphological and architectural modifications on the connective tissue (Ingber, 2008). In this way, tendon and muscular fascia respond to altered levels of physical activity by converting mechanical loading into tissue adaptation, for example, high-load resistance training induces an increase in Type I collagen synthesis that peaks three days post-exercise and returns to basal levels after five days (Langberg et al., 2000).

It is widely accepted that increasing training loads are necessary in order to improve an athlete's performance. The problem arises when this leads to diminishing rest interval lengths between training sessions and competition periods. As a matter of fact, increased loads are tolerated only through interspersed periods of rest and recovery-training periodisation (Kreher & Schwarz, 2012). In other words, collagen turnover normalisation of the muscular fascia and tendon down to basal levels requires a proper balance between training/competition intensity and recovery period length after exercise. Therefore, when this very relevant aspect is not properly considered, repetitive overuse and lack of rest bring about a failure of collagen turnover, which leads to collagen overproduction and undesirable structural changes (fascial restriction) (Chapter 1).

Moreover, it is well worth enquiring into the soft tissue's behavior when high mechanical demands are sustained by the athlete on an already highly strained fascial network. Interestingly, fibroblasts, cells with a high level of mechanosensitivity, aside from their reaction to biochemical cues, respond differently to different distinct degrees of pre-tension states within the fascial body network. Thus, the higher the fascial stiffness the higher the collagen synthesis and buildup within the extracellular matrix (Langevin et al., 2010). In other words, the same type of physical activity generates different adaptive responses from the fascial tissue according to the preceding strain and stiffness levels. In the short term, increasing training and competition loads would increase fascial tissue resistance so as to ensure optimal force transmission at each muscular contraction. However, in the medium term, the ensuing restructuring process would give rise to a stiffer fascial network, hence decisively modifying the soft tissue's viscoelastic behavior. In this context, the decreasing local elasticity limits the fascial system's capacity for deformation and force absorption, which magnifies the risk of musculoskeletal injury (Purslow, 2010).

Fascial stiffness in myofascial and tendon injury

Different potential risk factors have been proposed for acute musculoskeletal injuries (muscle strain). Amongst others, insufficient warm-up, strength imbalances, muscular fatigue and, to a significant extent according to the theoretical frameworks discussed above, an increase in myofascial stiffness or the existence of a previous muscle injury associated to fibrosis scar with no deformability stand out (Petersen & Hölmich, 2005).

Furthermore, muscle injury healing is a complex process including three overlapping phases: (1) degeneration and inflammation, (2) muscle regeneration and (3) fibrosis defined as the replacement of normal structural elements of the tissue by an excessive accumulation of non-functional fibrotic tissue (Jarvinen et al., 2005). The fibrotic phase depends on the contribution of particular growth factors, including transforming growth factor-β1 (TGF-β1), a potent stimulator of collagen

proliferation, which can induce myofibroblastic differentiation of fibroblasts and differentiation of myogenic cells into myofibroblasts in injured skeletal muscle, increasing skeletal muscle fibrosis after injury (Tomasek et al., 2002) (Chapter 1). Interestingly, recent findings suggest that TGF-β1 activation is partly controlled by tissue stiffness and myofibroblast contractile forces (Hinz, 2009). Therefore, based on the previous rationale, it is worth highlighting the influence of the muscle injury mechanical surroundings (high-tension state matrix) on the excessive proliferation of pathological collagen crosslinks presenting multidirectional arrangement. Thus, fibrotic scar tissue would decrease fascial tissue's capacity to deform and adapt (local elasticity) when subject to high-amplitude, high-velocity movements. This process, in turn, would distort mobility between the fascial interfaces and, ultimately, would lead to hypertrophic scarring with high risk of muscle re-injury.

Similarly, the increase of fascial stiffness directly influences the development of tendinous injuries, since the tendon is a specialised myofascial terminal structure. Thus, force generated by muscle is transferred to bones via tendons to produce movement. However, this force, from muscle to tendon, is not only transmitted by each myofibre, made up of sarcomeres arranged in series and equipped with a myotendinous junction (myotendinous force transmission), but also the existing fascial continuity, between epymysium, perimysium, endomysium and paratenon, epitenon, endotenon (Chapter 1). This provides an important functional continuity that also enables force transmission via the muscular supporting connective tissue (myofascial force transmission) (Huijing 2009). In detail, muscle fascia forms a continuous honeycomb tied together by interfaces or connective bonds, which, in turn, constitute an interfascial trabecular system that provides mechanically competent links and hence favours force transmission to the tendon through the musculoskeletal cell matrix (Passerieux et al., 2007). Additionally, the existence of intermuscular septa and other collagen-reinforced structures provides important stiff connections between agonist and antagonist muscles, from which force transmission is transmitted to the tendon. Contrary to a common misconception, tendons are extensible tissues which exhibit elastic and time-dependent properties and also take part in the overall function of the myofascia-tendon complex. In general, mechanical loading at physiological levels is beneficial to tendons that directly respond to physical activity by increased metabolic activity and collagen synthesis. However, the mechanical properties of tendons, including their Young's modulus (measure of the stiffness of an elastic material), may suffer modifications in response to excessive loading (Wang et al., 2012). In other words, mechanical loading rise on the tendon channeled through the fascial network, described above, renders the tendon more load-resistant but it also considerably decreases its stress-susceptibility (Kjaer et al., 2006) (Chapter 5). Therefore, as part of the tendinous injuries' treatment protocol, it seems essential to correctly balance and dissipate the forces transmitted to the tendon from the muscle fascia. This can be achieved by increasing the elastic capacity of the latter, thereby favoring tensional homeostasis and providing the proper balance between absorption and transmission of forces towards the tendon.

Contribution of fascial therapy

At this point, it is necessary to provide answers to the following questions: Can pre-tension states be modified by manual therapy? Could cell and tissue physiology be influenced using fascial therapy? Considering the high mechanosensitivity exhibited by fibroblasts, would it be possible to exploit this peculiarity according to the treatment's specific purpose? Going one step further, from a global perspective, how could these new concepts be introduced as part of the classic models for prevention, treatment and rehabilitation of musculoskeletal injuries?

Ideally, fascial tissue must be strong enough to transmit forces and elastic enough to absorb forces and to prevent tearing under externally applied strains (Purslow, 2002). At present, with regards to muscle injury treatment (during the phases of muscle regeneration and fibrosis) and tendinous injury treatment, different rehabilitation programmes focus on increasing resistance and fascial tissue capacity to sustain loads of muscular

contraction, through therapeutic exercise (Khan & Scott, 2009). Along these lines, a commonly suggested primary intervention involves pain-free protocols with a progressive approach: eccentric exercises inducing longitudinal arrangement of collagen fibres and overload running programmes (Petersen & Hölmich, 2005).

However, when the athlete is experiencing a state of high local and general fascial pre-tension, which is frequently observed in a sports context, it will prove necessary to include, within prevention and treatment protocols, techniques specifically addressed to increasing elasticity and deformation capacity of stiff fascial areas. To this same end, classical rehabilitation programmes comprise pain-free stretching practices and other techniques specifically directed at the restricted area, such as deep friction massage, Graston technique, shock wave therapy, and/or ultrasound (Hammer, 2008) (Sussmich-Leitch et al., 2012). However, from the authors' clinical experience involving amateur and elite professional athletes, these measures might prove insufficient. In this context, and according to the previously examined concepts, it becomes apparent that there is a need to apply skillful manual forces over the restricted areas in order to restore and improve the fascial system's capacity to absorb and dissipate repetitive mechanical loads.

Regeneration and fibrosis

During the initial phases of the healing process, within the area of ruptured and necrotised myofibres, there are a proliferation of inflammatory cells and myogenic satellite cells that activate, divide, differentiate and, finally, fuse (regeneration), owing to the buildup of connective tissue bridges between the injury ends (fibrosis) (Jarvinen et al., 2005). Initially the scar tissue is characterised by a disorganised and random arrangement of the new collagen fibres. The absence of parallelism of these fibres to their original force transmission axis is a feature common to scars missing mechanical stimuli. Thus, even though sustained immobilisation improves muscle fibre penetration into the connective tissue, their orientation is not parallel to the uninjured muscle fibres' main axis. On the other hand, early mobilisation favours collagen production and proper orientation, though dense scar formation in the injury area may prevent muscle regeneration. Moreover, the application of early motion exercises, after short immobilisation, encourages better muscle fibre penetration throughout the connective tissue and better orientation of regenerated muscle fibres.

In any event, it is important that exercises are pain free in order to prevent further injury during rehabilitation (Jarvinen et al., 2007). With the aim of assisting the proper development of this process during the initial phases of the treatment, matrices should be kept highly tensed so as to enhance collagen synthesis and the correct linear arrangement of the injured area. To this effect, it is suggested that the initial reflex contracture be maintained as an ideal tension habitat so as to increase biosynthetic activity and movement of fibroblasts towards the scar/bridge region. Additionally, the practice of pain free isometric and concentric strength exercises is recommended. In any case, collagen overproduction, during the proliferation phase, might limit myotubes penetration throughout the connective tissue scar and, subsequently, prevent a strong muscle fibre coupling between both injury ends. As described above, this is what happens during muscle injury treatment after early mobilisation, and also when scarring processes are rushed.

This normally occurs within a professional sport context, by the introduction of strength exercises lacking proper load management procedures during the initial healing phases, aiming at rapidly obtaining a scar with the highest possible level of functionality. In this context, eccentric strength training can stimulate the activation and proliferation of satellite stem cells that participate in the skeletal muscle regeneration. However, it also induces an excessive proliferation of collagen and dense scar tissue within the injured muscle. This gradual development of fibrotic scar tissue within the injured area hinders muscle regeneration and, ultimately, leads to an incomplete functional recovery characterised by a reduced contractile function and muscle extensibility.

In effect, considering that remodeling and reconstruction processes may stretch well into 12 months, it is frequently found that apparently healed myofascial injuries are, in fact, highly scarred, which increases the risk of re-injury (Baoge et al., 2012). In these cases, the pathological collagen crosslinks that take place are associated with increased local tension, and reduced elastic capacity, which are adjustments derived from the scar adaptation to the early multidirectional, high-speed and high-amplitude loads and movements. Therefore, in the medium-to-long term, this healing model's reliability seems somehow limited. Additionally, over the past few years it has been common practice in sports medicine to utilise biological agents, such as autologous growth factors (platelet rich plasma), that can accelerate the healing process by releasing high doses of growth factors to the damaged tissue (Creaney & Hamilton, 2008). However, as before, connective tissue proliferation excess, associated with the release of different growth factors, might decisively impair the achievement of the adequate regeneration-fibrosis balance and retractile scar formation, thereby resulting in the same functional deficiencies described above.

Consequently, the authors suggest manual treatment in this context (high-tension matrix), which is grounded in the need to accomplish a restoration of the pre-injury status of damaged tissue, avoiding excessive collagen proliferation and involving the use of the scar modeling technique. This manual procedure, described later, favours the rearrangement of the tissue's viscoelastic behavior and allows the release of the elastic energy accumulated (not dissipated) within the scar's surrounding area, thereby encouraging the extracellular matrix muscle to return from a high-tension to a low-tension state.

Tendon injury treatment

It is important not to isolate the tendinous structure during the design of rehabilitation programs. On the contrary, in addition to the localised treatment applied onto the collagen cross-linking and adhesions between the tendon and the surrounding peritendinous tissues, it is necessary to stress the importance of applying treatment to the rigid interfaces. In effect, as described above, excessive mechanical loads increase stiffness in fascial intermuscular septa.

This, in turn, intensifies force transmission and repetitive traction loading towards terminal regions. Tendons are mechano-responsive tissues, in so far as they adaptively change their structure and function in response to altered mechanical loading conditions (Chapter 5). This is why repetitive overuse initially causes cell matrix changes that thicken and harden the tendon (reactive tendinopathy). This fact becomes especially obvious throughout gestures that combine high articular amplitude movements and eccentric contractions, during which a stiff fascial network is continually tensed by external forces (distancing of bone levers) and internal forces (muscular contraction). At this stage, a proper load management procedure, based on the reduction of mechanical demands, would grant the tendon enough time to progressively adapt. Once injured, the tendon undergoes a slow and spontaneous healing process (tendon disrepair) that results in the formation of scar tissue and a loss of normal collagen fibre organisation. In this context, progressive exercise, particularly eccentric exercise, increases collagen production and restructures the matrix (Cook & Purdam, 2009) (Wang et al., 2012). Moreover, from the authors' clinical experience, prior to the execution of the eccentric and/or stretching exercises protocols, the introduction of different manual techniques, as described below, is proposed, to normalise the fascial network's tensional homeostasis and reduce the previously mentioned interfaces stiffness. Thus, the tendon, as a dynamic and mechanoresponsive tissue can favourably respond to controlled loading associated with matrix remodeling after injury. This is provided that, concurrently, the fascial system has been equipped with the capacity to dissipate and distribute through the continuity of the fascial network the excess of mechanical tension.

Scar modeling technique

This technique, developed by the authors, is used, in general, to treat fascial restrictions, and specifically, it is employed for scar therapy in chronic myofascial injuries. To that end, different mechanical stimuli are manually performed in a controlled way (directed manual mechanotransduction) (Martínez et al., 2013). Initially,

the combination of different forces can be used by means of manual application of compression, traction and torsion vectors that deform the fascial tissue, which allows the therapist to form a first impression of the resistance level (barrier) over the restricted area (Figure 19.1). Thus, the tissue is held in a certain line of tension over a sustained period of variable time (30–90 seconds), until a release of tension is perceived. At this moment, contact points and the tissue's deformation vectors are repositioned, until a new barrier is felt. Within this iterative process, these steps are successively repeated until a normalisation of the tension and stiffness of the scar area is eventually detected (Pilat, 2003). In this manner, the pursuit of tensional homeostasis by the therapist's manual treatments, guided by the release (jumps) of accumulated elastic energy in the restricted areas, would cause a 3D reorganisation of fascial interfaces on a macroscopic level (through interfaces between different fascial layers). This results in tensional normalisation on the microscopic level (tensional re-harmonisation between the cytoskeleton and extracellular matrix through receptor integrins). This re-harmonisation would enable cell function normalisation and would provide medium-term remodeling of the extracellular matrix (Martínez & Galán, 2013) (Chapter 1). Other authors consider the possibility of causing structural changes in fibrosis, through the decrease of cross-links between collagen fibres (Tozzi, 2012). Moreover, some benefits of myofascial therapies may be due to neurophysiological effects. In this sense, Schleip (2003) suggests that, in fascial techniques, the manual induction process would cause modulations at different levels of the nervous system, through stimulation of mechanoreceptors present in fascia and responsive to manual pressure and deformation. For example, therapeutic stimulation of free nerve endings in fascia may trigger a vasomotor reaction that leads to an increased hydration of the treated area (Chapter 4).

In conclusion, from a global rehabilitative approach, direct fascial techniques allow the collagen's restructuring capacity to increase prior to the execution of strength and stretching exercises. This is aimed at encouraging the longitudinal arrangement of the collagen's and fibroblasts' tension axes, the application of eccentric loads on deformable matrices presenting a smaller number of pathological crosslinks and better hydration within fascial interfaces. This makes more sense than performing loading therapy on rigid matrices with weak sliding capacity between fascial layers (Figure 19.2).

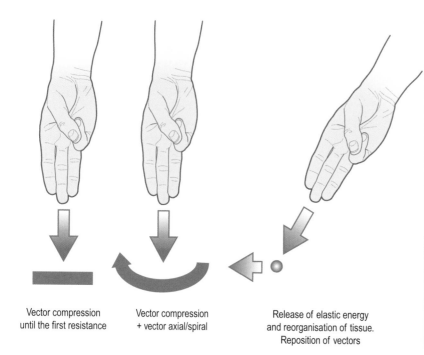

Vector compression until the first resistance

Vector compression + vector axial/spiral

Release of elastic energy and reorganisation of tissue. Reposition of vectors

Figure 19.1

Scar modeling technique based in axial and compressive vectors

Contact phase: initial vector compression maintained by the finger flexor tone of the second, third and fourth fingers. Stimulation phase using spiroid/circular vector to generate a maintained tension against a sense of resistance.

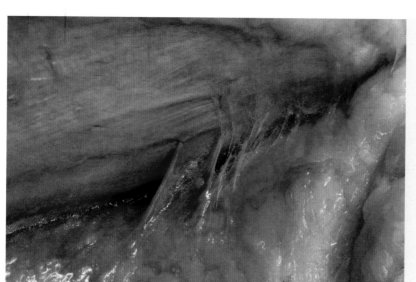

Figure 19.2

Thigh side in fresh corpse dissection

Pathological collagen crosslinks between superficial and deep fascia. The figure depicts the entrapment and perforation of a cutaneous nerve. The importance of hydration is highlighted.

(Courtesy of Andrjez Pilat)

Real time sonoelastography (RTSE) in myofascial injury

To validate therapeutic techniques it works well in the authors' experience to use ultrasound elastography for the assessment of mechanical tissue properties in real time, such as tissue stiffness and elasticity (Chapter 24). Interestingly, RTSE reveals the elasticity curve registering the myofascial tissue pretension during repair and fibrosis (sonoelastographic evolution control). This information is then used to conduct the proper treatment according to the variation of the mechanical properties response of myofascial tissue after fascial therapy is performed (Martínez & Galán 2013) (Figure 19.3).

Bone and joint injuries after sport trauma

For each type of bone and joint injury after sport trauma, rehabilitation programmes must be case specific and consider, provided no collateral risks are detected, the possibility of replacing complete immobilisation by early, controlled and progressive mobilisation with the purpose of increasing matrix synthesis and enhance new collagen fibre orientation parallel to the stress lines of the normal collagen fibres. However, because of the potential increased risk of adverse

events, and the insufficient background evidence so as to determine the exact starting point after surgery concerning mobilisation, some clinicians hold a conservative approach. Then again, arthrofibrosis is a well-known sequela of bone and joint injuries after sports trauma, when treatment choice has involved immobilisation and protection of the injured area for primary treatment or post-operative management (Kannus, 2000).

Historically, conventional rehabilitation programmes base their treatment of decreased range of articular motion on the application of stretching and passive and active articular mobilisations (anterior-posterior glide mobilisation). However, within this context, the connective tissue intimately related to the joint (capsule, ligaments, periarticular myofascia) dehydrates, loses its elastic capacity, and presents considerable disorganisation (intercrossing collagen fibres and capsule shrinkage). As a result, deformation and sliding capacity between fascial layers is limited and, consequently, intimate gliding and movement capacity between articular surfaces is also reduced (gliding, bearing, translation and/or rotation).

Therefore, it seems convenient to introduce, prior to the application of articular techniques, fascial tissue manipulation directly addressed to the fascial periarticular system. This therapy would

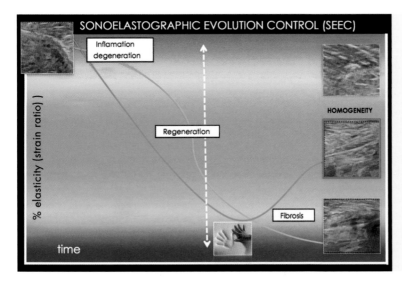

Figure 19.3

Schematic relationship between the physiological scarring process and the elastography chromatic scale

An elasticity curve that shows the ideal moment for scar modeling implementation in order to prevent fibrosis. The green line represents cicatrization with restitution of local elasticity after manual 'modeling' of the scar and the blue line shows cicatrization with elasticity loss and a high risk of relapse. (From Martínez & Galán et al., 2013, with permission)

comprise different alternatives, such as scar modeling technique, deep massage, deep frictions and neuromuscular techniques. This methodology, on the one hand, intends to induce the rehydration of the fundamental substance (thixotropic reaction), enabling collagen fibres to move friction-free against each other, and on the other to encourage the rupture of pathological collagen cross links. Subsequently, the execution of active progressive loading exercises is also suggested in order to enhance the organisation and arrangement of collagen fibres parallel to the main axes of mechanical tension.

Moreover, it is important to highlight that stiffness within the periarticular myofascial tissue may alter muscle tone regulation and negatively influence protocols designed for muscle strengthening, proprioceptive re-education and training for restoration of sport-based movements. All three are required during the treatment process involving these types of injuries. This is intimately related to the role of the fascial tissue as a substrate of proprioception (mechanosensitive signaling system) and to the function of mechanoreceptors (Stecco et al., 2007) (Van der Wal, 2009), specifically of muscle spindles, which are specialised structures of connective tissue inserted into the muscle fascia (endomysium and perymysium) (Chapter 1). They are characterised by being highly sensitive to even small tension variations throughout the fascial network. Therefore, considering that the main stimulus for these receptors is deformation, it can be inferred that an increase in stiffness and disorganisation within the fascial system, after performance of immobilisation protocols, may decisively alter the capacity of adaptation of such a system, thus undermining its adaptive response before different stimuli involving traction, torsion or compression forces. In conclusion, the authors emphasise the importance of applying manual structural techniques so as to model the periarticular fascial tissue, in order to normalise the stimulatory mechanism of mechanoreceptors, thereby enabling effective efferent motor responses during muscle strengthening and proprioceptive protocols.

Summary

If fibroblast behaviour depends on surrounding mechanical processes, it is relevant to try to fully understand these processes, not only during prevention and treatment of myofascial and tendon injury, but also in bone and joint injuries after sport trauma. Most of the existing rehabilitation protocols offer programmes involving progressive loading exercises. However, based on the authors' clinical experience with fascia, this widespread approach would not consider the pre-existing state of collapse and restriction of the fascial network associated with a repetitive overuse pattern common in the sport's field. Therefore, the authors would like to stress the benefits of initiating any rehabilitation process by using manual therapy on the restricted and fibrotic areas, aimed at encouraging the rearrangement and remodeling of fascial architecture.

References

Armsey, T.D. & Hosey, R.G. (2004) Medical aspects of sports: epidemiology of injuries, preparticipation physical examination, and drugs in sports. *Clin Sports Med.* 23(2): 255–279.

Baoge, L., Vanden Steen, S., Rimbaut, N., Philips, E. et al., (2012) Treatment of skeletal muscle injury: a review. *ISRN Orthopedics.*

Creaney, L. & Hamilton, B. (2008) Growth factor delivery methods in the management of sports injuries: the state of play. *Br J Sports Med.* 42(5): 314–320.

Cook, J. & Purdam, C. (2009) Is tendon pathology a continuum? A pathology model to explain the clinical presentation of load-induced tendinopathy. *Br J Sports Med.* 43: 409–416.

Fredericson, M., Cookingham, C.L., Chaudhari, A.M., Dowdell, B.C., Oestreicher, N. & Sahrmann, S.A. (2000) Hip abductor weakness in distance runners with iliotibial band syndrome. *Clin J Sport Med.* 10: 169–175.

Hammer, W.I. (2008) The effect of mechanical load on degenerated soft tissue. *J Bodyw Mov Ther.* 12(3): 245–256.

Hinz, B. (2009) Tissue stiffness, latent TGF-beta1 activation, and mechanical signal transduction: implications for the pathogenesis and treatment of fibrosis. *Current Rheumatology Reports* 11(2): 120–126.

Huijing, P.A. (2009) Epimuscular myofascial force transmission: a historical review and implications for new research. *J Biomech.* 42(1): 9–21.

Ingber, D.E. (2008) Tensegrity and mechanotransduction. *J Bodyw Mov Ther.* 12: 198–200.

Jarvinen, T.A., Jarvinen, T.L., Kaariainen, M. & Kalimo, H. (2005) Muscle injuries: biology and treatment. *Am J Sports Med.* 33(5): 745–764.

Jarvinen, T.A., Jarvinen, T.L., Kaariainen, M., Aarimaa, V. et al. (2007) Muscle injuries: optimising recovery. *Best Practice & Research: Clinical Rheumatology* 21(2): 317–331.

Kannus, P. (2000) Immobilization or early mobilization after an acute soft-tissue injury? *Phys Sportsmed.* 28(3): 55–63.

Khan, K.M. & Scott, A. (2009) Mechanotherapy: how physical therapists' prescription of exercise promotes tissue repair. *Br J Sports Med.* 43: 247–252.

Kjaer, M., Magnusson, P., Krogsgaard, M., Boysen Møller, J., Olesen, J., Heinemeier, K., Hansen, M., Haraldsson, B., Koskinen, S., Esmarck, B. & Langberg, H. (2006) Extracellular matrix adaptation of tendon and skeletal muscle to exercise. *J Anat.* 208(4): 445–450.

Kreher, J.B. & Schwartz, J.B. (2012) Overtraining syndrome: a practical guide. *Sports Health.* 4(2): 128–138.

Langberg, H., Skovgaard, D., Asp, S. & Kjaer, M. (2000) Time pattern of exercise-induced changes in type I collagen turnover after prolonged endurance exercise in humans. *Calcif Tissue Int.* 67(1): 41–4.

Langevin, H.M., Storch, K.N., Snapp, R.R., Bouffard, N.A. et al. (2010) Tissue stretch induces nuclear remodelling in connective tissue fibroblasts. *Histochemistry and Cell Biology* 133 (4): 405–415.

Martínez Rodríguez, R. & Galán del Río, F. (2013) Mechanistic basis of manual therapy in myofascial injuries. Sonoelastographic evolution control. *J Bodyw Mov Ther.* 17(2): 221–234.

McBain, K., Shrier. I., Shultz, R., Meeuwisse, W.H. et al. (2012) Prevention of sports injury I: a systematic review of applied biomechanics and physiology outcomes research. *Br J Sports Med.* 46(3): 169–173.

Magnusson, S.P., Langberg, H. & Kjaer, M. (2010) The pathogenesis of tendinopathy: balancing the response to loading. *Nat Rev Rheumatol.* 6: 262–268.

Passerieux, E., Rossignol, R., Letellier, T. & Delage, J.P. (2007) Physical continuity of the perimysium from myofibers to tendons: Involvement in lateral force transmission in skeletal muscle. *J Struct Biol.* 159: 19–28.

Petersen, J. & Hölmich P. (2005) Evidence based prevention of hamstring injuries in sport. *Br J Sports Med.* 39: 319–23.

Pilat, A. (2003) *Inducción Miofascial.* 1st ed. McGraw Hill Interamericana.

Purslow, P. (2002) The structure and functional significance of variations in the connective tissue within muscle. Comparative Biochemistry and Physiology – Part A: *Molecular & Integrative Physiology* 133(4): 947–66.

Purslow, P. (2010) Muscle fascia and force transmission. *J Bodyw & Mov Ther.* 14: 411–417.

Schleip, R., Findley, T., Chaitow, L. & Huijing, P. (eds.) (2012) *Fascia – The Tensional Network of the Human Body.* Churchill Livingstone Elsevier.

Schleip, R. (2003) Fascial plasticity – a new neurobiological explanation. *J Bodyw Mov Ther.* 7(1): 11–19, 7(2): 104–116.

Stecco, C., Gagey, O., Belloni, A., Pozzuoli, A., Porzionato, A., Macchi, V., Aldegheri, R., De Caro, R. & Delmas V. (2007) Anatomy of the deep fascia of the upper limb. Second part: study of innervation. *Morphologie.* 91(292): 38–43.

Sussmilch-Leitch, S.P., Collins, N.J., Bialocerkowski, A.E., Warden, S.J. & Crossley, K.M. (2012) Physical therapies for Achilles tendinopathy: systematic review and meta-analysis. *J Foot Ankle Res.* 5(15): 1146–1162.

Tomasek, J.J., Gabbiani, G., Hinz, B., Chaponnier, C., et al. (2002) Myofibroblasts and mechano-regulation of connective tissue remodelling. *Nature Reviews Molecular Cell Biology.* 3(5): 349–363.

Tozzi, P. (2012) Selected fascial aspects of osteopathic practice. *J Bodyw Mov Ther.* 16(4): 503–519.

Van der Wal, J. (2009) The Architecture of the Connective Tissue in the Musculoskeletal System—An Often Overlooked Functional Parameter as to Proprioception in the Locomotor Apparatus. *Int J Ther Massage Bodywork* 2(4): 9–23.

Wang, J., Guo, Q. & Li, B. (2012) Tendon biomechanics and mechanobiology – a mini review of basic concepts and recent advancements. *J Hand Ther.* 25(2): 133–41.

Further reading

Kjaer, M. (2004) Role of extracellular matrix in adaptation of tendon and skeletal muscle to mechanical loading. *Physiological Rev.* 84(2): 649–698.

Ophir, J., Céspedes, I., Ponnekanti, H., Yazdi, Y. et al. (1991) Elastography: a quantitative method for imaging the elasticity of biological tissues. *Ultrasound Imaging.* 13(2): 111–134.

CHAPTER 20

How to train fascia in football coaching

Klaus Eder and Helmut Hoffmann

Positive and negative influences on the myofascial system in football

Excellence in any sport, including football or soccer, demands a sport-specific level of physical conditioning, combined with corresponding technical skill, to ensure mastery of sport-specific patterns of movement, as well as the tactical insights needed to engage in competitive play.

Football, in particular, is characterised by a wide range of stereotypical patterns of movement that are sport, or discipline, specific. If these patterns of movement are performed cumulatively in sufficient number, over a prolonged period of time, it is reasonable to expect that these football-specific movement stimuli will provoke reactions that manifest themselves as adaptations of the particular biological structures involved (joints, ligaments, neuromeningeal and myofascial structures) to permit adequate 'processing' of the incident stresses and loads (Chapter 5). Over the past 20 years, in the course of delivering medical care to football players at virtually every performance level from the amateur to professional athletes who represent their countries internationally, we have empirically identified a wide diversity of changes to which football players are prone. In this context, because it involves the side-specific dominance of a kicking leg and a support leg, football is also characterised by corresponding asymmetric differences in adaptations and changes, particularly with regard to the myofascial system.

As a rule these adaptations maximise the quality of the sport-specific patterns of movement and thus serve to enhance the individual's performance in the particular sport. On the other hand, they are also often the cause of changes in muscular stress patterns within the sport and may, in certain circumstances, lead to abnormal loading or overloading of the musculoskeletal and myofascial structures involved. Knowledge of the football-specific changes affecting the musculoskeletal and myofascial systems enables coaches and the medical team to assess any structural and functional implications more easily and lays the groundwork so that athletes can engage in structure-specific preparation and recovery routines. The information below is intended to raise awareness among coaches and the medical team concerning the existence of football-specific adaptations and to ensure that these phenomena receive proper attention.

Football-specific changes and adaptations involving the musculoskeletal system

The following sections outline typical football-specific adaptations, with a special focus on myofascial changes that are encountered repeatedly in practice even in the absence of injuries. A correspondingly high probable incidence of such changes must be anticipated in the active football player (that may also persist for years afterwards) and it is important to bear this in mind when preparing for training and competitive matches. The following categories of change figure prominently in football and are deserving of attention:

Changes in the kicking leg due to ball contact

By definition, the game of football entails a varying number of contacts with the ball.

In this process, the mechanical stresses associated with ball contact, if generated in sufficient number and magnitude, provoke changes in the biological structures. During the course of evolution, nature has developed our musculoskeletal system, and especially our lower limbs as components of the pelvic-leg axis, specifically for locomotion, walking and running (Chapters 13 and 17). Our feet with their longitudinal and transverse arches are ingeniously designed to cushion the impact of our body mass with each step and to propel our body forward in the terminal phase of the gait cycle. On contact with the ball, a force is generated over a short period of time that is precisely opposed to the arched construction of the foot, giving rise to corresponding mechanical forces and stresses. With each individual kicking action, the mechanical reaction forces released by the ball mass are of a magnitude that remains well within the physiological range and generally does not exceed the stress tolerance of the structures involved. However, if this action is repeated a sufficient number of times over a prolonged period, possibly many years, the resultant stimuli then act as a form of microtrauma, eventually leading to changes in the musculoskeletal system. Such changes have been postulated and discussed ever since the mid-1980s, for example, by Hess (1985), and Lees & Nolan (1998).

To ensure appropriate preparation for the sudden and brief tensile stresses generated by ball contact, strengthening occurs at the insertion sites of the talonavicular ligament that is placed under tensile stress by the action of kicking. The increased numbers of more strongly developed Sharpey's fibres take up an increased amount of space and may then often even be visible radiologically as a talar beak and/or tibial peak, a phenomenon that results in reduced dorsiflexion mobility at the ankle joint.

Alongside and as a result of these direct changes to the ankle joint in response to kicking movements, football players are also likely to develop muscle changes that are characterised by varying degrees of right-left asymmetry (support leg vs kicking leg). The kicking movement of the leg axis in question represents an 'open kinetic chain' type of load in which the foot is moved with maximum forward velocity (moving point) and the hip remains relatively stationary (fixed

point). At the same time, every kicking movement necessarily imposes a 'closed kinetic chain' type of load on the non-kicking side. In this case, the non-kicking foot is planted on the ground (fixed point), while the structures above it throughout the pelvic-leg axis and torso are in motion (moving point) and need to be adequately stabilised against gravity by a complex set of coordination mechanisms. Similarly varied neuromuscular control actions then create the basis for long-term muscular adaptations to these football-specific movement patterns. In the long term, the active musculoskeletal system, as well as the myofascial system, may be assumed to adapt progressively to the characteristic movements that they are called upon to perform, and to the loads associated with those movements as they develop an optimised muscular response.

Reports describe muscle differences between the support leg in relation to the kicking leg (Knebel et al., 1988) (Ekstrand et al., 1983). Kicking the ball is a multiple-joint movement in which an, obviously, explosive extension movement at the knee is combined with active flexion of the hip and extension (plantar flexion) of the foot at the ankle joint. In general, these authors describe both an increased maximum strength capacity and an increased striking force during quadriceps extension on the kicking-leg side, accompanied by increased maximum strength and striking force of the knee flexors on the support-leg side (Figure 20.1).

Our own empirical observations on the degree of quadriceps muscle development in football players suggest additional neurophysiological aspects and considerations relating to long-term functional adaptations. Although football players have greater quadriceps strength on the kicking-leg side than on the support-leg side, examination of the thighs in most players shows that the thigh circumference tends to be slightly reduced in the area where the vastus medialis muscle is most fully developed. Evidently the variable 'muscular configuration' of the quadriceps is an adaptive response of the musculoskeletal system to years of locally varying, stereotypical functional demands (the kicking leg with its numerous open kinetic-chain loads,

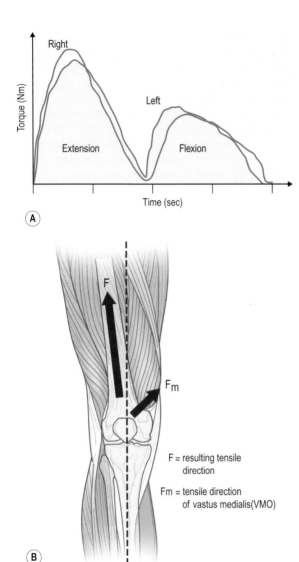

Figure 20.1 A & B

Agonist-antagonist relationship in the muscles of the knee joint.

have revealed that, despite the increased maximal strength of the kicking-leg quadriceps (peak isokinetic torque-time curves – Isomed 2000 System – around the belly of the vastus medialis muscle 10 cm proximal to the medial knee joint space), thigh circumference is 3.2 mm smaller on average; and 20 cm proximal to the medial knee joint space, thigh circumference was again 1.8 mm smaller on average.

From a neurophysiological standpoint, a 'chronic' vastus medialis deficiency in the kicking leg can be explained by the absence of any need during open kinetic-chain activity to stabilise the knee joint in terms of tibial rotation relative to the femur in response to gravitational effects. The long-term change in the innervation pattern gradually results in adaptation that is optimised for kicking the ball. The other side of the coin is that this process alters the relative contributions of the individual quadriceps muscles to the resultant quadriceps force. Deficiency of the vastus medialis tends to lateralise the quadriceps pull on the patella, thereby altering the kinematics of the femoropatellar joint. By contrast, the loads on the support leg during running and sprinting tend not to alter the physiological pattern of intra-articular kinematics. As a result, in statistical terms, degenerative changes in the femoropatellar joint are detected far more commonly on the kicking-leg side than on the support-leg side.

Support leg changes due to kicking technique

The changes in the kicking leg, described above, suggest that the contralateral support leg is obviously exposed to different loads during the kicking of a football ball. It is interesting that all football players, virtually irrespective of their performance level, tend to place their support leg in a very precise position when kicking the ball, with the instep or with the inside/outside of the foot. This results in a highly consistent pattern of stereotypical mechanical loads acting on the musculoskeletal structures. To ensure successful ball acceleration by following through with the kicking leg to transfer momentum effectively to the ball, the support leg must be planted correctly next to the ball on the ground. The following initial observations are important in this regard (Hoffmann, 1984):

in contrast to the support leg with its closed kinetic-chain loads). It is not uncommon for there to be clearly identifiable volume deficiencies in the territory of the vastus medialis muscle of the kicking leg in some players. Our own empirical measurements in 35 football players

- As far as possible, football players plant their support leg next to the ball with remarkable consistency and precision. Tests have shown that intra-individual differences from one ball contact to the next are less than 1 cm.
- Football players plant their support leg level with the ball (relative to the frontal plane).
- As the foot is planted on the ground, the body's centre of gravity shifts outward toward the support leg, usually moving beyond the left knee or even further laterally.
- The lateral distance of the support leg from the ball can vary markedly from one player to the next. Despite these pronounced differences, however, the individual solutions and movement patterns are performed with great precision (intra-individual consistency). However, the further the support leg is placed away from the ball, the greater the lateral shift in the body's centre of gravity. The joints along the pelvic-leg axis of the support leg have to stabilise and compensate for this position and this will then culminate in corresponding adaptive changes over time. These side-specific changes are most clearly identified in the ankle joint. The greater the lateralisation of the pelvic–leg axis, the greater the lateral and shear forces acting on the joints of the foot. Even in the absence of injuries and/or trauma, these forces have the potential to induce long-term adaptations.

These changes are then reflected not only in the stereotypical kicking actions that occur during training and competitive matches, but also in ordinary walking and running (Chapters 13 and 17). They document the adaptations of the pelvic–leg axis as a whole. Depending on individual predisposition, these changes will specifically impinge on the affected biological structures of the particular football player.

Adaptations of the lumbopelvic-hip region

The muscular adaptations, described above, that occur on the support-leg and kicking-leg sides in response to the demands of football also bring in their wake long-term changes throughout the lumbopelvic–hip region. Our own gait analyses (kinematic, dynamic and palpatory findings)

together with manual therapy assessments have highlighted the following aspects: the dominance of the powerful quadriceps and hip flexors (especially the iliopsoas muscle) on the kicking-leg side causes the pelvis to tilt posteriorly on that side (posterior pelvic tilt with inflare component). This in turn causes an anterior pelvic tilt (relatively upright ilium with outflare component) to develop on the contralateral support-leg side in an attempt to stabilise the body's centre of gravity in the long term. Additionally, these changes are often accompanied by a decreased range of motion in the sacroiliac joint on the kicking-leg side. This asymmetrical range of motion, combined with torsion of the hips, produces apparent lengthening of the support-leg axis and leads to functional pelvic obliquity. Furthermore, the new stress patterns are transmitted to the structures of the lumbar spine. As a result of the posterior pelvic tilt on the kicking-leg side, physical examination of football players often reveals that the lumbar spine is rotated posteriorly to the right due to increased tension on the iliolumbar ligaments.

Implications for the myofascial system

To summarise, football players can be expected to exhibit changes and side-specific adaptations affecting all the joints and ligaments of the lower limb, and hence the associated musculoskeletal structures together with the entire functional unit of the pelvic–leg axis with its associated myofascial chains. Varying in degree between different players, and depending on individual predisposition and the duration (years of training) and quantity (scope of training) of the loads and stereotypical movement patterns, these changes may become a source of problems. In consequence, some rethinking of priorities will be necessary, both when preparing for training/competitive matches and during the recovery (cool down) phase in order to optimise regeneration processes. Furthermore, alongside the classic and now conventional strategies (with their focus on joints, ligaments, and the musculoskeletal system), consideration should also be given to the myofascia and to relevant exercises that will enable such considerations to be translated into practice. In this context side-specific connective-tissue properties will also manifest themselves as a result of adaptation to

Table 20.1

Muscles of the myofascial inflare and outflare chains (adapted from Meert, 2003).

Myofascial inflare chain	Myofascial outflare chain
Torsion + flexion (e.g. left-sided chain)	(Torsion + extension (e.g. left-sided chain
Rectus capitis lateralis muscle, left Scalene muscles, left Sternocleidomastoid muscle, left Major and minor pectoralis muscles, left Intercostal muscles, left External oblique abdominal muscle, left Internal oblique abdominal muscle, right Diaphragm (transverse separating structure) Iliopsoas muscle, right Obturator muscles, right Adductor muscles, right Vastus medialis muscle, right Peroneal musculature, right Plantar fascia	Obliquus capitis muscles, left Longissimus capitis muscle, left Trapezius muscle (descending part), left Levator scapulae muscle, left External rotators, left shoulder Superior posterior serratus muscle, left Inferior posterior serratus muscle, left Diaphragm (transverse separating structure) Thoracolumbar fascia, quadratus lumborum muscle, left Psoas muscle, right Gluteal musculature, right; tensor fasciae latae muscle, right Vastus lateralis muscle, right Sartorius muscle, right Mediocrural musculature, right Plantar fascia

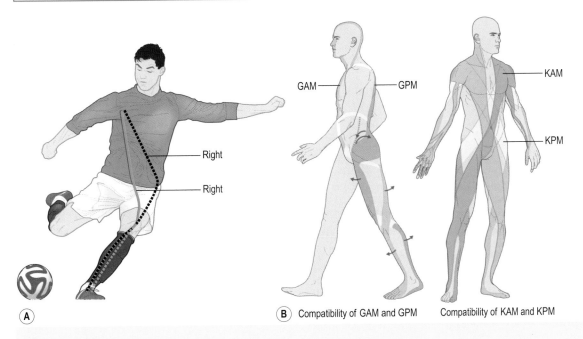

Figure 20.2 A & B

Football-specific stereotypical movements with associated myofascial chains.

the stereotypical stresses of training/competitive matches. Both connective tissue properties are often found to be reduced on the kicking-leg side. Both the straight anterior myofascial chain and the crossed anterior myofascial chain are found to be less taut and, because of this reduced firmness, paradoxically less elastic. The three-dimensional architecture of collagen 'network structures' is

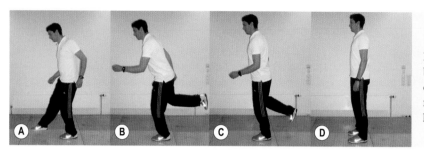

Figure 20.3 A–D

Football-specific complex stabilisation exercise involving contralateral torso rotation and reversal of support-leg/kicking-leg function.

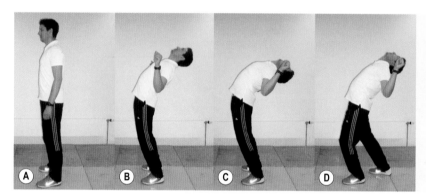

Figure 20.4 A–D

Stretching the straight anterior myofascial chain to prevent entrapment.

therefore altered in terms of firmness and elasticity (Chapter 10).

The lateral (outer) fascia of the thigh is also more clearly pronounced with increased firmness. A dominant straight posterior myofascial chain and crossed posterior myofascial chain are found on the support-leg side (Figure 20.2A & B).

Building up optimised fascial structures/networks in the medium and long term

On the basis of the anatomical, biomechanical and physiological principles previously outlined, practitioners generally have at their disposal a number of exercise and movement types that will encourage the medium- and long-term build-up and optimisation of the collagen structures involved (formation of a functionally elastic shear lattice). In broad terms, at the turnaround points of movements, where the agonists operating in synergy and the stretched antagonists meet, virtually isometric tension of the contractile elements is demanded. This enables further small

movements with directional change via the fascial (elastic) elements, as well as a developmental and directional stimulus. Preparatory counter movements of this type, close to the turnaround points of movements, may be combined with a variety of rotational components (3D arrangement of the fascial network) (Chapter 14). In terms of the previously described football-specific adaptations and changes involving the musculoskeletal system, the focus of the intended optimisation and build-up routines for the fascial network should counter the preferred stereotypical movements of the particular football player on the opposite side and be performed on a scale that is slightly greater in quantitative terms.

Alongside this more rapid form of dynamic stretching, consideration should also be given in this setting to the potential usefulness of slow dynamic stretching exercises. Whereas classic static stretching exercises in sports practice are mostly directed at specific muscles, so as to deliver a stretching/elongating stimulus to the myotensive contractile structures, increasing support is now being given to a school of thought that advocates chain-oriented tension transmission extending beyond individual muscles (i.e. beyond the immediately affected joints) and into myofascial chains. Transmission of tension states beyond the individual, anatomically definable muscles via the fascial network yields stretching exercises that benefit complex muscle chains. An additional focus of these stretching exercises targets anatomical predispositions to compression of neuronal/neuromeningeal structures that, in turn, may have devastatingly adverse and restrictive effects on neuromuscular efficiency (Bracht & Liebscher-Bracht, 2010). The football-specific demand profile, in particular, gives rise here to the complex and locally narrowed structures of the lumbopelvic-hip region: potential compression/entrapment phenomena localised here represent the true causal or primary lesion for a vast number of problems in football players (for example, footballer's groin). The exercises recommended by us in this setting take into account the methodological aspects of fascia training and thus make a contribution to the development and functionalisation of an optimised fascial network.

Taking account of the myofascial system when preparing for training and competition

Medium- and long-term individual measures

In order to meet the complex set of physical demands encountered in football, an individual therapeutically oriented strategy is required that will preserve the functionality and efficiency of the musculoskeletal system. Looking at the football-specific demand profile, we repeatedly find that the stereotypical movement patterns with high rotatory components acting on the pelvic-leg axes lead to unphysiological and excessive loading of the joints and ligaments, myofascia and neuromeningeal structures. Their viscoelasticity is reduced so the joints involved are no longer able to return to the 'resting position' after the stresses of movement. As a result adaptive postural patterns (compensation strategies) become established. These mechanical disturbances are accompanied by disordered circulation of the interstitial fluids, a state in which the smooth physiological gliding ability between myofascial and neuromeningeal structures is compromised. The possible consequences include hypoxia (nutritive deficiency) and painful adhesions in the various tissues. In our experience, changes of this type are localised in the various diaphragms of the body (the respiratory diaphragm, the urogenital diaphragm of the pelvic floor, the diaphragm of the knee formed by the popliteal fascia, and the diaphragm of the foot formed by the plantar fascia). The regular assessment and long-term treatment of these structures in order to maintain the functionality and efficiency of the entire musculoskeletal system, for example, form part of the remit of the medical therapy teams working with professional football squads.

Preparing for training and competition

Passive modalities: Elastic taping and kinesiotaping

In preparing for training/competitive matches, elastic tapes and kinesiotapes may be used to stabilise joints. Functional tapes replace and supplement ligamentous and osseous joint-stabilising factors and produce tensile and relaxing effects on the skin and subcutaneous receptors, thus selectively facilitating or inhibiting muscle tone/activity (neurophysiological and myotensive/myofascial improvement of joint stability via muscular joint stabilisation factors). See Eder/Mommsen (2007) and Mommsen/Eder/Brandenburg (2007) for further information on these techniques.

Active modalities

The purpose of all preparatory modalities/activities in this context can be subsumed under the following definition: optimal psychological and physical preparation for subsequent football-specific psychological and physical demands in order to achieve the current best possible level of performance.

In line with ideas originally outlined by Schlumberger (Eder & Hoffmann, 2006), these active modalities comprise, in general, the following key areas:

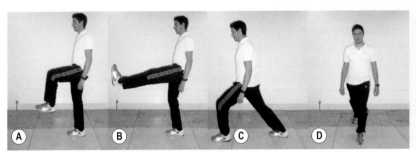

Figure 20.5

Example to illustrate dynamic stretching: hurdle walk.

- Boosting physiological metabolic activities using moderate running with varying intensity in order to raise core body temperature, increase general metabolic activities, and optimise neuromuscular control processes.
- Structure-specific preparation of the musculoskeletal system for football-specific movement sequences utilising dynamic stretching and taking account of myofascial structures (Chapter 14).
- Preparation for football-specific stereotypical movement patterns with progressively increasing complexity and intensity. In particular, football-specific cutting movements with directional changes of varying intensity should be integrated in this process, as well as phases of acceleration and deceleration, initially without the ball and then, as preparation advances, receiving the ball and running with it as well as situation-specific movement sequences (corners, free kick variations, etc.).

In terms of structure-specific preparation of the musculoskeletal system, in particular, the widespread practice of static stretching immediately prior to the stresses of training/competitive matches should be discarded (Chapter 9). Similarly, the exercise forms involving preparatory counter movement and rapid bouncing as a type of 'dynamic stretching' to shape and develop the fascial network are less suitable (if not actually unsuitable) as immediate preparation for the stresses of training/competitive matches. Instead, the suitable approach involves 'dynamic stretching'

that, as well as catering for the myotensive (muscular contractile) and neuromuscular (proprioceptive) movement prerequisites, also prepares the myofascial structures for the stresses and loads that are to follow.

In our experience plyometric exercise forms (Chapter 22), initially with a unidirectional character and then building up with a multidirectional three-dimensional character (linear and lateral as well as rotatory), have proved themselves useful for activating joint-specific capsular receptors to round off structure-specific preparation and can then transition into football-specific stereotypical movement patterns without and with the ball (Chapter 10).

Taking account of the myofascial system during recovery after the stresses of training/competitive matches

Generally recognised measures, after the stresses of training and competitive matches for the timely restoration and recovery of physical performance, have the following objectives:

- Replenishment of exercise-induced fluid and energy deficits (for example, muscle glycogen stores).
- Optimisation of physiological metabolic status (supply and removal in the context of biochemical regeneration processes) by promoting the circulation using moderate, low-intensity aerobic (alactic) movement types incorporating exercises that

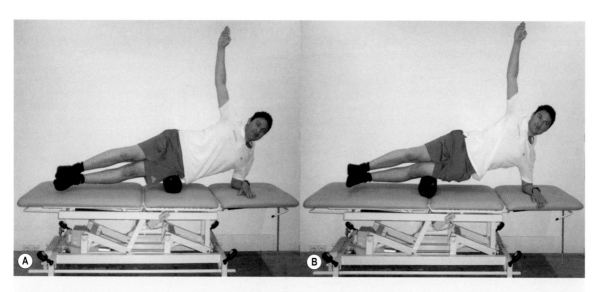

Figure 20.6 A & B

Myofascial auto-release techniques for the dorsolateral fascia of the kicking-leg thigh.

are not football-specific, such as cycling or aqua-jogging (characterised by reduced intra-articular load stresses on the joints).

- Possibly, physiotherapy to monitor the status of the joints and ligaments of the lower limb and spinal column.

These activities should be supplemented with special reference to the fascial network. To release fascial adhesions and resolve swellings that have developed following the stresses of training/competitive matches, myofascial auto-release techniques can be integrated into the regeneration strategy thereby promoting dynamic hydration of the collagenous ground substance (Chapter 15). Foam rollers are suitable for this purpose. The locally limited contact surface of these rollers permits a slow gradual rolling movement via the gravitational application of the athlete's bodyweight and so encourages a continuous further rolling movement along the course of the affected fascia. Here too, in the specific context of football, it is important to direct such efforts preferentially to the most commonly affected fascia. In our experience these are the lateral

structures of the kicking leg due to football-specific adaptations.

Conclusion

More recent scientific insights have brought about a paradigm shift in our understanding and appreciation of the function and importance of the fascial network. Alongside the classic targets of training, such as musculoskeletal function and performance, cardiopulmonary function and performance, and neuromuscular coordination and control, this radical change of perspective highlights the imperative to revise and reorientate training objectives, and their implementation and achievement, by adopting appropriate training modalities. In terms of fascial training, this requires measures and methods to develop and optimise a fascial network, as well as strategies to integrate fascial aspects into direct preparation for and recovery from the stresses of training/competitive matches, thus ensuring that the fruits of modern fascia research are incorporated into the football-specific training process.

References

Bracht, P. & Liebscher-Bracht, R. (2010) *SchmerzFrei Das SchmerzCode-SelbsthilfeProgramm, Vol. 1: unterer Rücken*. Bad Homburg v.d.H.: LNB Verlag.

Brüggemann, H. & Hentsch, H. (1981) *Röntgenologische Veränderungen bei Fußballspielern*. Orthopädische Praxis. 4: 335–338.

Eder, K. & Hoffmann, H. (2006) *Verletzungen im Fußball – vermeiden – behandeln – therapieren*. Munich: Elsevier Verlag.

Eder, K. & Mommsen, H. (2007) *Richtig Tapen – Funktionelle Verbände am Bewegungsapparat optimal anlegen*. Balingen: Spitta Verlag GmbH & Co. KG.

Ekstrand, J., Gillquist, J., Liljedahl, S.O. (1983) Prevention of soccer injuries. Supervision by doctor and physiotherapist. *Am J Sports Med*. 11(3): 116–120.

Hess, H. (1985) Fussball. In: Pförringer, *W. Sport – Trauma und Belastung*. Erlangen: perimed Fachbuch-Verlagsgesellschaft mbH

Hoffmann, H. (1984) *Biomechanik von Fußballspannstößen*. Frankfurt/Main: unpublished dissertation, University of Frankfurt/M.

Knebel, K.P., Herbeck, B. & Hamsen, G. (1988) *Fußball-Funktionsgymnastik. Dehnen, Kräftigen, Entspannen*. Reinbeck: Rowohlt Verlag.

Lees, A. & Nolan, I., (1998) The biomechanics of soccer: a review. *Journal of Sports Science*. 16(3): 211–234.

Meert, G.F. (2003) *Das Becken aus osteopathischer Sicht*. Munich/Jena: Urban & Fischer Verlag.

Mommsen, H., Eder, K., Brandenburg, U. 2007. *Leukotape K – Schmerztherapie und Lymphtherapie nach japanischer Tradition*. Balingen: Spitta Verlag GmbH & Co. KG.

Mueller-Wohlfahrt, H.-W., Ueblacker, P., Haensel, L. & Garrett, W. E. Jnr. (2013) *Muscle Injuries in Sports*. Stuttgart/New York: Georg Th-ieme Verlag.

Myers, T.W. (2001) *Anatomy Trains: Myofascial Meridians for Manual and Movement Therapists*. Edinburgh/London: Churchill Livingstone.

Wirhed, R. (1984) *Sport-Anatomie und Bewegungslehre*. Stuttgart-New York: Schattauer Verlag.

CHAPTER 21

Athletic coaching

Stephen Mutch

The connected fascial net

To paraphrase and expand on the wisdom of Benjamin Franklin, there are three certainties in life: death, taxes and collagen turnover.

Our bodies are constantly changing. Over a 24-hour period, our connective tissue will have changed, responded and adapted to any previous experience or demands placed on it. The universal network of fascia is architecturally shaped by a dominance of tensional strain, or biotensegrity, rather than by a dominance of compression (Schleip & Muller, 2012) (Chapter 1). Within this network are regions of densification and a connective tissue continuum that envelopes every muscle and organ of the body.

Humans truly are adaptive opportunists, with a resilient 'fascial suit' demonstrating an impressive capacity to change, match, react and respond to tasks of varying physiological or biomechanical demands in a bid to establish internal equilibrium. The constant sampling of the internal and external environment points to consistent evolution and each of us becoming a consummate stimulus-response individual being.

The inner fascial components of muscle ensure that there is functional integrity, with the continuity of the fascial 'net' underpinning the muscle components in times of fatigue, growth, trauma or repair (Purslow, 2010). Matt Wallden (2010) likens the three key components enveloping muscle tissue as 'a little like the struts that may support a brick bridge from bony landmark to bony landmark, and that is constantly under repair'; an ever-developing system whereby the muscle can maintain functional capacity, despite the consistent reparation of damaged tissue and necessary on-going growth. Extrinsic support to muscle is offered through supplemental force transmission that is provided by the endomysium, perimysium and epimysium (Chapter 1). Of all force generated from a 'muscle', 30–40% of it has been transmitted via the connective tissue rather than along the tendon (Huijing et al., 2003, 2007, 2011).

Healthy and resilient: Our ever-changing fascial suit!

Mechanotherapy

There has never been more focus on the need to carefully examine the rehabilitative practices and training for those involved in feats of human performance, whether in the realms of dance, sports or movement activities, such as yoga, Pilates or martial arts to give but three well-known examples. This also refers to those people who may be undertaking basic 'exercise' or movement activities for health in their homes, streets or gyms.

Every one of these activities, social, recreational or professional, will include a degree of performance, depending on many variables, but some consideration should be given for the on-going fitness of the fascial tissue which could yield huge gains in movement efficiency and comfort, even in those who may claim to exist in a relatively uninjured state. The good news is that there are some sound biomechanical and neurophysiological foundations for a change in approach to include fascial training to enhance resilience, wellness and robustness (Chapter 11).

To ensure the fascia better meets its demands, irrespective of changes in length, strength and ability to shear, it is the task of those humble construction workers of the connective tissue, the relatively unsophisticated myofibroblasts, to consistently adjust matrix remodelling. Renewal dynamics predict that there is an anticipated replacement of 30% of collagen fibres within six months and 75% in two years (Schleip & Müller, 2012). There is some form of remodelling of tissue architecture constantly. In response to specific training or activity there will be greater benefits: for example, the strain magnitude applied to human tendons needs to exceed the value of commonplace habitual activity for there to be tendon adaptation (Arampatzis et al., 2010) (Chapter 5).

However, the human body has become adept at utilising a variety of methods available to the myofascialskeletal system, in order to perform mechanical work in the lower limb. The animal kingdom has offered breathtaking examples of the benefits of utilising stored energy within the tendons and fascia of the legs and hind limbs. Kangaroos and gazelles can jump further and higher due to the release of kinetic energy stored in the tendons and fascia of their hind legs (Chapter 10). Human fascia has a similar storage capacity (Sawicki et al., 2009). Humans can use stored energy for locomotion when walking or running (Chapter 17). Movement is produced following the oscillatory actions of lengthening and shortening within the elastic fascia, whilst the leg muscles essentially remain at a constant length even when contracting (Fukunaga et al., 2002) (Kawakami, 2012).

Walking also offers an example of how elastic energy storage and return is optimised, in this instance in the Achilles tendon. Additionally there is a trade-off in power production between the hip and ankle due to the contrast in joint efficiency (Sawicki et al., 2009). Ensuring that there is adequate 'spring' to the ankle is a metabolic advantage, as a lack of suitable myofascial storage and return will increase the demand and reliance on the hip joint instead. This metabolic energy exchange is a reason why certain populations find that there is a significant 'performance' challenge to their regular walking, such as readily witnessed in the elderly, amputees, the neurologically compromised or those injured in sport.

This aspect of the ageing process is pertinent to the regenerating fascial 'body suit', as its architecture becomes more haphazard with more multidirectional fibres. This generates additional cross links within the fascia, causing a reduction in elasticity and increasing local adhesion that affects glide between tissues (Chapter 19). The inevitable loss of springiness in the tissues is reflected in gait and overall mobility.

Mechanotherapy is a term coined to demonstrate how movement can stimulate repair, facilitate tissue healing and influence remodelling via mechanotransduction (Khan & Scott, 2009). Mechanotransduction is a physiological process whereby cells sense and respond biologically to the application of mechanical stimuli (Chapter 2). Rather than remaining solely a strictly homeostatic function for the maintenance of healthy cell structure in the absence of injury, mechanotherapy offers up a physiological cellular function to clinical exercise prescription in the management of injury. The role of therapeutic exercise in any form is to apply mechanical loads to tissue in a way that provides physical, and cellular, benefits. The cumulative load should be within the envelope of function (Zanou & Gailly, 2013) (Chapter 5). Body tissues respond to mechanical stimuli in different ways, whether in states of health or disease, as will now be described. Tendon and muscle injuries require some initial respect for the early phase of healing and inflammation but are both receptive to controlled loading leading to cell proliferation, matrix remodelling, myotube alignment and a more complete recovery (Khan & Scott, 2009) (Chapter 19).

In the case of muscle tissue, load-induced responses are well established, with overload particularly stimulating the upregulation of mechanogrowth factor (or 'MGF'), which is a variant of IGF-I, and associated with cell proliferation and the remodelling of collagen. The process occurs as a result of other growth factors and cytokines, and is manipulated in the presence of controlled overload training, leading to hypertrophy and alignment of regenerating myotubes (Zanou & Gailly, 2013).

Tendons are capable of withstanding considerable loads, of up to eight times bodyweight, during human locomotion (Magnusson, Langberg & Kjaer, 2010) (Chapter 5). A feature of tendon is the ability to transmit contractile forces to bone in order to generate movement. The mechanical loading of tendon results in upregulation of IGF-I and increased synthesis and remodeling of collagen (Zanou & Gailly, 2013). Fibroblasts have the ability to move through the three dimensional collagen matrices, so exertional tractional forces could have effects on remote as well as local tissue organisation, depending upon the surrounding tissue mobility (Grinnell, 2008). After injury, tendons generally respond well to responsible loading, although this does vary with anatomical location and, in cases of tendon surgery, early excessive motion can be detrimental to overall repair (Killian et al., 2012).

Research is needed to examine the potentially beneficial effects of mechanotransduction on tissue response for articular cartilage and on osteocytes in bone, both recognised as being primary mechanosensors (Khan & Scott, 2010).

Scarring: A price worth paying for evolutionary survival?

Whilst scarless total regenerative tissue repair would be an idealistic conclusion to injury and the wound healing process for human beings, unfortunately repairing tissues do not exhibit identical structural, aesthetic and functional capabilities to their originals. Scars are the natural and inevitable outcome of a normal continuum of tissue repair (Bayat et al., 2003).

The remarkable adaptability of the body in health and disease has no better example than the astonishing organ that is human skin. Essentially skin is a highly specialised mechanoresponsive interface, with an ability to adapt to stretch due to a network of interrelated cascades that trigger collagen synthesis to ensure homeostatic equilibrium is restored (Zollner et al., 2012).

When there is tissue injury, however, wound healing has been developed out of these overlapping cascades of cytokine and inflammatory activity in an attempt to prevent infection and potential wound breakdown. The inevitable resultant scar tissue has been dubbed 'the price to pay for evolutionary survival following a wounding', due to this rapid biological optimal healing mechanism (Bayat, 2003).

Vranova et al. (2009) observed how studies on changes to skin behaviour have noted how functional changes in other systems may be brought about: in the respiratory, lymphatic and neuromuscular systems, for example. They investigated the potential changes in the mechanical behaviour of the skin, as a result of a large scar, and hypothesised that through the application of treatment there would be an improvement in skin behaviour observable by objective means of measurement.

This is of interest for the sporting population, where scar tissue is commonplace and post-operative scars are not unusual, as well as for anyone who has residual skin scars from surgery or accidents. Though skin varies in thickness from 0.5–5 mm, its visco-elastic nature is altered following trauma due to the multilayered nature, texture and lines of the local tissue morphology. In surgical situations, whilst the stretching of adjacent skin routinely facilitates wound closure, thick collagen bundles can be found with more space between them. Both the collagen and elastin are oriented in significantly more parallel patterns in post-operative samples than in non-operative tissue (Verhaegen et al., 2012).

Unlike cartilage, for example, skin is regenerated with relatively high quality tissue, the activity of fibroblasts being a key component of the biomechanical process due to dynamic cytoskeletal remodelling (Langevin et al., 2011). Also to be considered is the effect of scar tissue on the desirable smoothness of the shifting layers of the skin, with respect to the subcutis, to optimise range of motion (Chapter 19). The superficial fascial layer plays a role in the support and patency of structures, such as veins and lymphatic vessels, and ensures integrity of the skin (Stecco & Day, 2010).

There is a broad spectrum of scar types of the skin, ranging from atrophic (depressed scars), hypertrophic (raised scars), and keloid scars to scar contractures. These will also be influenced by the mechanophysiological conditions of the injured person or from surgical intervention, both elective and emergency cum traumatic (Ogawa, 2011). The raised keloid scar develops beyond the margins of the original wound, 'invading' previously normal skin, and continues developing without any spontaneous regression. It is usually only termed keloid after being present for a year (Bayat et al., 2003). These scars will often be found on highly mobile sites with high tension (Ogawa et al., 2012).

Tissue viscoelasticity shapes the dynamic response of mechanoreceptors and overuse, trauma or surgery can alter the capacity of endofascial collagen layers to glide upon one another appropriately. This in itself affects proprioception, in addition to alterations in the distribution of lines of force within the fascia and the surrounding musculoskeletal structures. The sliding is facilitated by hyaluronic acid, an anionic non-sulfated glycosaminoglycan that is essentially a lubricant. Produced by cells specialised in the biosynthesis and secretion of hyaluronic acid, these were termed 'Fasciacytes' by Stecco et al on examination of cadavers and ultrasound of volunteers' fascia in 2011. The complex molecules behave by forming a gel like composition within the ground substance but, by becoming more soluble, they can move from gel to fluid when heated, for example with certain direct treatment techniques or with exercise. An increased density of loose connective tissue and the aggregation of closely packed gel-like hyalonic acid can thus affect the sliding of two adjacent fibrous layers, altering the behaviour of the deep fascia and local muscles. Potentially, this is a reason for myofascial pain (Stecco et al., 2011).

Myofascial release has shown reductions on viscoelasticity, scar sensitivity and improvements in the range of motion (Chapter 19). Therefore, mechanotherapy or fascial fitness (Chapter 11) could also have far reaching effects on the viscoelasticity of the skin and, by extension, for the associated motor system with influence on global motor patterns, trigger points and neuromuscular stability (Vranova et al., 2009). Manual treatments are non-invasive, and

effective, even on fascial areas remote to pain, with an ability to modify the extracellular matrix and restore gliding (Stecco & Day, 2010). These effects may be on areas of fascial compromise, at a subdermal or superficial fascial level, as well as on the assortment of visible scar types on the skin.

By reducing skin tension around scars and wounds, mechanotherapy not only has the capacity to treat keloids and hypertrophic scars but may also prevent them if clinical approaches follow the mechanotransduction studies (Ogawa et al., 2012).

Changing methods of treatment, training and thinking on recovery

Exercise and the fitness of fascia

It seems indisputable that exercise can be beneficial in health and disease. There is, inevitably, a need for some caution, as whilst controlled loading can enhance healing in most settings a fine balance must be reached between loads that are too low (leading to a catabolic state) and too high, potentially leading to microdamage (Killian et al., 2012) (Chapter 5).

Cells and tissues will respond in different ways according to the manner in which force is applied (Standley & Meltzer, 2008). There appears to be a complex relationship between exercise and pro-inflammatory cytokine production. Repetitive or high amplitude cyclic stretch can lead to their increased production (Eagan et al., 2007). Brief static stretch or low amplitude mechanical input has been found to show anti-inflammatory outcomes and demonstrate a reduction in cytokines IL-3 and IL-6 (Meltzer & Standley, 2007) (Branski et al., 2007). Repetitive high amplitude mechanical inputs generally increase TGF□1, whilst static stress attenuates the increase in soluble TGF□1and type-1 procollagen following tissue injury (Bouffard et al., 2008). Brief stretching reduces TGF□1 mediated fibrogenesis (Benjamin, 2009).

This suggests that stretching and dynamic exercise could have a *direct impact* on tissue inflammation and the risk of fibrosis or scarring following an injury. There are, therefore, clear implications for potential treatment and rehabilitation of injury, as a result of this cellular change as a response to tissue stretch. An in vivo animal model study investigated this response for the peripheral connective tissues of the lower back region (Corey et al., 2012). They noted that 'a number of potentially interrelated local and systemic mechanisms may have contributed to the reduction in tissue inflammation observed'. As the stretch that was induced was of the whole, conscious animal, the authors considered that, in addition to local or peripheral mechanisms, centrally mediated effects – involving stimulation of the hypothalamic-pituitary-adrenal axis and systemic cortisol secretion – are potentially induced by stretching. Stress, during tissue stretch, could also activate descending pain inhibitory pathways, with inhibition of neurogenic inflammation via reduced secretion of neuropeptides (Substance P, CGRP) into the tissue.

The stimulation of fascial fibroblasts to lay down fibre architecture, with the potential for a more elastic storage capacity, is to be encouraged for Fascia Fitness (Chapter 10). This is affected through movements that will load the fascial tissues in multi-dimensional ranges of motion, with dynamic movements to facilitate elastic springiness (Fukashiro et al., 2006). These forms of Fascia Fitness exercise may be supplemental to traditional exercise or movement forms that will still yield fascial changes, for example, classic loaded weight training or, at the other end of the spectrum, the slow and melting postures of yoga (Schleip & Muller, 2012) (Chapter 11).

Active therapeutic stretch interventions, such as physical therapy or yoga (Chapter 12), may involve slow and gentle, but non-habitual body movements, and may capitalise on the central and peripheral effects (Bouffard et al., 2008) in addition to the effects of the local changes in tissue hydration. This is a critical subject, as two thirds of fascia is water (Schleip et al., 2005) (Chapter 3).

Loading, stretching or compression will inevitably squeeze water from the sponge-like connective tissues. (Those utilising the foam rollers as a form of self-management, take note.) This may be replaced with fresh fluid from surrounding tissue and the local vascular network. In healthy states, extracellular water of fascia is in a state of bound water rather than bulk water. It is the bulk water that represents a high percentage within ground substance in environments such as oedema, inflammation and in the presence of accumulated waste products and free radicals (Schleip & Muller, 2012). A partial rehydration seems likely to occur when the fascia is squeezed again, with an influx of bound water molecules enhancing the health of the ground substance at a stroke.

Altered hydration tissue status, associated with strain hardening tension, increases in the lumbodorsal fascia, in addition to active contractility of the myofibroblasts and fibroblasts, could even provide a significant contribution to lumbo-pelvic stability (Barker et al., 2004). This combination of factors may be significant as to why some forms of stretching have been thought to have had a direct anti-inflammatory effect on the peripheral connective tissues of the low back (Corey et al., 2012) and could lead to a better understanding of myofascial manipulation on viscoelastic tissue properties.

Functional examples within sport

It has been suggested that, for the appropriate exercise of fascial tissues for wellness and health, there are a few training principles that should be followed based on biomechanical and neurological considerations (Schleip & Muller, 2012) (Chapter 11). Fortunately many contemporary and, indeed, ancient movement practices have components that recognisably already have elements of these philosophies in their formats. A list, that is by no means exhaustive, would include yoga (Chapter 12), plyometrics (Chapter 22), rhythmic gymnastics, dance (Chapter 15), qi running, and martial arts (Chapter 16) as examples where these training principles apply in some part. The principles do not present an ideology, rather a framework for specifically targeting the optimal renewal of the fascial net. These principles can be applied in sport and movement as aspects of dynamic warm-ups prior to training or sporting activities. Furthermore,

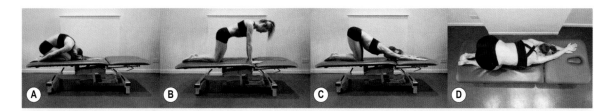

The 'Double Prayer' for Back Line

This has been successful for athletes in warm-ups for sport, or after being in a prolonged position for any length of time. Positions are not held statically nor is there any 'stretch' held.

Figure 21.1 A & B

In this first position the athlete tucks the head under, with arms by the side. Pelvis is lowered to the feet. Back line is extended with the head tucked. This is a brief transition position bringing hips to 90 degrees and shoulders, elbows and wrists all in line. (Figure 21.1 a& b).

Figure 21.1 C & D

With the hips remaining in 90 degrees, the arms slide forwards with forehead resting on the bed/floor. This serves to sink the thorax into the bed/floor as well generating thoracic extension, and a change in fascial movement along the back line incorporating an end point with the head position (Figure 21.1 c).

From this position then a side flexion movement allows for movement for the thoracic spine and lateral line fascial glide particularly at the thorax on pelvis (Figure 21.1 d). Instruction is to reach 'one hand over' (the other).

Finally a rotational movement for the thoracic spine from this position. Instruction is to reach 'one hand under (the other arm and the head turns to follow the hand that is now under the arm)'.

These last two additions to the basic Double Prayer are useful for sports demanding thoracic rotation and extension, such as racquet sports, table tennis, hockey, basketball and volleyball.

integrating neuromuscular training programmes into warm-ups has been hypothesised to improve joint position sense, enhance joint stability and develop protective joint reflexes (Herman et al., 2012).

Examples of multi-planar movements include those utilising the framework of fascial lines as described by Tom Myers (2001), with the Back Line as well as the Lateral (internal) and the Spiral Lines shown (Chapter 6). These have been beneficial in warm-ups for racquet or ball sports, swimming and in track and field. Additionally, in sports such as cycling, shooting or archery, for example, where there are episodes of limited dynamic movement or fixed positions for extended periods, these Fascial Fitness exercises (Chapter 11) have been advantageous before or after bouts of training and competition.

Preparatory counter movement, in the form of a slight pre-tensioning in the opposite direction, briefly increases the elastic tension in the fascial body suit, with the kinetic energy stored on the reverse side of the fascial net dynamically released via a passive recoil effect as the body moves back to the original position in a fluid motion.

Smoothness and softness of movement is also encouraged in the silent manner of the legendary Japanese warriors, the Ninja. Athletes can be encouraged to move, walk (Chapter 17) or even run in a flowing manner, each elegant change of direction preceded by a gradual deceleration of one movement followed by an effortless gradual acceleration without any jerkiness. A reminder to move with as 'little noise as possible' is required and will generate greater fascial spring qualities.

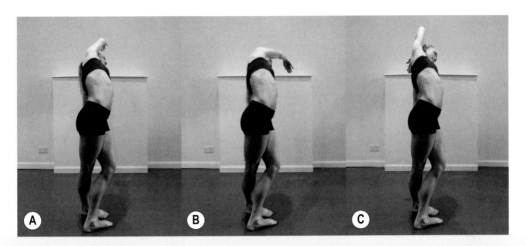

Figure 21.2 A–C
Lateral Line

Here a fascial fitness Lateral Line exercise is shown. Two images of each movement are shown, including one with a light weight as described in the text to enhance the movement via the Preparatory counter movement, in the form of a slight pre-tensioning in the opposite direction, briefly increasing the elastic tension in the fascial body suit.

Here a block of the pelvis and right hip is facilitated with a crossover from the left leg. The right lateral line is clearly being encouraged to glide with the instruction 'reach over your head' or 'bring your arm to your ear' (Figure 21.3 a). This is vividly shown from the side view (Figure 21.2 a).

With the last exercise the instruction is encouraging to 'reach in front' (Figure 21.2 c) and as seen from behind (Figure 21.3 c).

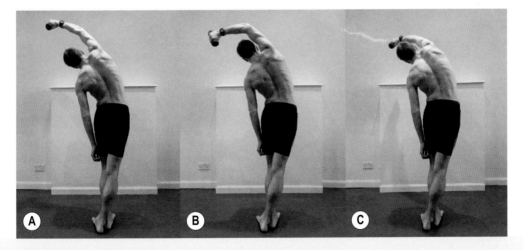

Figure 21.3 A–C

With the last exercise the instruction is encouraging to 'reach in front' (Figure 21.2 c) and as seen from behind (Figure 21.3 c)

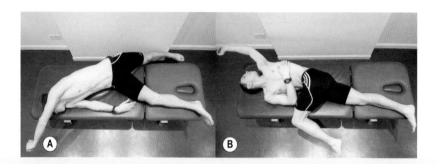

Spiral Line

Figure 21.4 A & B

1. In these images, the athlete is facilitating a spiral line utilising rotation with hip flexion and extension. He starts on his side by lifting the uppermost (left) hip as high as possible then moving the opposite arm out wide of the head which should turn to follow it (Figure 21.4 b).

   This is followed by the top (left) leg being taken backwards (into hip extension) with a straight knee whilst the left arm comes across the body thereby twisting the trunk around (Figure 21.4 a).

   This exercise can be performed on the floor as well as a bed or plinth. Athletes can benefit from thoracic rotation and extension in racquet sports, volleyball, table tennis, basketball, field and ice hockey.

2. There is an alternative method of mobilising the spiral line by manipulating the surface on introduction of the swissball in a gym or home setting.

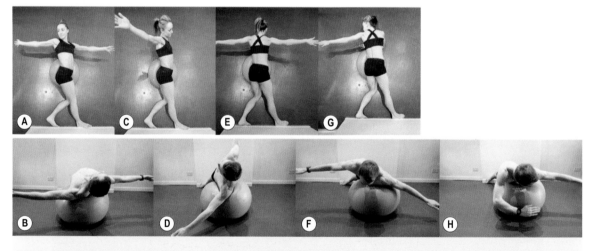

Figure 21.5 A–H

The athlete crosses top (right) leg over bottom at a wall for some stability, then opens both arms out to the side making a cross. The head follows the right arm which is going to move around with the twisting of the trunk. The hand and arm sweeps around the trunk beyond the 180 degrees and then finishes with that right arm coming under the body 270 degrees from the start position (Figures 21.5 A–H).

Flowing dynamic 'stretching' motions are also recommended. These are applied to long myofascial chains in multidirectional movements employing slight changes in angle to maximise the areas of the fascial network being exercised. At the end of these dynamic stretches, soft and gentle 'mini-bounces' and *micro-movements* may be incorporated exploring the outer reaches of the connective network.

A perceptual refinement of shear, gliding, and tensioning motions within superficial fascial membranes is encouraged: *a form of fascial proprioceptive refinement* that encourages the body and brain to respond to less predictable movements employing a variety of different qualities and strategies. The interplay of the brain and Central Nervous System, in reading and recording of the sensory-afferent information thus allows for appropriate movements and this training assists in this interactive processing and integration.

Ultimately, movement is a directed and directional energy conducted by vectors of force, with corresponding myofascial lengthening or spread in a sustainable manner that can be employed in daily functions as well as sports (Schleip & Müller, 2012). Tensile integrity represents efficiency and balanced dynamic postural equilibrium (Dellagrotte et al., 2008).

The employment of these principles should ensure 'wellness' for the fascial net, facilitating the optimal integration of a continually adapting fascial suit: one that has evolved ideally to suit your movement needs.

References

Arampatzis, A., Peper, A., Bierbaum, S. & Albrecht K. (2010) Plasticity of human Achilles tendon mechanical and morphological properties in response to cyclic strain. *J Biomech*. 43: 3073–3079

Barker, P.J., Briggs, C.A. & Bogeski, G. (2004) Tensile transmission across the lumbar fasciae in unembalmed cadavers: effects of tension to various muscular attachments. *Spine*. 29(2): 129–138.

Bayat, A., McGrouther, D.A. & Ferguson, M.W.J. (2003) Skin scarring. *BMJ*. 326: 88–92.

Benjamin, M. (2009). The fascia of the limbs and back – a review. *J. Anat*. 214: 1–18.

Bouffard, N., Cutroneo, K., Badger, G., White, S., Buttolph, T., Ehrlich, H.P., Stevens-Tuttle, D. & Langevin, H.M. (2008). Tissue stretch decreases soluble TGF-beta1 and type-1 procollagen in mouse subcutaneous connective tissue: Evidence from ex vivo and in vivo models. *Journal of Cellular Physiology*. 214: 389–395.

Branski, R.C., Perera, P., Verdolini, K., Rosen, C.A., Hebda, P.A. & Agerwal, S. (2007) Dynamic Biomechanical Strain Inhibits IL-1[beta]-induced Inflammation in Vocal Fold Fibroblasts. *Journal of Voice*. 21: 651–660.

Corey, S.M., Vizzard, M.A., Bouffard, N.A., Badger, G.J. & Langevin, H.M. (2012) Stretching of the Back Improves Gait, Mechanical Sensitivity and Connective Tissue Inflammation in a Rodent Model. PLoS ONE. 7(1): 1–8.

DellaGrotte, J., Ridi, R., Landi, M. & Stephens, J. (2008) Postural improvement using core integration to lengthen myofascia. *J Bodyw Mov Ther*. 12: 231–245.

Eagan, T.S., Meltzer, K.R. & Standley, P.R. (2007) Importance of Strain Direction in Regulating Human Fibroblast Proliferation and Cytokine Secretion: A Useful in Vitro Model for Soft Tissue Injury and Manual Medicine Treatments. *Journal of Manipulative and Physiological Therapeutics*. 30: 584–592.

Fredericson, M., White, J.J., MacMahon, J.M. & Andriacchi, T.P. (2002) Quantitative analysis of the relative effectiveness of 3 iliotibial band stretches. *Arch Phys Med Rehabil*. 83: 589–92.

Fukunaga, T., Kawakami, Y., Kubo, K. & Kanehisa, H. (2002) Muscle and Tendon Interaction During Human Movements. *Exercise and Sport Sciences Reviews*. 30(3): 106–110.

Fukashiro, S., Hay, D.C. & Nagano, A. (2006) Biomechanical behavior of muscle-tendon complex during dynamic human movements. *J. Appl.Biomech*. 22(2): 131–147

Grinnell, F. (2008) Fibroblast mechanics in three dimensional collagen matrices. *J Bodyw Mov Ther*. 12(3): 191–193.

Herman, K., Barton, C., Malliaras, P. & Morrissey, D. (2012) The effectiveness of neuromuscular warm-up strategies, that require no additional equipment, for preventing lower limb injuries during sports participation: a systematic review. *BMC Medicine*. 10(75): 1–12.

Huijing, P.A. (2007) Epimuscular myofascial force transmission between antagonistic and synergistic muscles can explain movement limitation in spastic paresis. *J Electromyogr Kinesiol*. 17(6): 708–724.

Huijing, P.A., Yaman, A., Ozturk, C. & Yucesoy, C.A. (2011) Effects of knee angle on global and local strains within human triceps surae muscle: MRI analysis indicating in vivo myofascial force transmission between synergistic muscles. *Surg Radiol Anat*. 33(10): 869.

Huijing, P.A. & Baan, G.C. (2003) Myofascial force transmission: muscle relative position and length determine agonist and synergist muscle force. *J Appl Physiol*. 94: 1092–1107.

Kawakami, Y. (2012) Morphological and functional characteristics of the muscle-tendon unit. *J Phys Fit Sports Med*. 1(2): 287–296.

Khan, K.M. & Scott, A. (2009) Mechanotherapy: how physical therapists' prescription of exercise promotes tissue repair. *Br J Sports Med*. 43: 247–252.

Killian, M.L., Cavinatto, L., Galatz, L.M. & Thomopoulos, S. (2012) The role of mechanobiology in tendon healing. *J Shoulder Elbow Surg.* 21(2): 228–37.

Langevin, H.M., Bouffard, N.A., Badger, G.J., Iatridis, J.C. & Howe, A.K. (2011) Dynamic fibroblast cytoskeletal response to subcutaneous tissue stretch ex vivo and in vivo. *Am J Physiol Cell Physiol.* 288: C747–C756.

Magnusson, S.P., Langberg, H. & Kjaer, M. (2010) The pathogenesis of tendinopathy: balancing the response to loading. *Nat. Rev. Rheumatol.* 6: 262–268 .

Meltzer, K.R. & Standley, P.R. (2007) Modeled Repetitive Motion Strain and Indirect Osteopathic Manipulative Techniques in Regulation of Human Fibroblast Proliferation and Interleukin Secretion. *J Am Osteopath Assoc.* 107: 527–536.

Myers, T. (2001) The Anatomy Trains. Churchill Livingstone.

Ogawa, R. (2011) Mechanobiology of scarring. Wound Repair Regen, 19 Suppl 1: 2–9.

Ogawa, R., Okai, K., Tokumura, F., Mori, K., Ohmori, Y., Huang, C., Hyakusoku, H. & Akaishi, S. (2012) The relationship between skin stretching/contraction and pathologic scarring: the important role of mechanical forces in keloid generation. *Wound Repair Regen.* 20(2): 149–157.

Purslow, P. (2010) Muscle fascia and force transmission. *J Bodyw Mov Ther.* 14: 411–417.

Sawicki, G.S., Lewis, C.L. & Ferris, D.P. (2009) It pays to have a spring in your step. *Exerc Sport Sci Rev.* July; 37(3): 130.

Schleip, R., Klingler, W. & Lehmann-Horn, F. (2005) Active fascial contractility: Fascia may be able to contract in a smooth muscle-like manner and thereby influence musculoskeletal dynamics. *Med Hypotheses* 65: 273–277.

Schleip, R. & Müller, D.G. (2012) Training principles for fascial connective tissues: Scientific foundation and suggested practical applications. *J Bodyw Mov Ther.* 1–13.

Standley, P.R. & Meltzer, K. (2008) In vitro modeling of repetitive motion strain and manual medicine treatments: potential roles for pro- and anti-inflammatory cytokines. *J Bodyw Mov Ther.* 12: 201–203.

Stecco, C. & Day, J.A. (2010) The Fascial Manipulation Technique and Its Biomechanical Model: A Guide to the Human Fascial System. *Int J Ther Massage Bodyw.* 3(1): 38–40.

Stecco, C., Stern, R., Porzionato, A., Maccho, V., Masiero, S., Stecco, A. & De Caro, R. (2011) Hyaluronan within fascia in the etiology of myofascial pain. *Surg Radiol Anat.* 33(10): 891–896.

Verhaegen, P.D., Schoeten, H.J., Tigchelaar-Gutter, W., van Marle, J., van Noorden, C.J., Middelkoop, E. & van Zuijlen, P.P. (2012) Adaptation of the dermal collagen structure of human skin and scar tissue in response to stretch: an experimental study. *Wound Repair Regen.* 20 (5): 658–666

Vranova, H., Zeman, J., Cech, Z. & Otahal, S. (2009) Identification of viscoelastic parameters of skin with a scar in vivo, influence of soft tissue technique on changes of skin parameters. *J Bodyw Mov Ther.* 13: 344–349.

Wallden, M. (2010) Chains, trains and contractile fields. *J Bodyw Move Ther.* 14: 403–410.

Zanou, N. & Gailly, G. (2013) Skeletal muscle hypertrophy and regeneration: interplay between the myogenic regulatory factors (MRFs) and insulin-like growth factors (IGFs) pathways. *Cell Mol Life Sci.* Apr in Press

Zollner, A.M., Tepole, A.B. & Kuhl, E. (2012) On the biomechanics and mechanobiology on growing skin. *J Theor Biol.* 297: 166–175.

Further reading

Benjamin, M., Kaiser, E. & Milz, S. (2008) Structure-function relationships in tendons: a review. *J. Anat.* 212: 211–228.

Bogduk, N. & MacIntosh, J.E. (1984) The applied anatomy of the thoracolumbar fascia. *Spine* 9: 164–170.

Brown, S.H. & McGill, S.M. (2009) Transmission of muscularly generated force and stiffness between layers of the rat abdominal wall. *Spine* 15; 34(2): 70–5.

Carvalhais, V.O.D., Ocarino, J.D., Araujo, V.L., Souza, T.R., Silva, P.L.P. & Fonseca, S.T. (2013) Myofascial force transmission between the latissimus dorsi and gluteus maximus muscles: An in vivo experiment. *J Biomech.* 46: 1003–1007.

Chaitow, L. (2013) Understanding mechanotransduction and biotensegrity from an adaptation perspective. *J Bodyw Mov Ther.* 17: 141–142.

Chaudhry, H., Schleip, R., Ji, Z., Bukiet, B., Maney, M. & Findley, T. (2008) Three-dimensional mathematical model for deformation of human fasciae in manual therapy. *J Am Osteopath Assoc.* 108(8): 379–390.

Cusi, M.F. (2010) Paradigm for assessment and treatment of SIJ mechanical dysfunction. *J Bodyw Mov Ther.* 14: 152–161.

Hashemirad, F., Talebian, S., Olyaei, G. & Hatef, B. (2010) Compensatory behaviour of the postural control system to flexion-relaxation phenomena. *J Bodyw Mov Ther.* 14(2): 418–423.

Hides, J., Stanton, W., Mendis, M.D. & Sexton, M. (2011) The relationship of transversus abdominis and lumbar multifidus clinical muscle tests in patients with chronic low back pain. *Manual Ther.* 16: 573–577.

Hinz, B., Celetta, G., Tomasek, J.J., Gabbiani, G. & Chaponnier, C. (2001a) Smooth muscle actin expression upregulates fibroblast contractile activity. *Mol Biol Cell.* 12: 2730–2734.

Hinz, B. & Gabbiani, G. (2003) Mechanisms of force generation and transmission by myofibroblasts. *Curr Opin Biotechnol.* 14: 538–546.

Hinz, B. (2007) Biological Perspectives. The Myofibroblast. One Function, Multiple Origins. *Am J Pathol.* 170(6): 1807–1819.

Hinz, B. (2010) The myofibroblast: paradigm for a mechanically active cell. *J Biomech.* 43: 146–155.

Hinz, B., Phan, S.H., Thannickal, V.J., Prunotto, M., Desmoulière, A., Varga, J., De Wever, O., Mareel, M. & Gabbiani, G. (2012) Recent Developments in Myofibroblast Biology: Paradigms for Connective Tissue Remodeling. *Am J Pathol.* 180(4): 1340–1355.

Hodges, P.W. & Mosley, G.L., (2003) Pain and motor control of the lumbopelvic region: effect and possible mechanisms. *J Electromyogr Kinesiol*. 13(4): 361–370.

Hodges, P.W. & Richardson, C.A. (1996) Inefficient muscular stabilization of the lumbar spine associated with low back pain. A motor control evaluation of transversus abdominis. *Spine* 21: 2640–2650.

Hodges, P.W. & Richardson, C.A. (1997) Contraction of the abdominal muscles associated with movement of the lower limb. *Phys Ther*. 77: 132–142.

Hodges, P.W., Richardson, C.A. & Jull, G. (1996) Evaluation of the relationship between laboratory and clinical tests of transversus abdominis function. *Physiother Res Int*. 1: 30–40.

Hodges, P.W., Holm, A.K., Holm, S., Ekstrom, L., Cresswell, A., Hansson, T. & Thorstensson, A. (2003) Intervertebral stiffness of the spine is increased by evoked contraction of transversus abdominis and the diaphragm: in vivo porcine studies. *Spine* 28: 2594–2601.

Hoffman, J. & Gabel, P. (2013) Expanding Panjabi's stability model to express movement: A theoretical model. *Med Hypotheses* Apr: 1–5.

Huijing, P.A. (2007) Epimuscular myofascial force transmission between antagonistic and synergistic muscles can explain movement limitation in spastic paresis. *J Electromyogr Kinesiol*. 17: 708–724.

Ianuzzi, A., Pickar, J.G. & Khalsa, P.S. (2011) Relationships between joint motion and facet joint capsule strain during cat and human lumbar spinal motions. *J Manip Physiol Ther*. 34: 420–431.

Kjaer, M., Langberg, H., Heinemeier, K., Bayer, M.L., Hansen, M., Holm, L., Doessing, S., Konsgaard, M., Krogsgaard, M.R. & Magnusson, S.P. (2009) From mechanical loading to collagen synthesis, structural changes and function in human tendon. *Scand. J. Med. Sci. Sports*. 19(4): 500–510.

Maas, H. & Sandercock, T.G. (2010) Force Transmission between Synergistic Skeletal Muscles through Connective Tissue Linkages. *J Biomed Biotech*. 1–9.

Masi, A.T., Nair, K., Evans, T. & Ghandour, Y. (2010) Clinical, Biomechanical, and Physiological Translational Interpretations of Human Resting Myofascial Tone or Tension. International *J Therap Massage Bodyw*. 3(4): 16–28.

Miyagi, M., Ishikawa, T., Kamoda, H., Orita, S., Kuniyoshi, K., Ochiai, N., Kishida, S., Nakamura, J., Eguchi, Y., Arai, G., Suzuki, M., Aoki, Y., Toyone, T., Takahashi, K., Inoue, G. & Ohtori, S. (2011) Assessment of Gait in a Rat Model of myofascial inflammation using the CatWalk System. *Spine* 36: 1760–1764.

Moseley, G.L., Zalucki, N.M. & Wiech, K. (2008) Tactile discrimination, but not tactile stimulation alone, reduces chronic limb pain. *Pain* 137: 600–608.

Schleip, R., Duerselen L., Vleeming A., Naylor, I.L., Lehmann–Horn, F., Zorn, A., Jaeger H. & Klingler, W. (2012) Strain hardening of fascia: static stretching of dense fibrous connective tissues can induce a temporary stiffness increase accompanied by enhanced matrix hydration. *J Bodyw Mov Ther*. 16: 94.

Schleip, R., Klingler, W. & Lehmann-Horn, F. (2005) Active fascial contractility: Fascia may be able to contract in a smooth muscle-like manner and thereby influence musculoskeletal dynamics. *Med Hypotheses*. 65: 273–277.

Schleip, R. & Klingler, W. (2007) Fascial strain hardening correlates with matrix hydration changes. In: Findley, T.W., Schleip, R. (Eds.), Fascia research – basic science and implications to conventional and complementary health care. Munich: Elsevier GmbH. 51.

Schuenke, M.D., Vleeming, A., Van Hoof, T. & Willard, F.H. (2012) A description of the lumbar interfascial triangle and its relation with the lateral raphe: anatomical constituents of load transfer through the lateral margin of the thoracolumbar fascia. *J Anat*. 221(6): 568–576.

Spector, M. (2002) Musculoskeletal connective tissue cells with muscle: expression of muscle actin in and contraction of fibroblasts, chondrocytes, and osteoblasts. *Wound Repair Regen*. 9(1): 11–8.

Stafford, R.E., Ashton-Miller, J.A., Sapsford, R. & Hodges, P.W. (2012) Activation of the striated urethral sphincter to maintain continence during dynamic tasks in healthy men. *Neurourol Urodyn*. 31(1): 36–3.

Standley, P.R. & Meltzer, K. (2008) In vitro modeling of repetitive motion strain and manual medicine treatments: potential roles for pro- and anti-inflammatory cytokines. *J Bodyw Mov Ther*. 12: 201–203.

Stecco, C., Porzionato, A., Lancerotto, L., Stecco, A., Macchi, V., Day, J.A. & De Caro, R. (2008) Histological study of the deep fasciae of the limbs. *J Bodyw Mov Ther*. 12: 225–230.

Taimela, S., Kankaanpaa, M. & Luoto. S. (1999) The effect of lumbar fatigue on the ability to sense a change in lumbar position. A controlled study. *Spine* 24: 1322–1327.

Tesarz, J., Hoheisel, U., Wiedenhofer, B. & Mense, S. (2011) Sensory innervation of the thoracolumbar fascia in rats and humans. *Neuroscience*. 194: 302–308.

Van der Waal, J. (2009) The Architecture of the Connective Tissue in the Musculoskeletal System—An Often Overlooked Functional Parameter as to Proprioception in the Locomotor Apparatus. *Int J Therap Massage Bodyw*. 2(4): 9–23.

van Wingerden, J.P., Vleeming, A., Buyruk, H.M. & Raissadat, K. (2004) Stabilization of the sacroiliac joint in vivo: verification of muscular contribution to force closure of the pelvis. *Eur Spine J*. 13: 199–205.

Vleeming, A., Schuenke, M.D., Masi, A.T., Carreiro, J.E., Danneels, L. & Willard, F.H. (2012) The sacroiliac joint: an overview of its anatomy, function and potential clinical implications. *J Anat*. 221(6): 537–67.

Vleeming, A., Snijders, C., Stoeckart, R. & Mens, J. (1997) The role of the sacroiliac joins in coupling between spine, pelvis, legs and arms. In: Vleeming et al. (Eds.), *Movement, Stability & Low Back Pain*. Churchill Livingstone. 53–71.

Willard, F.H., Vleeming, A., Schuenke, M.D., Danneels, L. & Schleip, R. (2012) The thoracolumbar fascia: anatomy, function and clinical considerations. *J Anat.* 221(6): 507–536.

Wipff, P-J. & Hinz, B. (2009) Myofibroblasts work best under stress. *J Bodyw Mov Ther.* 13(2): 121–127. RTIC.

Yucesoy, C.A. (2010) Epimuscular myofascial force transmission implies novel principles for muscular mechanics. *Exerc Sport Sci Rev.* 38(3): 128–134.

Yucesoy, C.A., Koopman, B.H.F.J.M., Baan, G.C., Grootenboer, H.J. & Huijing, P.A. (2003a) Extramuscular Myofascial Force Transmission: Experiments and Finite Element Modeling, *Arch Physiol Biochem.* Vol. 111, No. 4: 377–388.

Yucesoy, C.A., Koopman, B.H.F.J.M., Baan, G.C., Grootenboer, H.J. & Huijing, P.A. (2003b) Effects of inter- and extramuscular myofascial force transmission on adjacent synergistic muscles: assessment by experiments and finite-element modeling. *J Biomech.* 36(12): 1797–1811.

CHAPTER 22

Plyometric training: Basic principles for competitive athletes and modern Ninja warriors

Robert Heiduk

Introduction

The development of explosive strength is one of the major goals in competitive sport. It could be described as the ability to combine speed of movement with strength. There are several approaches for increasing explosive strength. The plyometric method is one of them. The range of different nomenclature for plyometric exercise, that are used interchangeably, makes it necessary to provide a clear definition. The objective of this chapter is to explain some basic biomechanical and neurophysiological information about plyometric training and especially the role of fascia, connective tissue. In addition, this chapter provides some guidelines for application and training programme design in competitive and recreational athletes.

Origin of plyometric training and terminology

The meaning of the term plyometric is composed of two Greek words: *plio*, meaning 'more' and *metric*, meaning 'to measure'. Measurable increase might be the most accurate way to explain the term plyometric (Chu, 1998). Commonly known as plyometrics, this category of exercise is mostly referred to as jump training. The earliest references using the word plyometrics have been found in 1966 in a soviet publication (Zanon, 1989). In the early 1960s, Soviet track and field coach Yuri Verkhoshansky experimented with maximal jumps and hops to increase power in his high level athletes. He found that 'depth' jumping, with landing and take off on both feet, would be effective for improving jump performance. He termed his new training

Shock Method. The name referred to the mechanical shock stimulation used to force the muscle to produce as much tension as possible (Verkhoshansky & Siff, 2009). Verkhoshansky's 'strange new system of jumps and bounds' quickly became very popular in the world of sport. In Germany it was popularised by Peter Tschiene, in South Africa by Mel Siff and in Italy by Carmello Bosco (Verkhoshansky & Siff, 2009). It has been suggested that the dominance of the eastern European countries in track and field, weightlifting and gymnastics during the 1970s, can be partially attributed to the Shock Method (Chu, 1998). In the USA it is most often called plyometrics. This term was coined by Verkhoshansky's colleague, track and field coach Fred Wilt, in 1975 (Chu, 1998).

The increased use of the term plyometrics in the fitness world led to the misconception of relating conventional jumps to plyometric training. Many types of activities in daily life and in sport include plyometric patterns, like throwing, jumping, hopping and bounding. However, these patterns are not on the same level, in terms of intensity, as plyometric training. The characteristic of true plyometric training is rapid eccentric loading as a result of increased muscle tension, elicited by the powerful stretch reflex and the explosive release of elastic energy stored in the fascial connective tissues (Chapter 10). In sports science, terms like reactive ability (Verkhoshansky & Siff, 2009), reactive strength (Schnabel et al., 2011), or stretch shortening cycle (SSC) (Komi, 2000) have become established as more precise definitions. Reactive strength is defined as the ability to couple eccentric and concentric muscle contraction in the shortest amount of time (Schnabel et al., 2011). Thus, a major goal of plyometric training is to compress the amount of time required between eccentric and concentric contraction. While this definition has only a muscle action orientated view and neglects the role of fascial connective tissues in displaying reactive ability, it would be more holistic to use the following definition:

Reactive Strength is the motor quality to show high power output within the Stretch-Shortening-Cycle (SSC). Sports science categorises reactive strength or the SSC as a separate motor quality. However, it relies strongly on maximum strength, innervation patterns of the muscles and the elastic recoil properties of fascial connective tissues (Schmidtbleicher & Gollhofer, 1985) (Chapter 10).

There are variations in time characteristics in different types of plyometric movement patterns. Güllich & Schmidtbleicher (2000) classify the reactive movements into a short (<200 milliseconds) and long (>200 milliseconds) SSC. Examples for a short SSC are sprinting with a ground contact time of 100 to 110 milliseconds, the long jump with 120 milliseconds and the high jump with 170 to 180 milliseconds (Bührle, 1989). The long SSC can be watched in the jump of a volleyball smash with ground contact times between 300 to 360 milliseconds.

Physiological key concepts and research findings

Compared to the pure concentric rate of force development, without a preceding eccentric movement phase, in the SSC a higher force is achieved (Komi, 2000). Currently there are two explanation models for this phenomenon. A neurophysiological model and a mechanical model. In the neurophysiological model it will be suggested, that the rapid pre-stretch of the muscle spindles during the eccentric phase, leads to a stretch reflex. As a result result, it develops a more powerful muscle contraction, due to the activation of more motor units (Komi, 1992). The faster the eccentric loading phase, the stronger the concentric muscle contraction (Böhm et al., 2006). A common example for a stretch reflex is the knee jerk reflex.

Rassier & Herzog (2005) consider the magnitude of force enhancement may come from three different factors: the magnitude of stretch, the rate of stretch and the duration of stretch. Bubeck (2002) adds, that under different loading conditions, the neuromuscular activation patterns change. This would indicate, that adaptations in an SSC are highly context specific. Some evidence suggests that the stretch reflex may be not

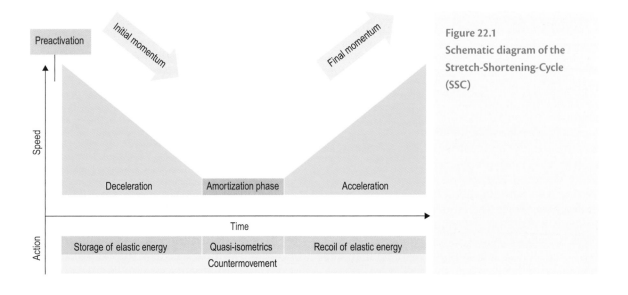

Figure 22.1
Schematic diagram of the Stretch-Shortening-Cycle (SSC)

activated in all muscles (Nardone et al., 1990). Monoarticular muscles, which cross one joint only, may be benefit more than biarticular muscles from the stretch reflex (Nicol & Komi, 1998).

The mechanical model proposes that the higher efficacy of movements within an SSC attributes to the storage of elastic energy in the elastic elements of the fascial tissues (Chapter 10). The spring-like release during the concentric phase has shown to produce higher force outputs (Komi, 2000). Figure 22.1 shows that a key factor in the SSC is the amount of coupling time between the eccentric and concentric phase, which is described as 'amortization phase' (Chu, 1998). If the amortization phase lasts too long, the energy being absorbed is lost as heat (Radcliffe & Farentinos, 1999).

Schmidtbleicher & Gollhofer (1985) found that in trained athletes the amortization phase was approximately 100 milliseconds, significantly shorter than in untrained subjects. Other researches suggests that the ideal coupling time lasts between 15–25 milliseconds (Bosco et al., 1981). Chu (1998) characterises the amortization phase as quasi-isometric muscle action. The muscle length does not change during this period. So, how might the immediate powerful movement be produced?

In contrast to the more muscle orientated neurophysiological view, the mechanical model suggests a storage of kinetic energy in the fascial tissues during the rapid prestretch in the eccentric phase. Some research indicates that the elastic recoil of the fascial elements seems to play a more vital role than was previously suggested (Chapter 10). Kawakami et al. (2002) confirm that during the eccentric phase of a counter movement plantar flexion, the gastrocnemius only works in a near-isometric manner, which means that hardly any length changes of the muscle fibres are observable in this phase (Chapter 1). The higher power output was attributed to the elastic recoil properties of the myofascial tissues.

In plyometric patterns like bouncing, Dean & Kuo (2011) observed that the elasticity of the fascial elements reduces the work needed from active muscle fibres, which leads to a decrease in energy expenditure. In running, plyometric training can increase energy efficiency and improve aerobic performance (Spurrs et al., 2003).

Ishikawa et al. (2005) investigated that different drop heights in depth jumps have a specific impact on fascial tissues. It seems that overly high eccentric loads limit the effectiveness of the catapult mechanism (Chapter 10). In addition, the interaction of the connective tissues may vary in different muscles. Zatsiorsky & Kraemer (2008) point out that the storage of elastic energy is only possible in more flexible tissues. Due to their superior muscle tension, in top-level athletes muscle stiffness exceeds the stiffness of fascial tissues. This leads to an increased elastic recoil in fascial tissues. Since muscle stiffness is proportional to its activation, it would reason that higher activation patterns were a main condition for energy storage in fascial tissues. Unfortunately research findings are inconsistent in this context.

Fouré et al. (2012) compared the influence of a 14-week plyometric training programme on the mechanical tissue properties of the myofascial complex and muscle activation patterns. After the training period, all subjects showed improvement in jumping performances. To their surprise, more experienced subjects showed a decrease in muscle activation and a higher efficiency in energy storage and recoil of the fascial tissues. Similarly, a comparison of a 12-week strength training versus plyometric training found no significant differences in EMG activation in jumping (Kubo et al., 2007). The researchers suggest that the gains in jump performance after plyometric training rely more on adaptations of the myofascial complex, rather than on neuromuscular changes.

Robert and Konow (2013) found, that tendons are able to buffer energy dissipation by muscle. This mechanism could lead to a reduced injury risk. Kuminasa et al. (2013) could show, that in contrast to Japanese distance runners, their Kenyan counterparts have a superior muscle-tendon architecture. This mechanical advantage could be one explanation, for the superior running efficiency of Kenyan distance runners.

The spring-like properties of the connective tissue vary for subjects of different genders, injury state and athletic background. This would be one explanation for the differences in the effects of plyometric training. It seems that there are movement and age specific differences in the behaviour of fascial tissues in plyometric training (Hoffrén et al., 2007) (Arampatzis et al., 2007). The same should be valid for muscle activation patterns.

In summary, research results in sport have to be interpreted very carefully. Distinctions in subjects of different performance levels are highly variable (Karavirta, 2011). Thus the success of training programmes for optimal individual adaptations strongly relies on personalisation.

Considerations for plyometric training

The implementation of proper plyometric training requires some preliminary considerations. At the beginning a specific goal should be defined. Like every other kind of exercise, the training effects are highly movement specific. A plyometric training programme for golfers is different to one for sprinters, jumpers, gymnasts, strength athletes or for rehabilitation. Moreover, the current ability level of the athlete has to be considered. A beginner needs a different training stimulus, to an intermediate, or a top-level athlete. Age, body weight, skill and previous injury play an important role (Holcomb et al., 1998). Starting with plyometric training, the development of a proper exercise technique under qualified instruction and supervision is paramount. The goal is to increase efficiency and avoid injury.

Injury prevention is a critical factor in plyometric training. High impulsive peak forces produce serious injury risks for the joints. Coaches should be aware that plyometric exercises can lead to muscle damage and collagen breakdown of the fascial tissues without decreases in skeletal muscle capacity (Tofas et al., 2008). Therefore risks may result from inappropriate or excessive use, rather than plyometric training itself (Verkhoshanky & Siff, 2009). Being technically correct and creating sensible progression seem to be the most important factors in injury prevention. In addition, the coach has to ensure a proper warm-up and the use of an adequate

landing surface (Borkowski, 1990). Wathen (1994) highlights that the quality of the landing surfaces plays a major role in performing plyometric drills. Allerheiligen & Rogers (1996) suggest spring loaded floors or rubber mats and caution against practicing on concrete or asphalt. Firm natural grass may be a sufficient training surface as well. However, overly soft surfaces diminish the effectiveness of plyometrics, as the mechanical stimulus on the body is lowered.

It is suggested that a carefully designed plyometric training regime, over the course of a season, may reduce the incidence of knee injury in athletes involved in sports with large jumping and cutting components (Hewett et al., 1999). In addition to the enhancement of the athlete's movement skills, the increased musculotendinous stiffness may be another possible factor for injury prevention (Spurrs et al., 2003).

Depth jumps are the most advertised form of plyometric training but also exert the highest loads on body structures (Allerheiligen & Rogers, 1996). Thus, these should only be used by a small percentage of athletes. People weighing more than 220lb (98kg) should not perform depth jumps from platforms higher than 18 inches (45 centimeters) (Chu, 1992).

Strength and conditioning practitioners should not design a plyometric training as a stand-alone programme. Every athlete needs an adequate strength base prior to starting plyometric drills. When strength is not adequate, it results in a loss of stability and forces are excessively absorbed by the joints. This leads to an increased risk of injury. For high-intensity drills, like depth jumps, literature suggests a strength ratio of 1.5–2.5 times body weight in the 1-RM (One Repetition Maximum) barbell-squat (Allerheiligen & Rogers, 1996) (Chu, 1992) (Gambetta, 1992).

These recommendations may not be appropriate for female athletes. There is no specific research to address this topic. Experience in daily sport practice suggests that for female athletes 1–1.5 times body weight in the 1-RM barbell-squat would be a suitable value. There is also a lack of research of recommendations for strength values in upper body plyometrics and for application in recreational athletes. For recreational athletes, the same principles apply but on a lower level. A healthy male should be able to squat with a weight of 0.8–1 times body weight for eight repetitions, perform 10 pull-ups and 20 push-ups. A healthy female should show eight repetitions of squats with 0.6–0.8 times body weight on the barbell, six pull-ups and 12 push-ups.

In addition, a sufficient amount of specific flexibility is needed to perform plyometric training safely (Chu, 1992). Davies & Matheson (2001) report the following contraindications to plyometrics: pain, inflammation, ligament and capsular sprains, muscle and tendon strains, joint instability, fascial tissue limitations based on post-operative conditions and a lack of strength base.

Training programme application for competitive athletes

First and foremost, for competitive athletes there is no general recipe that can be applied consistently to all athletes. Hence, at this point, it would make no sense to lay out a training regime because the requirements in each area of training are highly individual. However there are some basic rules that endure for all serious athletes.

Two different kinds of guidelines are useful to create an individual training programme. The first approach uses coaching principles which describe instructions in a greater context, such as educational aspects in order to ensure optimal training progressions. The four coaching principles in this approach are:

1. Move from simple to complex
2. From light to heavy
3. Technique first – quality over quantity
4. Avoid fatigue.

These principles suggest systematically increasing loads and the complexity of movements. Moreover, the principles promote the importance of movement quality instead of quantity – the coach has to ensure the perfect execution of the movement and must avoid fatigue. In the SSC, fatigue is absolutely counterproductive. It causes a stretch reflex decrease and a loss of elastic energy potential (Komi, 2000). This leads to a reduced muscle and joint stiffness, which can cause injury. Thus, turning plyometrics into a conditioning programme, which is usually designed to develop energy systems, is not advisable. One key to avoid fatigue is to keep a specific work-rest-ratio between sets. For rehabilitation, Chu & Cordier (2000) suggest a ratio of 1:5–1:10. When the exercise takes 10 seconds, 50–100 seconds rest would be appropriate. True Shock Training, for example, depth jumps, demands considerably longer rest periods. Depending on the intensity 3–10 minutes rest is advised (Bubeck, 2002) (Sialis, 2004).

The second approach determines the specific load. In plyometric training, intensity is determined by jumping height or effort, the usage of additional weight, or the style of exercise, like single or double leg exercises. Volume and frequency describe more quantitative variables, such as the amount of work within a training session, total number of jumps, number of sets and repetitions, work-rest-ratio between exercise and break within a training session and the number of sessions per week. According to the literature, a sufficient recovery time of 48–72 hours is needed (Chapter 1). This means a training frequency of approximately twice a week (Chu & Cordier, 2000). The coach should bear in mind that training alone is not the key. The combination of the

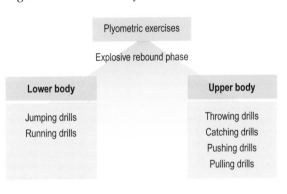

Figure 22.2
Classification of plyometric exercises

training stimulus and a sufficient recovery provide desirable results.

A classification of plyometric exercises (Figure 22.2) is helpful for designing a well-balanced training programme. This is also useful for the long-term timing of training, which is better known as periodisation. An example of a training session for competitive athletes might look like this:

1. mobility work and injury prevention
2. core activation
3. submaximal plyometrics
4. skill training
5. maximal plyometrics (rare)
6. strength training
7. energy system development.

Plyometric training for the recreational athlete

The 'higher-faster-stronger' approach does not necessarily fit into recreational health training. Recreational athletes who wish to increase their overall fitness and health, should ignore competition and focus more on elegance, pleasure and aesthetics. Under these conditions, the expression of emotions in movement becomes an important factor. Creativity plays a vital role. In movement, creativity claims the absence of standardised repetitive movement patterns and adds high variety to the training. Creative movement is a form of self-expression.

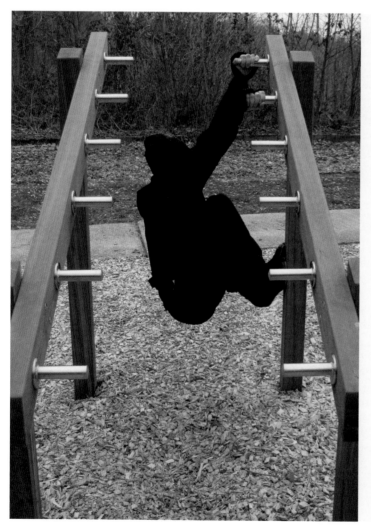

Figure 22.3

Squat bouncing

A basic exercise, which promotes complex flexibility and movement preparation of a Ninja. Take a deep squat position and hang up on a balustrade. While you keep tension in the upper body, you begin to bounce in this position. You should repeatedly change the body angle to target the fascial tissues.

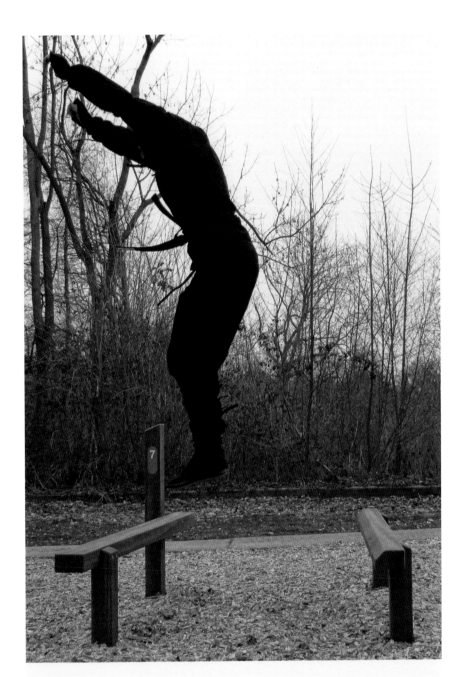

Figure 22.4
Precision jump

A parkour Ninja must be able to jump and land silently in exactly any position he wants. Practice first on larger objects with small jump distances. With increasing skill you will decrease the landing surfaces and increase the jump distance. Remember always to be silent!

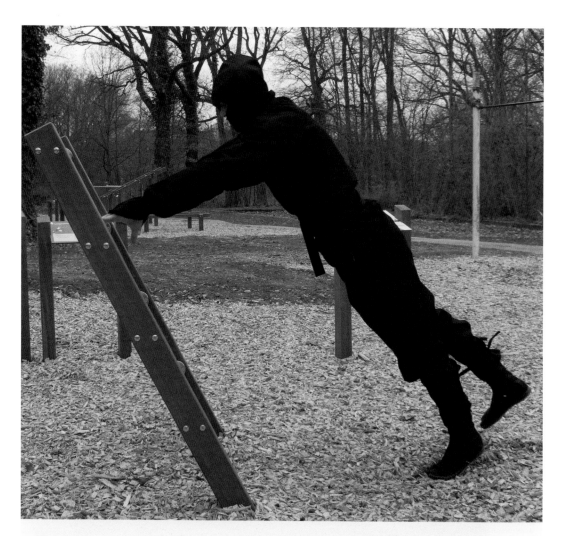

Figure 22.5
Plyometric pushup

This is a demanding challenge. The goal is to fall down into a push-up position and to reverse the movement as quickly as possible. You should always start at low falling heights. For the beginner, it is sufficient to start on a wall. For safety, always practice in a step position.

A perfect example can be found in playgrounds. If one watches children play, one will find that sprinting, bouncing (Figure 22.3), landing (Figure 22.4), hopping, swinging (Figures 22.6–22.8) and deceleration movements all contain components of the SSC. Thus, these movements should all be considered as sub-maximal plyometric training. Children often build a story around their games. This is a beautiful example of creativity as an inseparable continuum in natural movement.

In addition, 'playing' is ideal for the renewal of your fascial tissues. It always contains some strength, flexibility, speed and endurance

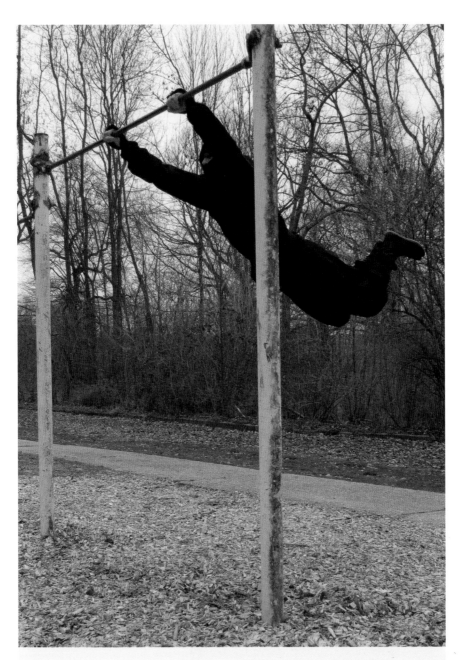

Figure 22.6
Bar swing

Plyometric stretching of the fascial tissues works best under full muscle tension. In the bar swing, the momentum provides an additional stimulus for the fascial complexes. For the Ninja, it is the basic stage before progression to bar exercises.

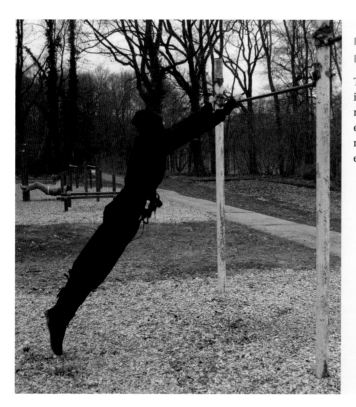

Figure 22.7
Bar jump

The bar jump is very important for overcoming obstacles. It allows the Ninja to use the momentum of the jump to create a rapid eccentric load. This 'monkey' style movement requires the courage to jump off in complete extension to catch the bar safely.

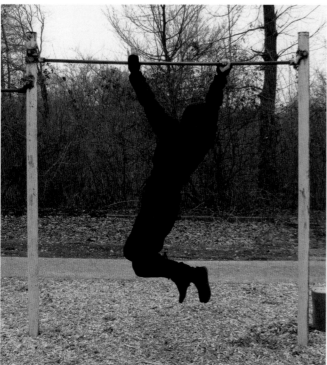

Figure 22.8
Bar deviation

Good upper body strength is required to master this skill. There is a Ninja secret using the fascial elastic recoil in deviation movements: If you bend your arms, you are using raw muscle strength. You should consider it as a one-handed swing instead. This advice will save muscle energy and allow the movement to appear more fluid and graceful.

components (Chapter 11). In contrast to the Western 'fitness monoculture', which strongly relies on an isolated view of separate body-systems, movement needs to be seen in a more holistic way. As mentioned previously, this strongly relies on the emotion in movement.

Themed training: The Parkour Ninja

A holistic approach could be achieved by themed training. If one feels inspired by a Ninja movie, the first step would be to imagine the main characteristics of a Ninja: black clothes, smoothness and silence, stealth and skill, super strength and amazing agility. These skills allow the Ninja to overcome all obstacles. In evolution, parkour can be considered a modern branch of Ninja movement skills. If we define parkour as art of efficent movement, all the Ninja principles still apply.

A basic composition of 'plyometric Ninja' exercises are presented in Figures 22.3–22.8.

All examples show, that in recreation-health training, there is no need for stringent programme variables. Find your own way to master different task specific skills. Interest and curiosity are the main factors in learning new skills.

In conclusion, the general considerations for plyometric training in recreational athletes are:

- Stop counting repetitions
- Break out of your pattern
- Inspire yourself
- Try something new
- Play around
- Be silent
- Listen to your body
- Aspire to fluidity and smoothness.

References

Allerheiligen, B. & Rogers, R. (1996) Plyometrics program design. National Strength and Conditioning Association (Eds.), *Plyometric and Medicine Ball Training*. 3–8. Colorado Springs: National Strength and Conditioning Association.

Arampatzis, A., Karamanidis, K., Morey-Klapsing, G., De Monte, G. & Stafilidis, S. (2007) Mechanical properties of the triceps surae tendon and aponeurosis in relation to intensity of sport activity. *J Biomech*. 40: 1946–1952.

Borkowski, J. (1990) Prevention of Pre-Season Muscle Soreness: Plyometric Exercise. *Abstracted in Athletic Training*. 25(2): 122.

Bosco C., Komi, P.V. & Ito, A. (1981) Pre-stretch potentiation of human skeletal muscle during ballistic movement. *Acta Physiologica Scandinavica*. 111: 135–140.

Bubeck, D. (2002) *Belastungsvariation und funktionelle Anpassungen im Dehnungs-Verkürzungs-Zyklus. PhD Thesis*. Fakultät für Geschichts-, Sozial- und Wirtschaftswissenschaften der Universität Stuttgart.

Böhm, H., Cole, G., Brüggemann, G. & Cole, H. (2006) Contribution of muscle series elasticity to maximum performance in drop jumping. *J Appl Biomech*. 22: 3–13.

Bührle, M. (1989) Maximalkraft-Schnellkraft-Reaktivkraft. In: *Sportwissenschaft*. 3: 311–325.

Chu, D.A. (1992) *Jumping into Plyometrics*. Champaign: Human Kinetics.

Chu, D.A. (1998) *Jumping into Plyometrics* (2nd ed.) Champaign, IL: Human Kinetics.

Chu, D. & Cordier, D. (2000) *Plyometrics in Rehabilitation*. In: Ellenbecker T.S. (Ed). Knee Ligament Rehabilitation. New York: Chuchill Livingstone. 321–344.

Davies, G.J. & Matheson, J.W. (2001) Shoulder plyometrics. *Sports Medicine and Arthroscopy Review* 9: 1–18.

Dean, J.C. & Kuo, A.D. (2011). Energetic costs of producing muscle work and force in a cyclical human bouncing task. *J Appl Physiol* 110(4): 73–880.

Fouré, A., Nordez, A., Guette, M. & Cornu, C. (2012) Effects of plyometric training on passive stiffness of gastrocnemii muscles and Achilles tendon. *Euro J Appl Physiol* 112(8): 2849–2857.

Gambetta, V. (1992) New plyometric training techniques: designing a more effective plyometric training program. *Coaching Volleyball*. April/May, 26–28.

Güllich, A. & Schmidtbleicher, D. (2000) *Struktur der Kraftfähigkeiten und ihrer Trainingsmethoden*. In: Siewers, M. (Ed.), Muskelkrafttraining. Band 1: Ausgewählte Themen – Alter, Dehnung, Ernährung, Methodik. Kiel: Siewers Eigenverlag. 17–71.

Hewett, T.E., Lindenfeld, T.N., Riccobene, J.V. & Noyes, F.R. (1999) The effect of neuromuscular training on the incidence of knee injury in female athletes. American *J Sports Med* 27: 699–705.

Hoffrén, M., Ishikawa, M. & Komi, P.V. (2007) Age-related neuromuscular function during drop jumps. *J Appl Physiol* 103(4): 276–283.

Holcomb, W.R., Kleiner, D.M., & Chu, D.A. (1998) Plyometrics: Considerations for safe and effective training. *Strength Cond J* 20: 36–39.

Ishikawa, M., Niemalä, E. & Komi, P.V. (2005) Interaction between fascicle and tendinous tissues in short-contact stretch-shortening cycle exercise with varying eccentric intensities. *J Appl Physiol*. 99(1): 217–223.

Karavirta, L. (2011) *Cardiorespiratory, neuromuscular and cardiac autonomic adaptations to combined endurance and strength training in ageing men and women*. Dissertation University of Jyväskylä, Finland.

Kawakami, Y., Muraoka, T., Ito, S., Kanehisa, H. & Fukunaga T. (2002) In vivo muscle fibre behaviour during counter-movement exercise in humans reveals a significant role for tendon elasticity. *J Physiol*. 540: 635–646

Komi, P.V. (1992) In *Strength and Power in Sport*. Stretch shortening cycle. Ed. Komi, P. V. Oxford: Blackwell Scientific. 169–179.

Komi P.V. (2000) Stretch-shortening cycle: a powerful model to study normal and fatigued muscle. *J Biomech*. 33: 1197–1206.

Kubo, K., Morimoto, M., Komuro, T., Yata, H., Tsunoda, N., Kanehisa, H. & Fukunaga, T. (2007) Effects of plyometric and weight training on muscle-tendon complex and jump performance. 39(10): 1801–1810.

Kunimasa, Y., Sano, K., Oda, T., Nicol, C., Komi P.V., Locatelli E., Ito, A. & Ishikawa, M. (2013) Specific muscle–tendon architecture in elite Kenyan distance runners. Scan. *J of Med & Sci in Sp*.

Nardone, A., Corra, T. & Schieppati, M. (1990) Different activations of the soleus and gastrocnemii muscles in response to various types of stance perturbation in man. *Exp Brain Res* 80: 323–332.

Nicol, C. & Komi, P.V. (1998) Significance of passively induced stretch reflexes on Achilles tendon force enhancement. *Muscle Nerve* 21: 1546–1548.

Radcliffe, J.C. & Farentinos, B.C. (1999) *High-Powered Plyometrics*. Champaign: Human Kinetics.

Rassier, D. & Herzog, W. (2005) Force enhancement and relaxation rates after stretch of activated muscle fibres. *Proceedings of the Royal Society B*: *Biological Sciences*. 272: 475–480.

Robert, T.J., Konow. N. (2013). How tendons buffer energy dissipation by muscle. *Exerc Sport Sci*. Rev., Vol. 41, No. 4, 186–193.

Schmidtbleicher, D. & Gollhofer, A. (1985) Einflussgrößen des reaktiven Bewegungsverhaltens und deren Bedeutung für die Trainingspraxis. In: Bührle, M. (Ed.), Grundlagen des Maximal- und Schnellkrafttrainings. Schorndorf: Hoffmann. 271–281.

Schnabel, G., Harre, D. & Krug, J. (Ed.) (2011) Trainingslehre - Trainingswissenschaft: Leistung-Training-Wettkampf. 2nd Ed. Aachen: Meyer & Meyer.

Sialis, J. (2004) *Innervationscharakteristik und Trainingsadaptibilitaet im Dehnungs-Verkuerzungs-Zyklus*. Stuttgart: University Stuttgart.

Spurrs, R.W., Murphy, A.J. & Watsford, M.L. (2003) The effect of plyometric training on distance running performance. *Euro J Appl Physiol* 89: 1–7.

Tofas, T., Jamurtas, A.Z., Fatouros, I., Nikolaidis, M.G., Koutedakis Y., Sinouris, E.A., Papageorgakopoulou N. & Theocharis, D.A. (2008) Plyometric Exercise Increases Serum Indices of Muscle Damage and Collagen Breakdown. *J Strength Cond Res* 22(2): 490–496.

Turner, A.M., Owings, M. & Schwane, J.A. (2003) Improvement in running economy after 6 weeks of plyometric training. *J Strength Cond Res* 17: 60–67.

Verkhoshansky, Y. & Siff, M.C. (2009) *Supertraining*. Sixth edition expanded version. Rome: Verkhoshansky SSTM.

Wathen, D. (1994) Literature review: explosive plyometric exercises. In: *National Strength and Conditioning Association* (Eds.), *Position Paper and Literature Review*: Explosive Exercises and Training and Explosive Plyometric Exercises. 13–16. Colorado Springs: National Strength and Conditioning Association.

Zanon, S. (1989) Plyometrics: Past and Present. *New Studies in Athletics* 4(1): 7–17.

Zatsiorky, V.M. & Kraemer, W.J. (2008) *Krafttraining – Praxis und Wissenschaft*. Third Edition. Aachen: Meyer & Meyer.

Further reading

Baechle, T.R. & Earle, R. (2008) *Essentials of Strength Training and Conditioning*. Third Edition. Champaign, IL: Human Kinetics.

Berthoz, A. (2000) *The Brain's Sense of Movement*. Cambridge: Harvard University Press.

Butler, D. & Moseley, L. (2003) *Explain Pain*. Adelaide: Noigroup Publications.

Coyle, D. (2010) *The Talent Code: Greatness Isn't Born. It's Grown*. London: Arrow.

Gambetta, V. (2007) *Athletic Development: The Art and Science of Functional Sports Conditioning*. Champaign: Human Kinetics.

Kurz, T. & Zagorski, M. (2001) *Science of Sports Training: How to Plan and Control Training for Peak Performance*. Second Edition. Vermont: Stadion Publishing.

McCredie, S. (2007) Balance: In Search of the Lost Sense. New York: Little, Brown and Company.

Yessis, M. (2008) *Russian Sports Restoration and Massage*. Michigan: Ultimate Athlete Concepts.

CHAPTER 23

Kettlebells and clubbells

Donna Eddy

This chapter discusses the fascial aspects of swinging a weight, namely a kettlebell. One kettlebell exercise or movement 'The Swing' (Scarito, 2008) will be thoroughly discussed (Figures 23.1–23.10). Writing this chapter became more interesting as the ideas and possibilities unfolded, simply because writing about kettlebells is bound to go against the grain of one school of kettlebell training or another (Jones, 2010) (Scarito, 2008) (Iardella, 2014) (Cotter, 2011).

The chapter includes a short discussion about clubbells (Figures 23.11–23.13), as they are evolving like kettlebells, into the mainstream fitness movement and will soon be seen as frequently as kettlebells in gyms, homes and in training videos. That said, having been introduced around 2001, kettlebells are considered new to the fitness industry and are still somewhat unknown to the home user (Armstrong, 2013).

The basis of including kettlebells in the practical application of fascial training is to highlight the integrative movement patterns that swinging a kettlebell provides and the potential to affect the connective tissue matrix through load tolerance (Chaudhry et al., 2008, cited in Chaitow, 2011) (Chapter 2). The force production, during the extended time the body is under tension to maintain the pendulous action when swinging the weight, enables this connection to be felt experientially (Figures 23.2, 23.5, 23.7, 23.9 and 23.13) (Schultz & Feitis, 1996).

Having a complex, not necessarily complicated, movement means there is no isolation of one body part or muscle, as is the focus of bodybuilding, which is the foundation of the typical gym training programme. Momentum is introduced to the movement, as the load of the kettlebell is 'outside' the centre of gravity of the person holding the weight. The entire body is recruited to direct and control this momentum, through body stabilisation and by accelerating and decelerating the tool (Fable, 2010). Swinging a weight means the entire body is involved and there are multiple options and angles for the weight to pass through, as opposed to a direct line used in push/pull exercises.

Variable lines of trajectory add to the complexity of the body's engagement. The benefit of this is clearly described by Schultz and Feitis (1996): 'Increased demand for movement furthers maturation of the connective tissue. As we use a [body] part it becomes more capable, more skilled. In turn, as we become more skilled, we explore a wider range of movement.'

The practical sequence included at the end of this chapter (Figures 23.1–23.13) moves from a closed chain structured swing, to an open chain flowing and segmentally engaging swing, which loads the entire structure in a systemic spiraling. This is also described by Myers & Schleip (2011) as a means to 'engage the longest possible myofascial chains' (Chapter 6). It is this engagement of the myofascial chains that provides the experiential difference of rotational inertia when executing The Swing (Tooling, 2012).

The one handed swing, (Figures 23.6–23.10) using a fascially focused technique, by adding rotation and some spinal flexion, highlights the 'contralateral activation [which] allows fascial integration' (Cotter, 2010) (Sonnon, 2009). By adding these rotational modifications to the traditional swing, the integration of the entire body is felt, especially in the 'Spiral Line', (Myers, 2001) (Chapter 6) when you swing the kettlebell or clubbell with one hand.

Load Tolerance (Schultz & Feitis, 1996) is experienced in real time when swinging a weight, as your body is being pulled by the force of the weight tractioning the joints and applying varying load forces during the entire movement. In this way, the entire body stabilises against the pull. The beauty of swinging the kettlebell is that you do not have to have a variety of weighted bells. Simply change the speed at which you swing and the forces shift accordingly (Maxwell, 2013).

For those familiar with Thomas Myers' work (Chapter 6), the availability to move the body in flowing arcs of movement and vector angles, is what is both valuable and unique about swinging a weight. These vector angles open a multitude of movement and exercise variations that are not an easily executed option with push/pull/pressing exercises. Also of note is the fact that it is not characteristic to 'muscle' the weight. With kettlebells, you swing the weight and integrate the movement throughout the body producing a fluid and graceful continuum (Maxwell & Newell, 2011).

In traditional training circles, eccentric loading is what we refer to when we discuss preparatory countermovements (Myers & Schleip, 2011) (Chapter 11). Being mindful of the loading and unloading provided by swinging through arcs, means negating gravity at certain points of the movement. As a result, there is a unique, full range inclusion of opposing actions. This is felt and seen in The Swing as full flexion to full extension of the lower half of the body (Figures 23.1, 23.8, 23.10 and 23.12).

I like to describe the opposing actions as interconnected tension and activation. One part of your body is eccentrically loading, preparing to contract with force the preparatory countermovement, whilst another area is contracting with force. Everything else is activated providing stability to support this fluid movement. Learning this is one of the unique challenges with kettlebell swinging. It is during this time under tension that the Ninja principle comes in to play (Myers & Schleip, 2011) (Chapter 11). One cannot be smooth and quiet like a Ninja if one is clanging and banging, slapping things around. Smooth, seamless motion is necessary for graceful weight swinging and it is through graceful motion that fascial training effects are achieved.

For trainers wishing to teach The Swing to their clients, be sure to look at the client's range of motion through the hips. The flexion of the hips during the down swing needs to be initiated with the pelvis anteriorly rotating, similar to the stiff leg deadlift action. Hamstring length is also a factor to ensure the spine is not flexing to gain this bottom position. To come out of the back or bottom position, clients need to focus on pressing their heels into the floor and activate the glutes to allow the hips to open. Once the body comes to a straight upright alignment and the bell is coming off the thighs, the client also needs to activate the quads to stabilise the entire lower body. The stability from global activation of the legs and the lower body spreads the effort throughout the entire body, rather than loading the spine and finishing the extension, the top position of the The Swing, with spinal effort (Cotter, 2011).

To set it out in practical terms, and simplify many of the relatively new terms fascial training introduces, we can count off the points from 'How to build a better Fascial Body' from the Fascial Fitness Workshop notes (Myers & Schleip, 2011) (Chapter 11), in relation to swinging a weight (kettlebell or club).

1. **Engages long Myofascial chains:** Entire backline/posterior chain for The Swing and when doing the exercise with one hand, the spiral line is felt more significantly (Chapter 6).

2. **Stretches load with multi-vectorial variations:** Felt at the end of range/the transition point.

3. **Employs elastic rebound:** Seen as graceful changes in direction for the kettlebell (Chapter 10).

4. **Uses preparatory countermovement:** The Swing takes you through full flexion of hips and extension of the shoulders, before opening into full extension of hips and partial flexion of the shoulders. Full flexion may be experienced if you wish.

5. **Encourages full proprioception:** The weight is swinging with a pendulous momentum so one must be vigilant and mindful whilst in motion. You cannot muscle the weight mindlessly.

6. **Respects matrix hydration:** Due to the tractioning effect of the displaced centre of mass with both kettlebell and club whilst training,

the joints' capsular fluids remain in tact. In addition, the emphasis is placed on resting between sets and having days of rest between training sessions.

7. **Fosters gently perseverance:** This chapter is entirely based on the development of one exercise in all its possibilities and variations. Emphasis is placed on moving slowly through the movement possibilities, as this is critical for safe and effective exercise results.

8. **Respects constitutional differences:** The beauty of The Swing is that it mimics a fundamental daily movement, the squat and the movement from sitting to standing. This is a movement from which everyone can benefit, when appropriate modifications are made.

9. **Proceed with caution:** This goes without saying, if you have followed all points above. Gentle perseverance with The Swing is needed before moving onto a more technical movement.

10. **Cultivates your fascial garden:** Starting with a fundamental movement, like The Swing, is a great step towards having a 'functional' body. Being functional moves you closer to our natural state and is a vital component to injury prevention and successful rehabilitation, if required (Forencich, 2003).

Clubs

Clubs allow even greater variation of movement than kettlebells. You could think of kettlebells as a progression from dumbbells and barbells, and therefore, clubs as a progression from kettlebells. Kettlebells came into mainstream fitness quite recently, with the training of instructors beginning in the USA in 2001 (Armstrong, 2013). Clubbell swinging, however, is still a relatively under-utilised form of exercise. As a result, there is a timeline consideration with the progression of these tools in the fitness industry. The growing trend towards functional movement also needs to be considered (Forencich, 2003). This shift towards more functional movement may be experienced with clubbells: you can swing outside your legs, which is virtually impossible with kettlebells due to their bulbous belly, and you can do overhead swinging. This opens up greater ranges of movement, which are not available with the kettlebell (Maxwell, 2013).

With clubs you can also 'circumnavigate' the body, opening rotations and angles not available with any other training tool (Maxwell, 2013). This circumnavigation is not part of The Swing discussed and presented here but is a movement option that opens and integrates all aspects of the body not available with traditional training tools and techniques.

As with the kettlebell, when working with the club the training load and effects are translated throughout the entire body. The goal of The Swing is to move smoothly (Sonnon, 2006). To move smoothly, whilst swinging either a club or a kettlebell, requires integrated stabilisation, which is achieved by using the pendulum effect provided by the displaced centre of mass. This allows the dynamic recoil action of the fascia to be tensioned and challenged throughout the exercise. Having smooth, fluid movement requires focus on timing your movement and performing with rhythm (Steer, 2009) (Chapter 10).

With both kettlebells and clubs, there are many health promoting benefits such as opening the hips, activating the glutes, decompressing the shoulders and providing a stimulating cardiovascular challenge all in one exercise (Heins, 2014). It is often the case that there will be less soreness after training and less overuse type injuries due to the integrated nature of weight swinging (Maxwell, 2013). As demonstrated in the various swing options (Figures 23.1–23.13), the entire posterior chain is activated. Alternatively, it can be said that the activation of the posterior chain is the focus for successful completion of The Swing movement.

The beauty of this integrated engagement is that it mimics a fundamental daily movement, the squat as well as the action of sitting and standing. The Swing, when executed properly, is an exercise that can be described as an all inclusive health promoting, corrective and stimulating exercise. With today's need to compensate for prolonged sitting, the activation of the glute muscles, and the prominence of connective tissue activation, through the effect of elastic recoil (Chapter 10), provides this

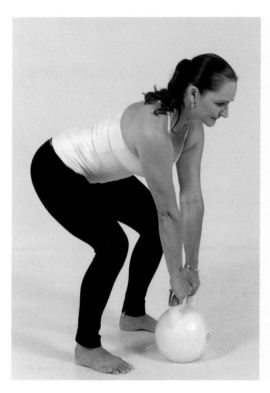

Figure 23.1

Two-handed strict swing – start position

In kettlebell circles this is the standard swing. Bell between legs with handle square in both hands. Use a deliberate hip action rather than 'squat' action to drive the swing. Lengthened, straight spine and arms through the movement is the traditional swing action.

Cues:

• Start with kettlebell slightly in front of toes, feet square and squat down holding the handle of the kettlebell with both hands.

• Note the straight back alignment and straight arms.

• Engage abdominals and squat a little deeper to initiate the lift of the bell.

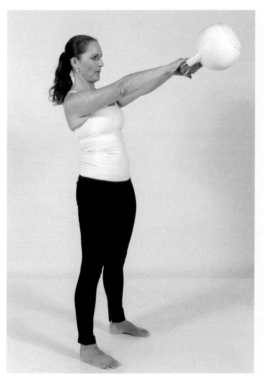

Figure 23.2

Two-handed strict swing – mid/top transition position

Cues:

• As the bell comes forward from between the legs, drive the lift of the weight with feet pressing firming into the floor and the glutes squeezing to open the hips.

• Arms remain straight and shoulder blades pressed down as the weight comes up to shoulder height.

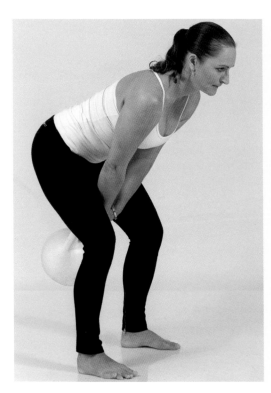

Figure 23.3

Two-handed strict swing – back position

Cues:

- The weight has come back down from the top position and swings between the legs.
- The focus is flexion at the hips rather than a deep knee bend.
- The kettlebell is high in this back position and the hands are high in the groin.
- Feel the weight pulling on the arms, keep them straight and the spine too.
- From this bottom position, the sequence starts again and you press the feet into the ground to start the upswing.

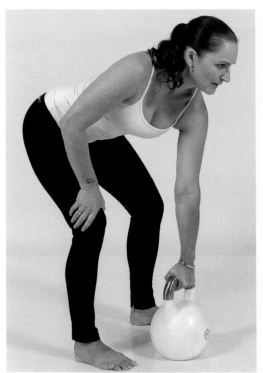

Figure 23.4

Single-hand strict swing – start position

As with the two-handed Swing, now using only one hand brings forth the challenge of resisting rotational pull from the unilateral load.

Cues:

- Start with the kettlebell slightly in front of toes, feet and legs square, squat down holding the handle of the kettlebell in one hand.

As with the two handed version:

- Note the straight back alignment and straight arm.
- Engage abdominals and squat a little deeper to initiate the lift of the bell.

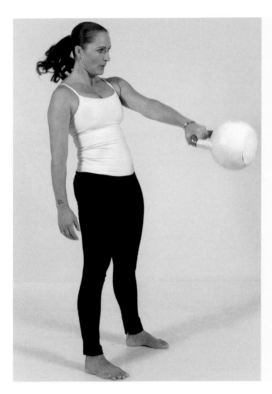

Figure 23.5

Single-hand strict swing – mid/top transition position

Cues:

- As the bell comes forward from between the legs, drive the lift of the weight with feet pressing firmly into the floor and the glutes squeezing to open the hips.
- Arms remain straight and shoulder blades pressed down as the weight comes up to shoulder height.

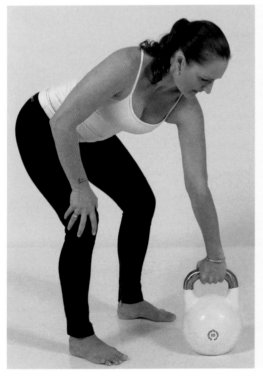

Figure 23.6

Single hand soft rotation swing – start position

Unlike the strict swing, with this version you allow the weight and line of pull (into rotation) to happen naturally. Your grip on the handle and the position of the handle set you up for this rotational pull to occur.

Cues:

- Start with kettlebell slightly in front of toes, feet/legs square and squat down to be holding the handle of the kettlebell with one hand.
- Note the straight back alignment yet soft arm position with the handle of the kettlebell rotated approximately 45° from square.
- Engage abdominals and squat a little deeper to initiate the lift of the bell.

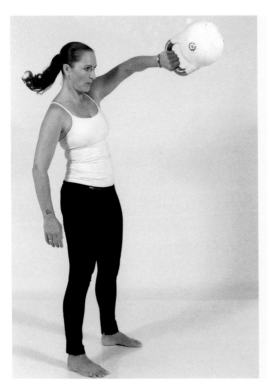

Figure 23.7
Single hand soft rotation
swing – mid/top transition position

Cues:

- As the bell comes forward from between the legs, drive the lift of the weight with feet pressing firmly into the floor and the glutes squeezing to open the hips.
- Arm is slightly bent to draw the bell up close to the body, rather than out as with the original version. As with the strict version, shoulder blades are pressed down as the weight comes up to shoulder height.

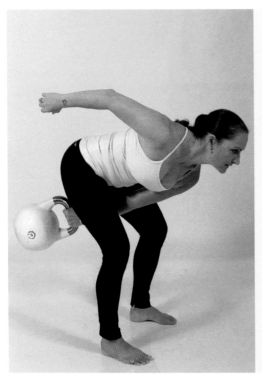

Figure 23.8
Single hand soft rotation
swing – back position

Unlike the strict swing, with this version you allow the weight and line of pull (into rotation) to happen naturally. Your grip on the handle and the position of the handle set you up for this rotational pull to occur.

Cues:

- The weight has come back down from the top position and swung between the legs.
- The focus is the flexion at the hips rather than a deep knee bend.
- The kettlebell is high in this back position and the hand is high in the groin.
- Feel the weight pulling on the arm, keep the arm and the spine straight. The arm and hand remain slightly rotated, so you lead with the thumb as the bell passes back between your legs.
- From this bottom position, the sequence starts again and you press the feet into the ground to start the upswing.

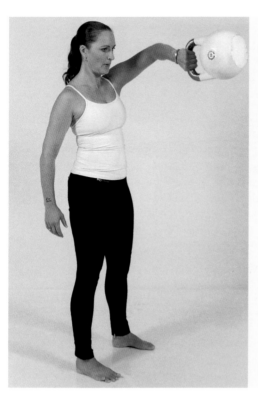

Figure 23.9

Single hand soft spiral

swing – mid/ top transition position

Cues:

- Start position for this version is same as Figure 23.6. Follow the set up cues in Figure 23.6.
- As the bell comes forward from between the legs, drive the lift of the weight with feet pressing firming into the floor and the glutes squeezing to open the hips.
- Arm is bent and you draw the bell up close to the body, lead and lift the elbow as the weight comes forward. As with the strict version, shoulder blades pressed down as the weight comes up to shoulder height.

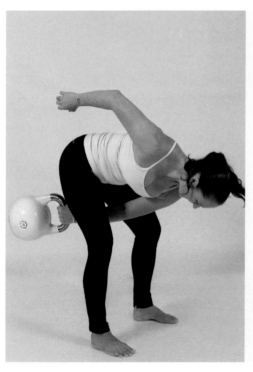

Figure 23.10

Single hand soft spiral

swing – back position

Cues:

- The weight has come back down from the top position and swing between the legs.
- The focus is the flexion at the hips rather than a deep knee bend.
- The kettlebell is high in this back position and the hand is high in the groin.
- Feel the weight pulling on the arm, allow the arm to remain slightly bent. The arm and hand remain slightly rotated, so you lead with the thumb as the bell passes back between your legs. Allowing the arm to remain bent in this version also encourages a soft spine, so allow the weight to flex the spine as it reaches the back/transition position.
- From this bottom position, the sequence starts again and you press the feet into the ground to start the upswing.

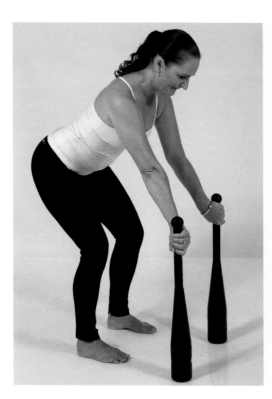

Figure 23.11

Two-handed club swing – start position

This is the standard Clubbell Swing. Club travels outside the legs with one club in each hand. Hip action rather than 'squat' action to drive the swing. Lengthened, straight spine and arms throughout the movement.

Cues:

- The clubs are upright a foot length away from your toes and sit shoulder width apart.
- The grip is with the thumbs down, so the hands are internally rotated. To start the movement, stand up straightening the legs and allow the weight of the clubs to draw them back past the outside of your legs.
- Feel the weight pulling on the arms, keep them straight and the spine too.
- From this bottom position, the swing phase of the sequence starts, and you press the feet into the ground to start the upswing.

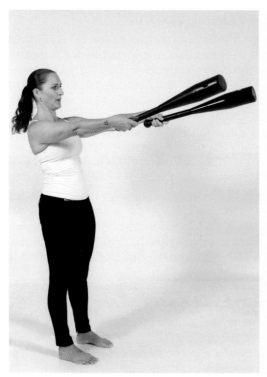

Figure 23.12

Two-handed club swing – mid/top transition position

Cues:

- As the clubs come forward from behind the body, drive the lift of the weight with feet pressing firmly into the floor and the glutes squeezing to open the hips.
- Arms remain straight and shoulder blades pressed down as the weight comes up to shoulder height. Unlike the kettlebell, there is a slight shift in the wrist position to accent the length of the lever.
- As the clubs reach their weightless point, just before transitioning back down, press the thumbs down to laterally flex the wrists, optimising the length of the arm and the entire swing.
- Remain upright and straight, arms and knees, until the clubs reach your sides. It is only as the clubs pass your knees that you flex at the hips to get into the back position.

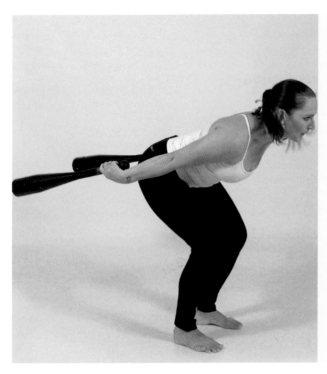

Figure 23.13
Two-handed club swing – back position
Cues:

- The weight has come back down from the top position and swings beside the legs. The body and legs are upright and straight until the clubs reach the sides of the body.

- The focus is the flexion at the hips rather than a deep knee bend.

- The clubs fall into formation with the head and torso following a lengthened line from the crown of head through the tailbone to tip of club, in this back position, as the chest comes towards the thighs, arms are straight.

- Feel the weight pulling on the arms, keep them straight and the spine too.

- From this bottom position, the sequence starts again and you press the feet into the ground to start the upswing.

restorative compensation (Schultz & Feitis, 1996). Allowing for constitutional differences, anyone can use and benefit from The Swing, when appropriate modifications are made.

A misconception in the fitness industry is that kettlebells are only for the 'hardcore' trainer or that kettlebells are only for those who do Olympic lifting. Kettlebells are a fantastic tool to introduce integrated movements. Training with a kettlebell is accessible to anyone willing to try something new (Ranes, 2009). Men and women alike can and do benefit from learning how to swing kettlebells.

Use and safety considerations

The Swing (Figures 23.1–23.5) demonstrates the most structurally fixed version of the exercise. 'Structurally fixed' means strict on posture and form whilst maintaining structural alignment as close to anatomically upright as possible (Eddy, 2013) It is a common fault to have this great alignment whilst swinging the weight, to then slump and compromise the spine when putting the weight down. To ensure alignment is kept at all times during your kettlebell practice, your session should only go to fatigue of the body, rather than failure (Beecroft, 2010).

The more advanced version of The Swing (Figures 23.6–23.10) requires a soft posture with greater proprioceptive connection than the aforementioned 'structurally fixed' version. For those new to kettlebell swinging, these 'soft' variations may look easier or look as though there is no control of the torso. These soft posture versions are considered more advanced. They are more technical to perform due to the multidirectional action and use of elastic recoil (Schultz & Feitis,1996) (Chapter 10).

The subtle variations of the soft version (Figures 23.6–23.10) are of similar neural and spatial complexity and, therefore, deciding which version to practice, or 'play' with, comes down to personal 'feel'. Ask yourself, 'How does the movement feel for my body when I play with it?' This will help your decision, or you may wish to alternate between the two soft versions.

This leads us to the weight of the kettlebell. What *should* the weight be to perform The Swing? As with any exercise or movement practice, err on the side of caution and start light. 8–10kg is considered light in kettlebell training and, depending on your movement experience, level of strength and co-ordination, you may go above or below this (Herschberg, 2011).

It is always best to seek instruction in person by attending a class, workshop or seeking a trainer. You cannot become proficient by only following a DVD or online video (Fable, 2010). Having a professional to watch, guide, correct and direct you will ensure that you are getting the most out of your time and your body, safely. The weight you use to perform The Swing needs to be heavy enough for you to feel the pull of the bell as it swings, yet light enough that you are in control of the bell at all times.

Ensure that you look after your wrists, hands, spine and shoulders, as these are the key areas where problems and injuries can arise. Bracing with the shoulders rather than muscling the bell up with the bicep is one simple focus that will allow you to maintain alignment and perform The Swing safely (Beecroft, 2010). Gripping the

bell handle too tightly can cause tearing to the skin. The weight of the bell is outside the hand and the handle slides during The Swing, or should be allowed to slide inside your grip, to follow the swing and arc of movement (Stehle, 2013).

Modifications to The Swing, in addition to the four versions in Figures 23.1–23.10, come down to physical restrictions. These include structural abnormalities, pregnancy and post injury rehabilitation. These modifications would need to be suggested by a qualified teacher or instructor.

Contraindications for performing The Swing include all the usual medical conditions and injury states that preclude you from any form of physical activity. These conditions include, but are not exclusive to, pregnancy, high blood pressure, physical pain from a previous injury, balance or coordination issues and youths under the recommended training age (Mayo, 2012). If you currently fit in to one of these categories, it would be best to seek medical advice prior to starting these new training methods.

References

Armstrong, D. (2013) DragonDoor Support. support@dragondoor.com [email received 9 May 2013]

Beecroft, M. (2011) Level One and Two Russian Kettlebell Workshops and RKC Preparation Course, Sydney AUS.

Beecroft, M. (2010) Level 1 Kettlebell Workshop and HKC Preparation Course. November, Sydney.

Chaitow, l. (2011) The role of fascia in Manipulative Treatment of Soft Tissues. http://chaitowschat-leon.blogspot.com.au/2011/11/role-of-fascia-in-manipulative.html [Accessed: 13 December 2012]

Cotter, S. (2010) Practical Session: Kettlebells. Elixr Health Club, Sydney AUS.

Cotter, S. (2011) IKFF Kettlebell Lesson 2 with Steve Cotter – Depth of Squat in Swing. http://www.youtube.com/watch?v=rt3Vq3g0Usc [Accessed: 19 May 2013]

Cotter, S. (2011) *Kettlebell Basics.* Underground Wellness USA.http://www.youtube.com/watch?v=TAYZ9gKZaI0 [Accessed: 9 Feb 2013]

Eddy, D. (2013) Kettlebells for Fascia Fitness. http://www.youtube.com/watch?v=CMZUXhis4Gw [Accessed: 23 May 1013]

Fable, S. (2010) The Kettlebell comeback. Idea fitness Journal. http://www.ideafit.com/fitness-library/kettlebell-comeback [Accessed: 29 March 2013]

Forencich, F. (2003) *Play as if your life depends on it. Functional Exercise and living for Homo sapiens.* USA: Go Animal.

Herschberg, J. (2011) What weight kettlebell should I get? http://www.livestrong.com/article/231757-what-weight-kettlebell-should-i-get/ [Accessed: 8 May 2013]

Heins, S. (2014) Clubs vs. kettlebells. Live chat with Shane Heins. http://daretoevolve.tv/forum/webinar-live-chats-hang-outs/live-chat-clubs-vs-kettlebells/ Accessed: 24 Sept 2014]

Iardella, S. (2014) Debating the kettlebell swing: the Russian vs the American swing. http://Irdellatraining.com/debating-the-kettlebell-swing-the-russian-vs-the-american-swing [Accessed: 24 Sept 2014]

Jones, B. (2010) Clarifying Hardstyle. Pittsburg PA [Accessed: 25 January 2013] http://www.dragondoor.com/articles/clarifying-hardstyle/

Mayo, S. (2012) Strength training: Ok for kids? http://www.mayoclinic.com/health/strength-training/HQ01010 [Accessed: 3 April 2013]

Maxwell, S. & Newell, K. (2011) Interview with the greats. http://www.newellstrength.com/interviews/ [accessed 13 December 2012]

Maxwell, S. (2013) Practical Session: Kettlebells and Clubbells. January & March Sydney.

Myers, T. (2001) *Anatomy Trains. Myofascial Meridians for Manual and Movement Therapists.* Churchill Livingstone.

Myers, T. (2009) 2nd ed. *Anatomy Trains. Myofascial Meridians for Manual and Movement Therapists.* Churchill Livingstone.

Myers, T. & Schleip, R. (2011) Fascial Fitness. New Inspirations from Connective Tissue Research. Workshop notes: slide 'How to Build a better Fascial Body'.

Ranes, C. (2009) Kettlebell Swing – Before and After – 8 weeks. https://www.youtube.com/watch?v=hvERPjkDeeE [Accessed: 22 May 2013]

Scarito, P. (2008) Kettlebell Basics. The two arm Kettlebell swing. http://www.youtube.com/watch?v=6u_nqS-nM2S8 [Accessed: 11th February 2013]

Schultz, R. & Feitis, R. (1996) *The Endless Web. Fascial Anatomy and Physical Reality.* California, U.S.A: North Atlantic books. 23.

Sonnon, S. (2006). The Bigbook of Clubbell Training. 2nd Ed. RMAX.tv Productions. Atlanta USA.

Sonnon, S. (2008). Kettlebell Foundation Series. RMAX.tv Productions. Atlanta USA.

Sonnon, S. (2009) Practical Session: Kettlebells. Bellingham Sports Club, Bellingham USA.

Steer, A. (2009) Clubbells 101. Choosing and Using your Clubbells. e-book. www.clubbellcoach.com [Accessed: 10 January 2011]

Stehle, M. (2013) 10 dangerous kettlebell mistakes. https://www.onnit.com/blog/10-dangerous-kettlebell-mistakes/ [Accessed: 17 May 2013]

Tooling, (2012) Tooling U-SME. USA http://www.too-lingu.com/definition-570110-120333-rotational-inertia.html [Accessed: 3 April 2013]

Further reading

Cobbett, G & Jenkin, A. (1905) *Indian Clubs.* G. Bell & Sons. http://archive.org/details/indianclubs00jenkgoog

Forencich, F. (2003) *Play as if your life depends on it. Functional Exercise and living for Homo sapiens.* USA: Go Animal.

Kehoe, D. (1866) *The Indian Club exercise.* New York: Peck & Snyder http://openlibrary.org/books/OL17998405M/The_Indian_club_exercise

Schultz, R.L. & Felitis, R. (1996) *The Endless Web. Fascia Anatomy and Physical Reality.* USA: North Atlantic Books.

Steer, A . (2009) Clubbells 101. Choosing and Using your Clubbells. e-book. www.clubbellcoach.com

Assessment technologies: From ultrasound and myometry to bio-impedance and motion sensors

Christopher Gordon, Piroska Frenzel and Robert Schleip

Introduction

While many therapists, coaches and movement teachers rely on their subjective palpatory and visual perception of fascial tissue dynamics, rapid developments in technology are offering useful diagnostic and assessment tools which can be used to examine different physical and physiological features of fascial tissues. This chapter will discuss four different techniques, which appear to be the most useful and promising for fascia oriented professionals:

- diagnostic ultrasound (for the assessment of tissue thickness, shear motion and stiffness)
- bio-impedance (changes in fluid content)
- myometry (measuring tissue stiffness and elasticity)
- motion sensors (movement quality).

Diagnostic ultrasound

Except for medical doctors, up until very recently clinicians and coaches within the field of sports and movement therapy rarely used any ultrasound equipment for their own assessments. However, new technological advances have made portable ultrasound equipment an increasingly useful diagnostic tool within this field. Practitioners focusing on segmental stabilisation, via muscular activation training, have successfully used ultrasound in their daily practices to assess proper (or lacking) activation of muscle layers related to 'core stability', such as the transversus abdominis or the multifidus muscles (Hodges et al., 2003). Similarly, proper activation of pelvic floor muscles is often assessed by observing positional changes of the bladder during specific loading manoeuvres (Lee, 2001).

For clinical assessment of fascial properties, the study by Langevin et al. (2011) provided an important impetus. Here, it was shown via ultrasound measurement that patients with chronic low back pain tend to express significantly less 'shear strain' (corresponding to the ability to slide in relation to one another) between different layers of their lumbar fasciae compared with pain-free control persons. Since then several practitioners have been applying ultrasound imaging so as to assess potential therapeutic changes in the degree of potential adhesions between adjacent fascial layers.

Ultrasound may also be used effectively to measure the thickness of fascial tissues. An impressive clinical study by Stecco et al. (2014) showed that in patients with chronic neck pain the thickness of the sternocleidomastoid fascia corresponded with the amount of pain and disability and also with the degree of therapeutic improvement after a myofascial manipulation treatment. Furthermore, a fascial thickness of 1.5 mm was found as a reliable cut-off point in this study for the diagnosis of fascia-generated neck pain (see Figure 24.1).

A fairly new development in this field is ultrasound elastography. Here, a mechanical vibration of the respective tissue is induced, for which the detected resonance frequency allows an indirect assessment of the tissue stiffness. The softer a fascial tissue is, the slower its induced vibratory frequency. This non-invasive technology is already used to assist in the detection of liver fibrosis, breast cancer, prostate cancer as

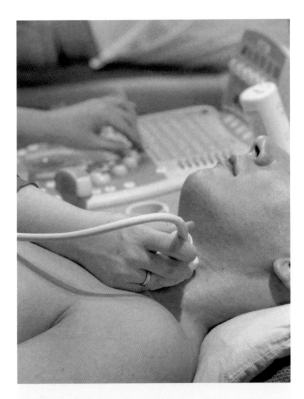

Figure 24.1

Use of diagnostic ultrasound to visualise and assess fascial properties

Use of portable ultrasound allows for the measurement of the thickness of various fascial membranes positioned close to the surface. For example, a thickness of 1.5 mm of the sternocleidomastoid fascia was found to be a useful cut-off point for making a diagnosis of myofascial neck pain (Stecco et al., 2014). (Photo © Afalter-Fotolia.com).

well as plantar fibrosis (Sconfienza et al., 2013). Our department at Ulm University is currently involved in a larger study to determine what 'normal' variations of fascial stiffness are within pain free patients of different age and gender groups for several important fascial layers in the human body. Once completed it may be easier to assess whether a specific fascial stiffness or softness is within normal values or not. Nevertheless, for comparative measurement within the same person (for example, before/after an exercise or

therapeutic intervention, or between different sides) ultrasound elastography can already serve as a useful diagnostic tool for fascia-oriented clinicians (Martínez Rodríguez & Galán del Río, 2013) (Chapter 19). Unfortunately prices for new equipment are still comparatively high, between $4000 and $10000 for diagnostic elastography and several times higher for ultrasound elastography as of June 2013. However, the respective technological industry has started to target physiotherapists, and others, as a new customer group. This has created the necessity to develop more affordable versions, with impressive imaging quality incorporated into smaller therapeutic practices.

Assessment of tissue properties via Indentometry

Introduction

At The Center for Integrative Therapy, we conduct clinical research (Gordon et al., 2011) in affiliation with the Fascia Research Group of the University Ulm and with the University of Tübingen, Germany. We have been amazed, how helpful it has been to collect data from our patients for quality management and the evaluation of our work standards. It has helped us, as a team, to determine what techniques are worth improving and what techniques need further critical research or thought. Sometimes it has even resulted in dropping certain approaches altogether. As a result, we have learned that objective evaluation can be a very inspiring and empowering process for all concerned.

The assessment toolkit

The algometer: pain pressure threshold

The use of the Pressure Algometer (Park et al., 2011) allows the clinician/trainer to not only test tissue sensitivity, but also to evaluate the client's pain threshold. Considered a subjective/objective measurement parameter, the clinician/trainer applies increasing amounts of pressure with the algometer to a related muscle area, for example a trigger point, (Myburgh et al., 2008) and asks the client to signal when the pain is uncomfortable. By doing this, the client gets an impression of the scale of pain, described from 0 to 10 with 10 representing unbearable pain. The clinician/trainer then repeats the procedure on several points around the problem area, before and after treatment, and records the results. Tenderness pressure is measured in pounds (lbs), and tissue penetration is measured in millimetres (mm).

The MyotonPro

The MyotonPro is a novel myometer (Aird, Samuel & Stokes 2012) that gives numerical feedback on biomechanical tissue properties such as stiffness and elasticity. This method of myometry for measuring tissues close to the skin, up to 1.5–2 cm depth, consists of creating an external mechanical impulse. The muscle's response is then recorded, in the form of an acceleration graph, and, subsequently, the tone, elasticity and stiffness is computed.

The Myotonometer

An alternative objective measurement device to the MyotonPro, this myotonometer was developed to quantify muscle tone, measuring and analysing muscle tone and stiffness. Protocols also allow quantification of the level of severity of the spastic paretic condition. Valid, reliable and quantifiable measures of muscle tone are obtained easily and quickly. Clinical trials have shown that myotonometric measurements can distinguish between injured and non-injured muscles (post injury) and quantify muscle imbalances.

Benefits of constant assessment

There are many benefits to monitoring treatment effectiveness. The most obvious advantage is being able to track client progress, as shown above. The trainer has a better tool for communication with the client by being able to show objective evidence of treatment progress. This means less reliance would be placed on subjective patient accounts of improvement, or lack thereof, and more on objective assessment tools, which measure an array of parameters.

Objective assessment allows for monitoring the quality and effectiveness of treatments. Clinicians can improve techniques through self-assessment, which leads to better methodologies and advancements in this field of health. Evidence-based studies are also beneficial for practices to substantiate treatments offered.

Outlook

This form of holistic approach is very promising in that evidence-based assessment can help the trainer/coach track the effectiveness of his/her work. This leads to many positive outcomes, in that quality management can now be objectively and subjectively assessed.

Another interesting field of application is in athletics. By conducting measurements pre- and post-training, it is possible to determine relative changes in the body tissues. Measurements can be conducted on a preventive basis on athletes

Device	Advantages	Disadvantages
MyotonPro	• Quick, non-invasive, objective and reliable measurements. • Muscle contraction detection through 1.5–2 cm of fat tissue.	• To date, available only for scientific purposes • Works only for superficial Myofascial tissues, depth 1.5–2cm • Relatively high cost of 4,000 Euros
Myotonometer	• Measures muscle strength and tone	• Difficult to buy on the market • Few reliability studies
Algometer with depth gauge	• Measures quickly, simply and reliably in depth of tissues up to 5–6 cm • Subjective and objective feedback • In pounds and millimetres • Low cost	• Needs good logistics and dialogue with client to acquire data quickly and efficiently

Table 24.1

Device comparison table

and/or entire teams on a regular basis. Regular assessments can reveal any imminent 'dangers', allowing preventive measures to be taken.

Conclusion

Evidence-based validation of our work can help to gain greater clarity and objectivity in our daily working routine. We hope that by reading this chapter our enthusiasm and inspiration will inspire readers to follow suit.

Electrical bioimpedance

Introduction

Tissue hydration is frequently used as a hypothetical explanation for the benefits of many different types of bodywork. The role of hydration in fascia was recently examined by Schleip et al. (2012) (Chapters 1 and 3). Here they showed that an increase in tissue stiffness may, at least, be partially caused by a temporarily altered matrix hydration. In sports, bioelectrical impedance analysis (BIA) is used to determine the body composition. It has shown that athletic performance is influenced by and dependent on the distribution and total amount of fat-free mass and body fat (Pichard et al., 1997). It was also used to detect hydration changes before and after treatment (Frenzel et al., 2013) and to help to determine influences that might change fluid distribution, for example, positioning (Kim et al., 1997). Lower impedance was shown along collagenous bands (Ahn et al., 2010). Along these bands some of the Traditional Chinese Medicine (TCM) meridians could be represented. It is, therefore, of great interest to have a measurement tool that detects fluid distribution within the body.

Bioelectrical impedance analysis (BIA) is described as an easy, non-invasive, relatively cheap, portable, rapid and operator independent method with excellent inter observer reproducibility to assess changes in hydration status. Furthermore BIA can reliably estimate the body compartments, total body water (TBW) and fat free mass (FFM), in healthy subjects and in patients with stable water and electrolyte balance under standardised conditions (O`Brien et al., 2002) (Kyle et al., 2004a) (Kyle et al., 2004b).

How does impedance measurement work?

Physiological fluids within the body contain ions. Therefore, an alternating current can flow through the body. If the body fluids are more viscous the electrical flow is opposed. Referring to an electrical model this behaviour is called resistance. In addition, the electrical current charges the cell membranes, which are therefore working as capacitors (capacitors are elements which store electrical energy in an electrical field) (Foster & Lukaski, 1996.) The measured (bio-) impedance (Z) is the sum of the ohmic resistance of all fluids in the body (TBW), called resistance (R), and the capacitive resistance due to the body cells which is called reactance (Xc)(De Lorenzo & Andreoli, 2003) (Kyle et al., 2004a). The formula is $Z = (R^2 + Xc^2)^{1/2}$ (Oldham, 1996).

Compared to muscle and blood, bone and fat are poorly conductive in the body. Therefore, if there is more bone and fat, the body is less conductive. Furthermore, as the alternating current induced is very low it is not noticeable for the subject (Foster & Lukaski, 1996) (Schüler, 1998). In addition, the applied frequencies are too high to stimulate muscles or the heart (Anderson, 1988).

Often it is of interest to be able to separate the measured impedance (Z) into resistance (R) and reactance (Xc). Therefore impedanciometry also measures a phase angle (PhA) enabling separation of Z into R and Xc. PhA further indicates the water distribution between the intra (ICW) and extra cellular (ECW) spaces. PhA is also an indicator of cell health: a high PhA reflects strong cell function and a low PhA is associated with increased morbidity and nutritional risk in subjects (Kyle et al., 2004a; 2012).

Body compartments

Measuring the body as a one compartment system, when measuring body weight for example, means that distribution shifts or imbalances within the body cannot be detected. In other words the weight can be the same in a subject with a lot of muscles and one with a lot of fat. Analysing different compartments (see Figure 24.2) of the body separately allows the description of distribution imbalances between the portions. For example, an independent measurement of fat free

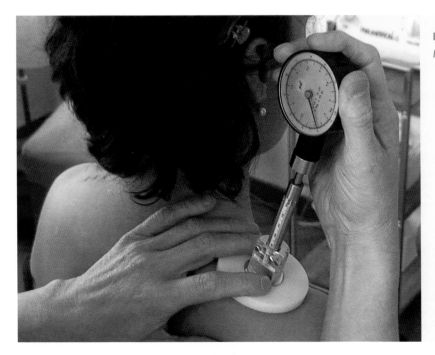

Figure 24.2
Myometry with the Algometer

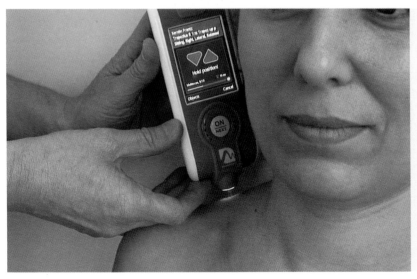

Figure 24.3
Myometry with the MyotonPro

mass (FFM) and total body water (TBW) permits detection of dehydration, which is frequent in the elderly or athletes after heavy training (Jaffrin & Morel, 2008).

Whole-body impedance measurement is typically performed in supine position with four surface electrodes placed on one side of the body. Two current source electrodes are placed on the backside of foot and hand and two detecting electrodes are positioned on the backs of the wrist and ankle (Foster & Lukaski, 1996) (Kyle et al., 2004a). A minimum distance of 3 cm should be kept between the current and the detecting electrode (Figure 24.3) as within this space an in-homogeneity of the electrical field occurs, leading to uneven distribution of the current within the measured segment. In other words, the bigger the distance the more current homogeneity in the measured segment and the better the segments capture (Schüler, 1998).

Electrical measurements and body/tissue properties

Equations

The human body can be seen as a set of several, most of the time five, cylinders, for example, limbs and trunk (Chertow et al., 1995) (Jaffrin & Morel, 2008). With the help of Ohm´s law the volume of a measured cylinder (segment) can be calculated when the conductive length (approximated by height) and the resistance (impedance) of the segment are known, following the formula: $V = L^2/R$ (V = volume; L = length; R = resistance) (Segal et al., 1991) (De Lorenzo & Andreoli, 2003). To adjust this comparison to real body geometry an appropriate coefficient needs to be introduced which takes, among others, the specific resistivity of the conducting tissue and the anatomy of the segment into account. An empirical relationship between the impedance quotient (height^2/R) and lean body mass (LBM) is known (Kyle et al., 2004a). In order to include one or more variables such as age, gender, weight, height or ethnic background to calculate fat free mass (FFM), total body water (TBW) and body fat, mathematical equations need to be generated which correlate the measurements to the volume of the compartment of interest. These equations are found by comparing resistance measurements with other methods of body analysis (Houtkooper et al., 1996) (Gudivaka et al., 1999). (For detailed lists of equations please see Houtkooper et al., 1996 and Kyle et al., 2004a.)

Frequency and BIA-methods

In living tissue, the dispersion of the electrical current is dependent on its frequency (Van Loan et al., 1993). Due to the capacitive character of cell membranes, zero- or low-frequency current flows around the cells only in the extra cellular water (ECW) whereas infinite- or high-frequency current also passes through the cell membrane and the intra cellular water (ICW) (Kyle et al., 2004a) (Jaffrin & Morel, 2008) (Medrano et al., 2010). The ideal frequency range cannot be reached

when measuring with surface electrodes and the frequency is limited to 5-1000 kHz. Hence they need to be extrapolated by using a graph, which is called the Cole-Cole plot (Cole & Cole, 1941) (Jaffrin & Morel, 2008). At 50 kHz the current passes through total body water (TBW) but depending on the tissue the distribution between intra cellular water (ICW) and extra cellular water (ECW) differs (Kyle et al., 2004a).

In BIA several measurement methods are performed. Single frequency BIA (SF-BIA) measures Z at one frequency (typically 50 kHz) and includes empirical regression models, which permit the estimation of fat free mass (FFM) and total body water (TBW) with reasonable accuracy in normally hydrated subjects (Gudivaka et al., 1999). Multi-frequency BIA (MF-BIA) combines impedance data from 2–7 frequencies with regression equations and seems to be sensitive to changes in the extra cellular water (ECW) or in the ECW/TBW ratio, which may indicate oedema and/or malnutrition (Kyle et al., 2004a) (Baracos et al., 2012).

Bioelectrical spectroscopy (BIS), like MF-BIA, also includes mathematical modelling and mixture equations (Kyle et al., 2004a). Body composition spectroscopy (BCS) works like BIS but uses BMI corrected parameters (Moissl et al., 2006). Bioelectrical impedance vector analysis (BIVA) is a graphical model of SF-BIA where the R-Xc-graph is compared with 50%, 75% and 95% tolerance ellipses calculated in a healthy population of same gender and race (Piccoli et al., 1996) (Piccoli et al., 2000) (Kyle et al., 2004a).

Electrical circuits

Another complex factor when describing the human body using an electrical model is that the behaviour of biological tissue needs to be compared with electrical circuits in which capacitance (body cells) and resistance (TBW) can be combined in series or parallel. In both combinations the same impedance can be measured but the component value will differ (Foster & Lukaski, 1996). Several models of R and Xc in series, in parallel and in combined circuits were established with additional variations in applied frequencies and constants which are specific to each model. All these models try to correlate the electrical signal to the volume of water in the compartment of interest (Gudivaka et al., 1999).

What are the difficulties with BIA?

The disadvantage of seeing the body as a set of cylinders, when measuring whole-body impedance (sum of arm, trunk and leg) is that the trunk is contributing disproportionally less (no more than 8%) to Z than the limbs. This is because small changes in the cross-sectional area of the limbs will show a relatively large impact on Z. Compared to the total volume of the body, these changes are relatively small and so large volume changes of the trunk can show little or no change in the geometry (Organ et al., 1994). This effect is not evident in subjects with balanced water distribution. Here, every segment measured is representative for the whole body situation (De Lorenzo and Andreoli, 2003). However, it highlights that variations of lean body mass (LBM) or body cell mass (BCM) (of the limbs or the trunk) or large liquid volume changes in the abdominal cavity (for example ascites) are not well captured by whole body impedance (Kyle et al., 2004a) (Fig. 24.4).

To overcome this limitation segmental BIA measurement is performed. De Lorenzo and Andreoli (2003) found this approach to be a relatively accurate method in assessing body composition in healthy subjects. Furthermore, it measures fluid distribution and its changes in both healthy and unhealthy subjects.

Another limitation of BIA is that the compartments' total body water (TBW), intra cellular water (ICW), extra cellular water (ECW), fat free mass (FFM) and body cell mass (BCM) are, themselves inter-correlated (Schoeller, 2000). In over-hydrated patients, for example, relevant protein malnutrition can be hidden in the fat free mass (FFM) due to an expansion of the extra cellular water (ECW) (Kyle et al., 2004a). To overcome this inter-correlation, BIA may be performed before and after a body fluid distribution altering intervention, for example, a local pressure applied on the tissue (Kotler et al., 1996). If the intervention changes the resistivity in the body water, for example, injection of crystalloid fluid, this approach would lead to potential error (Schoeller, 2000).

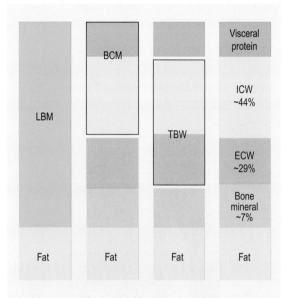

Figure 24.4

The approximate compartment distribution (after Kyle et al., 2004a)

Fat = body fat = weight minus FFM (Kyle et al., 2004a)

Lean Body Mass (LBM) = Fat Free Mass (FFM) = is everything that is not body fat (Kyle et al., 2004a).

Extra Cellular Water (ECW)

Body Cell Mass (BCM) = includes all non-adipose cells as well as the aqueous compartment of the fat cells (therefore size estimation is difficult) (Kyle et al., 2004a). It is the protein rich compartment which is affected in catabolic states (Baracos et al., 2012).

Intra Cellular Water (ICW)

Total Body Water (TBW) = ECW+ICW, strongly related to FFM, in healthy individuals it contains ~73% water (hydration-average varies with age) (Kyle et al. 2004a).

Summary

BIA works well in healthy subjects and in patients with chronic disease, as long as the appropriate validated equation regarding age, sex and race is chosen (Kyle et al., 2004b). For more detailed information on recommendations regarding clinical application of BIA see Kyle et al. (2004b).

Portable motion sensors

Within the fitness industry, it has become fashionable to wear easily portable electronic devices for assessing performance-oriented features such as heart rate variability, caloric output, number of

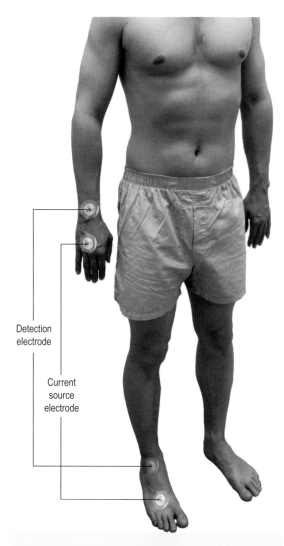

Detection
electrode

Current
source
electrode

Figure 24.5

Standard electrode position for whole-body impedance measurement

steps and distances, speed and acceleration. It is expected that this technological field will become one of the fastest growing markets within digital consumer products. For the field of fascia-oriented movement, approaches that measure speed and acceleration appear to be promising developments.

In the treatment of both Achilles tendinopathies as well as plantar fasciosis, clinical research has shown that slow eccentric contractions of the calf muscles are beneficial (for example, stepping slowly downwards with the heel while standing tiptoe on a stair). While most clinicians assumed that it is the eccentric contraction which is responsible for this effect, recent investigations from Kjaer et al. (2014) suggest that it is only the slow speed of the execution of the exercise that accounts for the beneficial results and not the eccentric or concentric activation (Chapter 5). Most people tend to move faster in concentric contraction compared with eccentric activations in this exercise. However, when closely supervised and encouraged to lift their heel with the same slow speed as they show during the standard dropping-down application, patients demonstrated exactly the same amount of improvement.

Similarly, there are also indications that a super-slow execution of foam roller treatments (for example, in cases of a painful hardening of the iliotibial band, a.k.a. runner's knee) may stimulate the locally treated fibroblast towards an increased expression of the enzyme MMP-1 during subsequent hours (Zheng et al., 2012). This would create an anti-fibrotic effect, or a general softening effect on scars and similar tissue contractures, via such super-slow treatment applications. It remains to be seen whether, and in what manner, small digital motion sensors can be developed to assist clients in conducting their self-treatments within their therapeutically recommended speed.

Even more promising is the use of tiny accelerometers. In general, a small mass is suspended inside a small box. The tool measures the displacement at the sensor itself and typically all three planes of movement. These displacements arise from changes in inertia and thus

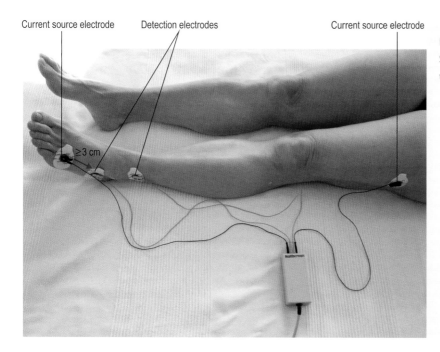

Current source electrode   Detection electrodes   Current source electrode

≥3 cm

Figure 24.6
Segmental measurement of
the foot

any acceleration or deceleration in the measured direction. Based on the advancements in micro-electronics, there have been rapid improvements in recent years in the development of wireless inertial sensors that can be worn on the body and that are small enough not to impede normal motion dynamics. These sensors respond to minute changes in inertia during an accelerating or decelerating movement. Costs have reduced dramatically in recent years (ranging from $20 to $250 for end user products and from $2 to $600 for technicians/scientists). Today, already, many smartphones include built-in accelerometers for daily usage.

Several running shoe companies have started to implant such sensors in their shoes. The monitoring device is then either worn as a wristband, wristwatch or is included as a software app in a related smartphone programme. Similar devices are available which can be easily attached to a belt or placed in a pocket. After some initial calibration steps, the related software programmes are usually capable of detecting the person's activity level, for example, whether they are resting, stair climbing or walking.

In plyometric training, they have also been used to evaluate training effects in terms of improved acceleration (Ruben et al., 2010). Together with appropriately developed algorithms in the accompanying software, they already allow recognition of their 'owner' by their individual movement signature: for example, in walking, stair climbing, etc. (Godfrey et al., 2008) (Strath et al., 2012).

It seems plausible that they may also be useful additions for detecting to what degree a person performs an exercise with fascia-friendly sinusoidal speed changes rather than in a jerky manner (Chapter 11, Fig. 11.2). In this respect such tiny motion sensors could also serve as protective support for the avoidance of strain injuries in dynamic movements. For runners, such sensors could possibly replace a skilled human ear to give biofeedback about the respective 'Ninja' quality on a given day (Chapter 11). They could also give recommendations to the runner about the proper insertion of brief walking pauses (i.e. when the initial elastic rebound quality gets lost in exchange for a more heavily-pounding movement quality).

References

Ahn, A.C., Park, M., Shaw, J.R., McManus, C.A., Kaptchuk, T.J. & Langevin, H.M. (2010) Electrical impedance of acupuncture meridians: the relevance of subcutaneous collagenous bands. *PLoS one* 5(7): e11907.

Aird, L., Samuel, D. & Stokes, M. (2012) Quadriceps muscle tone, elasticity and stiffness in older males: Reliability and symmetry using the MyotonPRO. *Arch Gerontol Geriatr.* 55(2): e31–e39.

Anderson, F.A., Jr. (1988) *Impedance Plethysmography in Encyclopedia of Medical Devices and Instrumentation.* John Wiley & Sons, 3: 1632–1643.

Baracos, V., Caserotti, P., Earthman, C.P., Fields, D., Gallagher, D., Hall, K.D., Heymsfield, S.B., Müller, M.J., Napolitano Rosen A., Pichard, C., Redman L.M., Shen, W., Shepherd, J.A. & Thomas, D. (2012) Advances in the science and application of body composition measurement. *J Parenter Enteral Nutr.* 36(1): 96–107.

Chertow, G.M., Lowrie, E.G., Wilmore, D.W., Gonzalez, J., Lew, N.L., Ling, J., Leboff, M.S., Gottlieb, M.N.,Huang, W. & Zebrowski, B. (1995) Nutritional assessment with bioelectrical impedance analysis in maintenance hemodialysis patients. *J Am Soc Nephrol.* 6(1): 75–81.

Cole, K.S. & Cole, R.H. (1941) Dispersion and absorption in dielectrics I. Alternating current characteristics. *J Chem Phys.* 9: 341–351.

De Lorenzo, A. & Andreoli, A. 2003. Segmental bioelectrical impedance analysis. *Curr Opin Clin Nutr Metab Care.* 6(5): 551–555.

Frenzel, P., Schleip, R. & Geyer, A. (2013) Effects of stretching and/or vibration on the plantar fascia. In: A. Vleeming, C. Fitzgerald, A. Kamkar, J. van Dieen, B. Stuge, M. van Tulder, L. Danneels, P. Hodges, J. Wang, R. Schleip, H. Albert, B. Sturesson eds. *Conference proceedings of the 8th Interdisciplinary World Congress on Low Back& Pelvic Pain.* Dubai 2013. 546–547.

Foster, K.R. & Lukaski, H.C. (1996) Whole-body impedance–what does it measure? *Am J Clin Nutr.* 64(3): 388S–396S.

Godfrey, A., Conway, R., Meagher, D. & OLaighin, G. (2008) Direct measurement of human movement by accelerometry. *Med Eng Phys.* 30(10): 1364–1386.

Gordon, C., Schleip, R., Gevirtz, R.N. & Andrasik, F. (2011) Eine neue integrative Kombinationstherapie. *PT-Zeitschrift für Physiotherapeuten* 63(10): 72–77.

Gudivaka, R., Schoeller, D.A., Kushner, R.F. & Bolt, M.J.G. (1999) Single-and multifrequency models for bioelectrical impedance analysis of body water compartments. *J Appl Physiol.* 87(3): 1087–1096.

Hodges, P.W., Pengel, L.H., Herbert, R.D. & Gandevia, S.C. (2003) Measurement of muscle contraction with ultrasound imaging. *Muscle Nerve* 27(6): 682–692.

Houtkooper, L.B., Lohman, T.G., Going, S.B. & Howell, W.H. (1996) Why bioelectrical impedance analysis should be used for estimating adiposity. *Am J Clin Nutr.* 64(3): 436S–448S.

Jaffrin, M.Y. & Morel, H. (2008) Body fluid volumes measurements by impedance: A review of bioimpedance spectroscopy (BIS) and bioimpedance analysis (BIA) methods. *Med Eng Phys.* 30(10): 1257–1269.

Kim, C.T., Findley, T.W. & Reisman, S.R. (1997) Bioelectrical impedance changes in regional extracellular fluid alterations. *Electromyogr Clin Neurophysiol.* 37(5): 297–304.

Kjaer, M. & Heinemeier, K.M. (2014). Eccentric exercise: Acute and chronic effects on healthy and diseased tendons. *J Appl Physiol.* Epub ahead of print; DOI: 10.1152/japplphysiol.01044.2013

Kotler, D.P., Burastero, S., Wang, J. & Pierson, R.N. (1996) Prediction of body cell mass, fat-free mass, and total body water with bioelectrical impedance analysis: effects of race, sex, and disease. *Am J Clin Nutr.* 64(3): 489S–497S.

Kyle, U.G., Bosaeus, I., De Lorenzo, A.D., Deurenberg, P., Elia, M., Gómez, J.M., Heitmann, B.L., Kent-Smith, L., Melchior, J.-C., Pirlich, M., Scharfetter, H., Schols, M.W.J. & Pichard, C. Composition of the ESPEN Working Group. (2004a) Bioelectrical impedance analysis-part I: review of principles and methods. *Clin Nutr.* 23(5): 1226–1243.

Kyle, U.G., Bosaeus, I., De Lorenzo, A.D., Deurenberg, P., Elia, M., Gómez, J.M., Heitmann, B.L., Kent-Smith, L., Melchior, J.-C., Pirlich, M., Scharfetter, H., Schols, M.W.J. & Pichard, C. (2004b) Bioelectrical impedance analysis-part II: utilization in clinical practice. *Clin Nutr.* 23(6): 1430–1453.

Kyle, U.G., Soundar, E.P., Genton, L. & Pichard, C. (2012) Can phase angle determined by bioelectrical impedance analysis assess nutritional risk? A comparison between healthy and hospitalized subjects. *Clin Nutr.* 31(6): 875–881.

Langevin, H.M., Fox, J.R., Koptiuch, C., Badger, G.J., Greenan-Naumann, A.C., Bouffard, N.A., Konofagou, E.E., Lee, W.N., Triano, J.J. & Henry, S.M. (2011) Reduced thoracolumbar fascia shear strain in human chronic low back pain. *BMC Musculoskelet Disord.* 12: 203.

Lee, D. (2011) *The Pelvic Girdle: An integration of clinical expertise and research.* 4th ed. Edinburgh, Elsevier.

Martínez Rodríguez, R. & Galán del Río, F. (2013) Mechanistic basis of manual therapy in myofascial injuries. Sonoelastographic evolution control. *J Bodyw Mov Ther.* 17(2): 221–234.

Medrano, G., Eitner, F., Walter, M. & Leonhardt, S. (2010) Model-based correction of the influence of body position on continuous segmental and hand-to-foot bioimpedance measurements. *Med Biol Eng Comput.* 48(6): 531–541.

Moissl, U.M., Wabel, P., Chamney, P.W., Bosaeus, I., Levin, N.W., Bosy-Westphal, A., Korth, O., Müller M.J., Ellegård, L., Malmros, V., Kaitwatcharachai, C., Kuhlman, M.K., Zhu, F. & Fuller, N.J. (2006) Body fluid volume determination via body composition spectroscopy in health and disease. *Physiol meas.* 27(9): 921–933.

Myburgh, C., Larsen, A.H. & Hartvigsen, J. (2008) A systematic, critical review of manual palpation for identifying myofascial trigger points: evidence and clinical significance. *Arch Phys Med Rehabil*. 89(6): 1169–1176.

O'Brien, C., Young, A.J. & Sawka, M.N. (2002) Bioelectrical impedance to estimate changes in hydration status. International journal of sports medicine. 23(5): 361–366.

Oldham, N.M. (1996) Overview of bioelectrical impedance analyzers. *Am J Clin Nutr*. 64(3): 405S–412S.

Organ, L.W., Bradham, G.B., Gore, D.T. & Lozier, S.L. (1994) Segmental bioelectrical impedance analysis. *J Appl Physiol*. 77(1): 98–112.

Park, G., Kim, C.W., Park, S.B., Kim, M.J. & Jang, S.H. (2011) Reliability and usefulness of the pressure pain threshold measurement in patients with myofascial pain. *Ann Rehabil Med*. 35(3): 412–417.

Piccoli, A., Piazza, P., Noventa, D., Pillon, L. & Zaccaria, M. (1996) A new method for monitoring hydration at high altitude by bioimpedance analysis. *Med Sci Sports Exerc*. 28(12): 1517–1522.

Piccoli, A., Pittoni, G., Facco, E., Favaro, E. & Pillon, L. (2000) Relationship between central venous pressure and bioimpedance vector analysis in critically ill patients. *Crit Care Med*. 28(1): 132–137.

Pichard, C., Kyle, U.G., Gremion, G., Gerbase, M. & Slosman, D.O. (1997) Body composition by x-ray absorptiometry and bioelectrical impedance in female runners. *Med Sci Sports Exerc*. 29(11): 1527–1534.

Ruben, R.M., Molinari, M.A., Bibbee, C.A., et al. (2010) The acute effects of an ascending squat protocol on performance during horizontal plyometric jumps. *J Strength Cond Res*. 24(2): 358–369.

Sconfienza, L.M., Silvestri, E., Orlandi, D., Fabbro, E., Ferrero, G., Martini, C., Sardanelli, F. & Cimmino, M.A. (2013) Real-time sonoelastography of the plantar fascia: comparison between patients with plantar fasciitis and healthy control subjects. *Radiology*. 267(1): 195–200.

Schleip, R., Duerselen, L., Vleeming, A., Naylor, I.L., Lehmann-Horn, F., Zorn, A., Jaeger, H. & Klingler, W. (2012) Strain hardening of fascia: static stretching of dense fibrous connective tissues can induce a temporary stiffness increase accompanied by enhanced matrix hydration. *J Bodyw Mov Ther*. 16(1): 94–100.

Schoeller, D.A. (2000) Bioelectrical Impedance Analysis What Does It Measure? *Ann N Y Acad Sci*. 904(1): 159–162.

Schüler, R. (1998) *Apparative Gefäßdiagnostik*. Ilmenau: ISLE Verlag. 17–23.

Segal, K.R., Burastero, S., Chun, A., Coronel, P., Pierson, R.N. & Wang, J. (1991) Estimation of extracellular and total body water by multiple-frequency bioelectrical-impedance measurement. *Am J Clin Nutr*. 54(1): 26–29.

Stecco, A., Meneghini, A., Stern, R., Stecco, C. & Imamura, M. (2014) Ultrasonography in myofascial neck pain: randomized clinical trial for diagnosis and follow-up. *Surg Radiol Anat*. 36(3): 243–253.

Strath, S.J., Pfeiffer, K.A. & Whitt-Glover, M.C. (2012) Accelerometer use with children, older adults, and adults with functional limitations. *Med Sci Sports Exerc*. 44 (1Suppl1). S77–S85.

Van Loan, M.D., Withers P., Matthie, J. & Mayclin, P.L. (1993) Use of bioimpedance spectroscopy to determine extracellular fluid, intracellular fluid, total body water, and fat-free mass. *Basic Life Sci*. 60: 67–70.

Zheng, L., Huang, Y., Song, W., Gong, X., Liu, M., Jia, X., Zhou, G., Chen, L., Li, A. & Fan, Y. (2012) Fluid shear stress regulates metalloproteinase-1 and 2 in human periodontal ligament cells: Involvement of extracellular signal-regulated kinase (ERK) and P38 signaling pathways. *J Biomech*. 45: 2368–2375.

Further reading

Deurenberg, P. (1996) Limitations of the bioelectrical impedance method for the assessment of body fat in severe obesity. *Am J Clin Nutr*. 64(3): 449S–452S.

Genton, L., Hans, D., Kyle, U.G. & Pichard, C. (2002) Dual-energy X-ray absorptiometry and body composition: differences between devices and com-parison with reference methods. *Nutrition*. 18(1): 66–70.

Medrano, G., Eitner, F., Walter, M. & Leonhardt, S. (2010) Model-based correction of the influence of body position on continuous segmental and hand-to-foot bioimpedance measurements. *Med Biol Eng Comput*. 48(6): 531–541.

Pirlich, M., Schütz, T., Ockenga, J., Biering, H., Gerl, H., Schmidt, B., Ertl, S., Plauth, M. & Lochs, H. (2003) Improved assessment of body cell mass by segmental bioimpedance analysis in malnourished subjects and acromegaly. *Clin Nutr*. 22(2): 167–174.

Scharfetter, H., Monif, M., László, Z., Lambauer, T., Hutten, H. & Hinghofer-Szalkay, H. (1997) Effect of postural changes on the reliability of volume estimations from bioimpedance spectroscopy data. *Kidney Int*. 51(4): 1078–1087.

Segal, K. R. (1996) Use of bioelectrical impedance analysis measurements as an evaluation for participating in sports. *Am J Clin Nutr*. 64(3): 469S–471S.

CHAPTER 25

Palpation and functional assessment methods for fascia-related dysfunction

Leon Chaitow

Introduction

Fascia provides structural and functional continuity between the body's hard and soft-tissues. It is a ubiquitous elastic–plastic, sensory component that invests, supports, separates, connects, divides, wraps and gives both shape and functionality to the rest of the body, while allowing gliding, sliding motions, as well as playing an important role in transmitting mechanical forces between structures (Chapter 1). At least, that is how fascia behaves when it is healthy and fully functional. In reality, due to age, trauma or inflammation, for example, fascia may shorten, becoming painful and restricted and fail to painlessly allow coherent transmission of forces, or smooth sliding interactions, between different layers of body-tissues (Langevin et al., 2009).

Adaptation

One way of viewing fascia-related dysfunction, that occurs gradually over time, happens suddenly following trauma or inflammation or which may be part of inevitable age-related changes, is as physiological or biomechanical adaptation or as compensation. Neuro-myofascial tissue contraction may result in varying degrees of pain-inducing binding, or 'adhesions', between layers that should be able to stretch and glide on each other, potentially impairing motor function (Grinnel, 2009) (Fourie & Robb, 2009) (Chapter 2).

A process evolves that can be neatly summarised as 'densification' of, previously, more pliable tissues including fascia. This involves interference with complex myofascial relationships, altering muscle balance, motor control and proprioception (Stecco & Stecco, 2009). These slowly evolving adaptive processes may become both habitual and built-in. For example, in an individual with a chronically altered postural pattern involving a forward head position, protracted shoulders, a degree of dorsal kyphosis and lumbar lordosis, there will be both a range of soft-tissue changes, fibrosis, etc., as well as the evolution of ingrained, habitual, postural patterns that are usually difficult to modify unless the chronic tissue features are altered via exercise and/or therapeutic interventions. Myers (2009) has expressed this progressive adaptive phenomenon as involving a process in which chronic tissue loading leads to 'global soft tissue holding patterns', where clear postural and functional imbalance and distress are both visible, as well as being palpable.

A shorthand summary of such processes may describe them as being the result of:

- Overuse, for example, repetitive actions
- Misuse, for example, postural or ergonomic insults
- Disuse, for example, lack of exercise
- Abuse, for example, trauma
- Or any combination of these.

Whatever the single or multiple contributing features may be, the end result is of structural and functional modifications that prevent normal activity, result in discomfort or pain, and which, themselves, make further adaptive demands as the individual attempts to compensate for restrictions and altered use patterns.

Assessment objectives

When evaluating possible interventions, whether therapeutic or exercise related, it is important to ascertain which tissues, structures, patterns and mechanisms may be involved? For example, is there any evidence of soft-tissue change, involving hypertonicity or fibrosis? Is there joint or neurological involvement? Are the tissues inflamed? In other words: why is this happening? What causative or maintaining features are identifiable? What actions might usefully be taken to modify, improve, and correct the situation?

As a starting point, in order to encourage rehabilitation, areas of restriction need to be identified and assessed so that they can be encouraged towards normality. The question as how best to identify such pathophysiological changes is, therefore, one of the key challenges that face practitioners, before manual and/or movement therapies or modalities can be safely applied. Fortunately, a range of palpation and assessment tools is available to help achieve the identification and localisation of dysfunction, as will be described later in this chapter.

Gathering evidence

Clinical decision-making needs to be based on a combination of the unique history and characteristics of the individual combined with objective and subjective information, gathered from assessment, observation, palpation and examination. The findings of such information gathering endeavours need to be correlated with whatever evidence exists, research studies, experience, etc. that offers guidance, regarding different therapeutic choices. The objectives of palpation and assessment are, therefore, the gathering of evidence regarding function and dysfunction, so that informed clinical decisions can be made, rather than being based on guesswork. What's too tight? What's too loose? What functions are impaired? Which kinetic and structural chains are involved? What are the causes? What can be done to remedy or improve the situation?

There are many functional assessment methods and protocols, as well as a variety of palpation methods that can assist in this search for information, and answers. Some of these have been tested for reliability, others are used extensively, without any clear evidence that they are reliable.

This leads to a key recommendation: that no single piece of 'evidence' gained from observation, or from the results of functional tests and assessment, or from palpation, should be used alone as evidence to guide clinical choices. It is far safer to rely on combinations of evidence that support each other and which point towards rehabilitation and/or treatment options.

Therapeutic options

When the sliding/gliding motion potential of fascia is reduced, is painful or has been lost, restoration of normal function requires attention to the causative, as well as the maintaining, factors associated with the dysfunctional fascial layers. This chapter focuses on evaluation, palpation and assessment of fascial changes that may be contributing to functional or pain-related symptoms. The intent of using such findings is to decide on the best ways of encouraging more normal function. There are, of course, multiple strategies that aim to improve, correct or rehabilitate such dysfunction but their underlying ambitions can briefly be summarised as follows:

- To reduce adaptive load: for example, to modify overuse, or misuse, or other features that are contributing to the problem
- To enhance functionality: for example, to improve posture, breathing function, nutrition, sleep, exercise patterns, as well as the local mobility and stability of tissues
- To focus on symptom reduction: which might be a poor, potentially short-term, choice unless and until adaptive demands are reduced and/or function improved.

Postural assessment

A general evaluation of posture and movement patterns offers initial clues as to areas that are either under-active or over-active in their ranges of motion or functionality.

Information gathering

1   A general evaluation of postural and movement patterns offers an overview of what is functional and which tissues, structures and areas require further investigation (see Therapeutic options)
2   Testing particular key muscles for relative shortness, as well as for functional efficiency, allows a more focused evaluation as to where restrictions exist.
3   Within identified areas, such as shortened muscles, local areas of dysfunction may be isolated by means of direct palpation (see notes on ARTT later in this chapter)

Crossed syndromes (see Figure 25.1)

Patterns of imbalance, such as the upper and the lower crossed syndrome patterns have classically been interpreted as demonstrating hypertonic extensor muscles overwhelming inhibited abdominal flexors (Janda, 1996).

Greenman (1996) explained this perspective as follows: 'Muscle imbalance consists of shortening and tightening of muscle groups (usually the tonic "postural" muscles), and weakness of other muscle groups (usually the phasic muscles), and consequent loss of control on integrated muscle function. The lower crossed syndrome involves hypertonic, and therefore shortened, Iliopsoas, rectus femoris, TFL, the

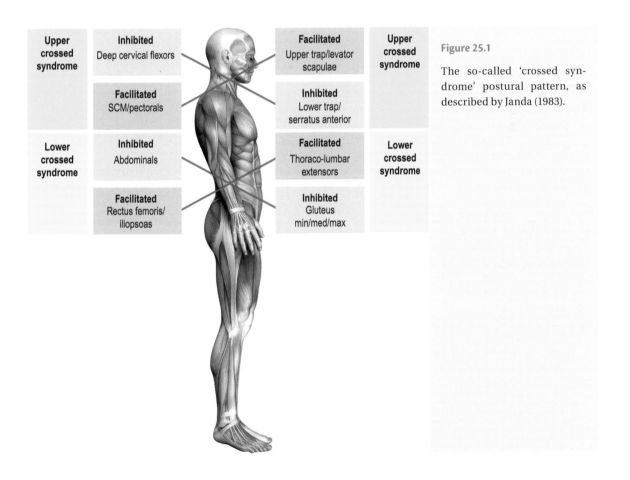

Figure 25.1

The so-called 'crossed syndrome' postural pattern, as described by Janda (1983).

short adductors of the thigh and the erector spinae group with inhibited abdominal and gluteal muscles. This tilts the pelvis forward on the frontal plane, while flexing the hip joints and exaggerating lumbar lordosis.' In addition, it is not uncommon for quadratus lumborum to shorten and tighten, while gluteus maximus and medius

weaken. The upper crossed syndrome involves, among other muscles, hypertonic cervical extensors, upper trapezius, pectorals, thoracic erector spinae, with inhibited deep neck flexors and lower fixators of the shoulders.

Key et al. (2010) note that this pattern may involve 'a posterior (pelvic) shift with increased anterior

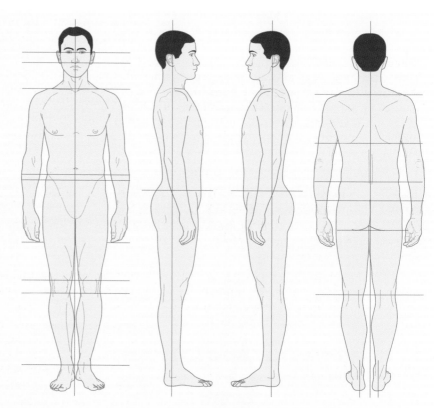

Figure 25.2

Postural evaluation recording form

Visual assessment for overall postural impression (i.e. not diagnostic)

The individual being assessed is standing.

Static assessment

1. **Posterior view**
   Note: symmetry and levels of shoulders and scapulae and any evidence of winging, head position, any spinal curvature as well as relative fullness of paraspinal msucles, position of pelvis, fat folds (creases) at waist and gluteals, symmetry and position of knees, feet, malleoli, achilles tendons, arms and any obvious morphological asymmetry such as scars or bruises.

2. **Lateral view**
   Note: status of knees: relaxed or locked in extension, spinal curves: exaggerated or reversed, head position: forward or balanced, evidence of abdominal ptosis ('sagging') or any obvious morphological asymmetry such as scars or bruises.

3. **Anterior view**
   Note: shoulder levels: is there symmetry at the midsternal line, head tilt, deviation of clavicles, asymmetry of pelvis: are crests level, patella symmetry and any obvious morphological asymmetry such as scars or bruises.

Do the imbalances you observe suggest a pattern where there may be restrictions, structures involving 'crossed-syndrome' patterns, rotations, side-shifts, or particular fascial chain involvement? If so, investigate further using palpation as well as functional assessments (see below).

Active assessment

Now observe the individual walking away from and back towards you, as well as from the side. Do this slowly and more rapidly, as you evaluate stride, balance/symmetry, weight transfer, unusual patterns of movement. Record the findings of your impressions. Observe a variety of potentially significant normal movements, particularly those that the individual complains of as being painful or limited, and, in addition, look closely at any abnormal patterns when the individual is 'long-sitting' (Figure 25.5) or bends forward, backwards and reaching upwards, as well as the breathing pattern.
Ask yourself:

- What needs to change to help improve/normalise this person's posture?

- What is tight, loose, rotated, off-centre, unbalanced, folded, crowded and/or compressed and where might restrictions exist that relate to such observations?

- What fascial structures might be involved in such restrictions that, if released, would allow for a postural lengthening, opening out, or unfolding to occur?

sagittal rotation or tilt', together with an anterior shunt/translation of the thorax, and the head. In such instances diaphragmatic control and altered pelvic floor function might result.

The soft tissue palpation puzzle: Problems are not necessarily where they appear to be!

In the descriptions of crossed syndromes, individual muscles are named. However, it has become obvious in recent years that the concept of individual muscles is flawed. The multiple fascial connections between 'named' muscles and other muscles means that their action is not independent. Force is transmitted in many directions offering muscles additional leverage and functionality, as well as adding load to sometimes-distant muscles. Individually named muscles can, no longer, be considered to be discrete and separate, operating individually. Huijing (1999) has pointed out that agonists and antagonists are coupled structurally and mechanically via the fascia that

connects them, so that when force is generated by a prime mover it can be measured in the tendons of antagonist muscles.

Franklyn-Miller and colleagues (2009) have shown that, for example, a hamstring stretch produces 240% of the resulting strain in the iliotibial tract and 145% in the ipsilateral lumbar fascia compared with the hamstrings. Strain (load) transmission, during contraction or stretching, therefore affects many other tissues beyond the muscle being targeted, largely due to fascial connections. Importantly, this suggests that apparent muscular restrictions, such as 'tight hamstrings', might not originate in the affected muscle but elsewhere. In the case of hamstring restriction, there may be fascial dysfunction in the tensor fascia lata, or the ipsilateral thoracolumbar, creating, encouraging or maintaining hamstring symptoms. This sort of fascial interconnectedness exists throughout the body so, as knowledge accumulates as to what structures are linked to others via fascia and at which orientation, understanding

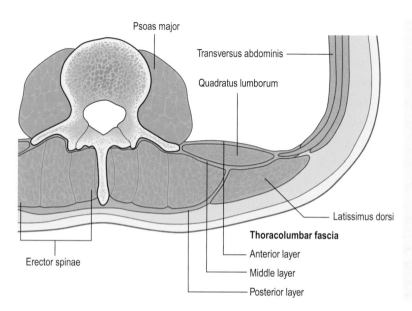

Psoas major

Transversus abdominis

Quadratus lumborum

Latissimus dorsi

Thoracolumbar fascia

Anterior layer

Middle layer

Posterior layer

Erector spinae

Figure 25.3

A transverse view of the fascial wrapping that binds together key muscles including quadratus lumborum, psoas, erector spinae, latissimus dorsi and transversus abdominus. (Gray's Anatomy)

sources of dysfunction should become more predictable.

Palpation and assessment and load-transfer: The thoracolumbar fascia

Palpation and assessment strategies need to take account of this load-sharing phenomenon. The scale of the palpation puzzle can be seen in the illustration of the huge number of potential links available from just one massive fascial structure, the thoracolumbar fascia. This ties together the erector spinae, latissimus dorsi, quadratus lumborum, psoas, transversus abdominus, and diaphragm muscles, as well as countless other minor muscle structures (Figures 25.3 and 25.4).

Unraveling the puzzle

As we focus attention on the assessment of relative shortness in named muscles, we need to maintain awareness that multiple fascial connections exist that bind together muscles with different names into a virtual interconnecting tensegrity structure (Chapter 6). An important distinction needs to be made in our search for culprit areas of restriction. There is a need to identify both the *location* of restriction, for example shortened hamstrings,

as well as the *source* of the restriction that, as has been explained, could be in the hamstrings but also possibly in the thoracolumbar fascia, or elsewhere.

Testing particular key muscles for relative restriction/loss of full range of motion, as well as for functional efficiency, allows a more focused evaluation as to where restrictions exist. There are strategies that can help to identify areas that may be responsible for dysfunction:

1. General observation: for example of normal posture and movement, such as standing and walking as described above (see Active assessment).

2. Observation of functional movements or postures: for example walking (Chapter 17), long-sitting (see Figure 25.5), bending, as well as Janda's (1996) Hip Abduction and Hip Extension tests.

3. Specific tests for muscle shortness: (see Table 25.1, Postural Muscle Assessment Sequence).

4. Direct manual palpation: see palpation exercises described later in the chapter.

Functional assessment: Hip abduction test, hip extension test

There are hundreds of functional assessment methods that offer evidence of overuse, inhibition,

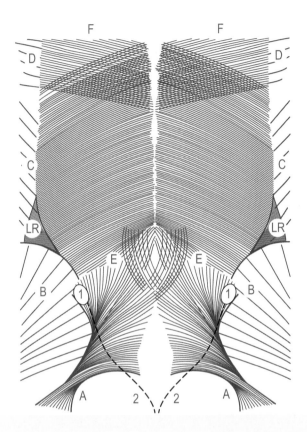

Figure 25.4

The deep layer of the thoracolumbar fascia and different fibre directions of attachments to:

A Sacrotuberous ligament connecting to hamstrings

B Fascia of gluteus medius

C Fascia of internal oblique

D Serratus posterior inferior

E Erector spinae muscles

LR Lateral raphe provides attachment for part of external oblique and latissimus dorsi, as well as distributing tension from the surrounding hypaxial and extremity muscles into the layers of the thoracolumbar fascia (Willard et al., 2012)

All of these fascial layers and structures interconnect with each other via the thoracolumbar fascia which, as seen in Figure 25.3, invests the erector spinae groups as well.

1. Posterior superior iliac spine

2. Sacrum

Note multiple directions of force transmission in sacral region. Palpated tenderness may help to identify directions of restrictive tension with potential influence on specific muscles. Note that there exist direct fascial connections between the upper extremity, the trunk, and the lower extremity. Multiple indirect, less obvious, fascial connections allow for force transmission of load, with profound clinical implications. (Barker et al., 2004)

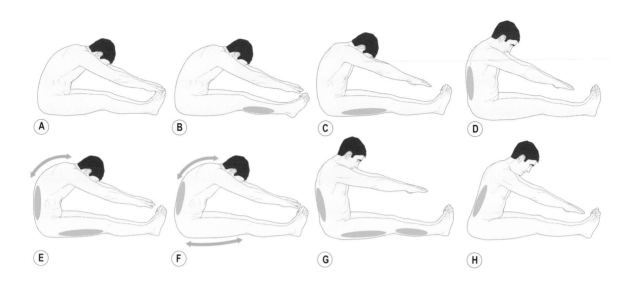

Figure 25.5 A–H

Long-sitting flexion: observation of patterns of restriction when flexibility is limited

Tests for shortness of the erector spinae and associated postural muscles.

A Normal length of erector spinae muscles and posterior thigh muscles.

B Tight gastrocnemlus and soleus; the inability to dorsiflex the feet indicates tightness of the piantar-fiexor group.

C Tight hamstring muscles, which cause the pelvis to tilt posteriority.

D Tight low-back erector spinae muscles.

E Tight hamstrings; slightly tight low-back muscles and overstretched upper back muscles.

F Slightly shortened lower back muscles, stretched upper back muscles and slightly stretched hamstrings.

G Tight low-back muscles, hamstrings, and gastrocnemius/soleus.

H Very tight low-back muscles, with lordosis maintained even in flexion.

restriction and other aspects of dysfunction, as well as, potentially, discomfort or pain, when being demonstrated, due to space constraints, just two examples are described below.

Hip abduction test

This assessment can be performed by including palpation, however, it is possible that adding digital touch to the muscles being evaluated would add sensory motor stimulation that might reduce the reliability of any findings. Observation alone is encouraged initially, with direct palpation being added subsequently (Figure 25.6A).

The aim of this test is to screen for stability of the lumbopelvic region. The patient should be side lying with the superior leg resting on the lower leg, which is flexed at the hip and knee. The upper-most leg should be in line with the torso. The patient is requested to slowly lift the leg toward the ceiling. If normal, the leg should abduct to 20° with no internal or external rotation, or hip flexion, and without any ipsilateral

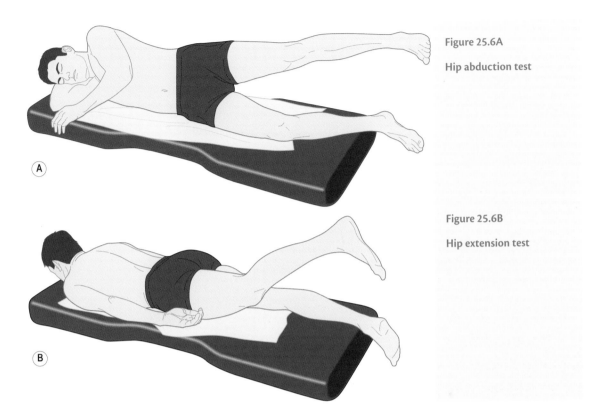

Figure 25.6A

Hip abduction test

Figure 25.6B

Hip extension test

'hip-hike' (pelvic cephalad elevation). There should be an initial moderate contraction of the lumbar erector spinae and/or quadratus lumborum, in order to stabilise the pelvis. However, this should not involve any obvious contraction merely an indication of toning.

The test is regarded as positive if any of the following are observed:

1. Ipsilateral external hip/leg rotation which suggests over activity and probable shortening of piriformis.

2. Ipsilateral external pelvic rotation, which suggests piriformis and other external hip rotator over activity and probable shortness.

3. Ipsilateral hip flexion, which suggests over activity and probable shortening of the hip flexors, including psoas and/or tensor fascia latae.

4. Cephalad elevation of the ipsilateral pelvis before 20° of hip abduction, which suggests over activity and shortening of quadratus lumborum.

5. An obvious hingeing should be noted at the hip, rather than in the waist area if gluteus medius

and tensor fascia lata are working optimally, and quadratus lumborum is not overactive.

6. Any pain reported in performance of the abduction movement. For example, discomfort noted on the inner thigh may represent adductor shortness.

7. Any combination of the above.

Hip extension test

The aim of this test is to evaluate coordination of a number of muscles (Figure 25.6b) during prone hip extension. The patient should lie prone with the arms at the side and feet extending beyond the table end. The patient is then requested to lift a specific leg toward the ceiling. An initial toning contraction of the thoracolumbar erector spinae, to stabilise the torso before the limb extends, is considered normal, if the action is achieved by coordinated activity of the ipsilateral hamstrings and gluteus maximus.

The test is considered positive if any of the following are observed:

Table 25.1

Postural muscle assessment sequence

The table lists the main muscles of the body that are prone to shortening when overused, misused (for example, poor posture), or abused (traumatised)(Janda 1996).

The letters E L R represent: E = equally-bilaterally-short, L = left short, R = right short.

The other abbreviations relate to lack of flexibility of: LL= low lumbar, LDJ = lumbodorsal junction, LT = lower thoracic, MT = mid-thoracic, UT = upper thoracic. Details for assessment of these muscles can be found in Palpation & Assessment Skills, Chaitow (2010).

Name: _____

E = Equal (circle both if both are short)
L or R are circled if left or right are short
Spinal abbreviations indicate low-lumbar, lumbo dorsal junction, low-thoracic, mid-thoracic and upper thoracic areas (of flatness and therefore reduced ability to flex – short erector spinae)

1. Gastrocnemius E L R

2. Soleus E L R

3. Medial hamstrings E L R

4. Short adductors E L R

5. Rectus femoris ELR

6. Psoas E L R

7. Hamstrings
   a) upper fibres E L R
   b) lower fibres E L R

8. Tensor fascia lata E L R

9. Piriformis E L R

10. Quadratus lumborum E L R

11. Pectoralis major E L R

12. Latissimus dorsi E L R

13. Upper trapezius E L R

14. Scalenes E L R

15. Sternocleidomastoid E L R

16. Levator scapulae E L R

17. Infraspinatus E L R

18. Subscapularis E L R

19. Supraspinates E L R

20. Flexors of the arms E L R

21. Spinal flattening:
    a) seated legs straight LL LDJ LT MT UT
    b) seated legs flexed LL LDJ LT MT UT

22. Cervical spine flexors short? Yes No

1. Knee flexion of the leg being extended suggests over activity and probable hamstring shortness.

2. Delayed or absent ipsilateral gluteus maximus firing. Absence of a meaningful contraction of gluteus maximus at the outset of the extension movement is considered significant, as this should be a prime mover. Inhibition may indicate over-activity of the erector spinae group and/or of the ipsilateral hamstrings.

3. False hip extension occurs, where the hinging/pivot point of the leg, during the first 10° extension, occurs in the low back rather than at the hip itself, suggesting over activity of the erector spinae and inhibition of gluteus maximus.

4. Early contraction of the contralateral periscapular musculature suggests a functional low back instability, involving recruitment of the upper torso as compensation for inhibition of the intended prime movers.

Observed posture, together with observation of movement patterns, as well as in long-sitting, hip abduction and hip extension tests, offers clues as to which muscles/groups of muscles may be overactive and potentially shortened, and which may be inhibited. This information can be refined by testing specific muscles for shortness, as indicated in Table 25.1.

Having identified muscles with reduced range of motion, local areas, or areas distant from them, may be sought that could be affecting them. These may then be usefully assessed (see discussion of thoracolumbar fascia above).

ARTT palpation features of local dysfunction

Fascial, or general musculoskeletal dysfunction, involving pain and/or restriction for example, is commonly associated with a number of predictable features that can be summarised using the acronym **ARTT**

- **A** stands for **A**symmetry, since one-sided fascial dysfunction is more usual than bilateral.

- **R** stands for **R**ange of motion restriction. In almost all cases of fascial or general musculoskeletal dysfunction, there will be a reduction in the range of movement available to the tissues involved.

- **T** stands for **T**enderness or sensitivity/pain, which is a common but not universal. Fryer et al. (2004) have confirmed that sites in the thoracic paravertebral muscles, identified by deep palpation as displaying 'abnormal tissue texture', also showed greater tenderness than adjacent tissues characteristic of dysfunction. Fascial dysfunction frequently involves a particular quality of sharp, cutting or 'burning' sensation, when moved, compressed or stretched.

- **T** stands for **T**extural or **T**issue changes. Dysfunctional tissues are commonly associated with hypertonicity, fibrosis, induration/hardening, oedema or other palpable modifications from the norm. Fryer et al. (2005) examined the possibility that tissue texture irregularity of paravertebral sites might be due to greater cross-sectional thickness of the paraspinal muscle bulk. Diagnostic ultrasound (Chapter 24) showed that this was not the case. Changes in the 'feel' of fascia, when dysfunctional, have been described as 'densification': a word that neatly summarises what is commonly palpated. Fryer et al. (2007) examined the EMG activity of deep paraspinal muscles, lying below paravertebral thoracic muscles with 'altered texture', that were also more tender than surrounding ones. This demonstrated increased EMG activity in these dysfunctional muscles, i.e. they were hypertonic.

All four elements of ARTT are not always apparent when dysfunctional tissues are assessed/palpated. However, it would be unusual for there to not be at least two, and ideally three, of these characteristics in evidence when fascia is functioning other than optimally.

ARTT exercise

Have the patient stand flexing from the waist, as you stand in front, viewing the paraspinal musculature from the head. One side of the paraspinals will commonly be more 'mounded' than the other. Note the level at which this occurs and have the individual lie prone.

In this example let's assume it is the lower thoracic/upper lumbar area on the left. At this stage you will have established that the 'A' (asymmetry) in ARTT is identifiable. Now palpate both left and right sides of this area of the back in order to evaluate the relative tone on each side. The more mounded side, left in this example, will inevitably be felt to be 'tighter', more hypertonic.

Testing for the 'R' element of ARTT is easily achieved by gently attempting to lengthen the paraspinal tissues, either via simply pressing into them, or by trying to flex the tissues laterally with thumb, finger or hand. There will be reduced range of motion on the hypertonic shortened side.

Once you have sensed the difference in tone, one side to the other, palpate a little deeper into the musculature, possibly from a slightly lateral angle rather than vertically, and sense any differences you can identify in the texture of the tissues. It should usually be possible to sense greater rigidity and possibly, depending on chronicity, some fibrotic elements on the hypertonic side. If so, you will have established one of the 'T' (texture, or tissue) elements of ARTT.

Pressure applied into the tissues, on each side should establish that, in most instances, the hypertonic side will be tender (producing the second 'T') in ARTT.

Translating ARTT into fascial assessment is less obvious than when applying it to muscles or joints, since many fascial restrictions may be deep and not directly palpable. However, superficial fascia and loose areolar tissues are easily evaluated, as described below.

Exercises: Skin and fascia palpation

Ideally the exercises below should be practiced on 'normal' tissue as well as on areas where dysfunction is apparent or suspected. In addition, practice on tissues that are overlying large muscle masses and also where there is minimal muscle between the palpating contact and underlying bone. The more variety of tissues, and individuals of different ages and physical condition, that are involved in palpation exercises the more rapidly palpatory literacy will be achieved (Chaitow, 2010).

Exercise 1

Skin drag

- Before starting the exercise itself remove any watches or jewellery.
- With no pressure at all, only the very lightest of touch of one or two finger pads, stroke the skin of the area where the watch had been, so that you move from skin that was not covered by the strap, to cross over that area and back again several times.
- Do you notice an obvious difference, as you cross this more 'moist' area, compared with the dryer areas?
- Increased skin hydrosis (sweat) changes should be palpable. What you are feeling is known as 'drag' and you are using drag palpation to identify increased hydrosis, which is often associated with hypertonicity, tissue dysfunction and fascial resistance to sliding.
- When you are comfortable that you can recognise the feeling of drag and using no pressure at all, only the very lightest of touch of one or two finger pads, stroke the skin of your anterior thigh (for the purpose of this exercise), in various directions.
- Then do the same on the lateral thigh, overlying the densest aspects of the iliotibial band.
- Try to sense and identify areas of drag. These will be far less obvious than the area under a watchstrap but should make themselves known when smooth finger-movement, over the skin, becomes slightly 'rough'.

Exercise 2

Sliding and rolling superficial fascia

- Place two or three finger pads on the skin of the anterior thigh with minimal compressive force (grams only) and slide it (the skin together with superficial fascia, to which it is bound) towards the knee, until you feel resistance. Then return to where you started and slide the skin towards the hip.
- Compare the ease of movement in one direction with the other.

- Was there greater resistance in one direction or the other?
- Perform the action over areas that displayed 'drag' sensations, as well as those that did not.
- Now perform the same actions on the lateral surface of that leg, overlying the iliotibial band. Compare ease of movement with the anterior surface, or areas free of, as well as displaying 'drag'.
- After exploring one leg, perform the same evaluations on the other leg, as well as in other easily accessible areas of the body, such as the anterior and the lateral calf area, comparing and remembering the different 'feel' of these tissues as you lift, slide and roll them.
- Compare your findings. Was there greater resistance to sliding skin/superficial fascia in some locations compared to others and did this correlate with drag?
- Was there greater resistance on one surface of the leg, or aspect of the leg, compared with the other?
- What differences did you notice when trying to perform the same exercises on areas with little muscle-cover or where there were dense fascial layers (iliotibial band)?

Exercise 3

Testing skin elasticity

- Now gently hold a pinch of skin between your index and middle finger pads, and your thumb in an area already tested for skin 'slideability', as in Exercise 2.
- Lift this to sense its degree of elasticity, which will differ greatly in different areas of the body.
- What you are holding is skin and superficial fascia, together with some of the adipose/areolar/loose connective tissue that lie between those layers and the underlying dense connective tissue. This 'loose' material includes a variety of cells and substances, such as proteoaminoglycans, which facilitate the 'slideability' of the various layers of tissue, on each other (Chapter 3).
- When this facility is reduced or lost, dysfunction, restriction and pain are almost inevitable consequences.

Repeat this light pinch-and-lift in various parts of the thigh, both where there is a thick layer of muscle and also where there is minimal muscle and more fascial tissue.

- Now see if you can 'roll' the skin' and superficial fascia between fingers and thumbs, in the different areas you are testing, in various directions.
- Did you notice that where reduced sliding (Exercise 2) was observed, skin is less easy to lift/stretch and roll?
- In general, the greater the degree of underlying hypertonicity and shortening, the greater will be the resistance to free sliding on underlying structures of the skin/superficial fascia.
- In many instances, there will be a correlation between drag, and lack of easy sliding capacity, and loss of elastic quality (Chapter 10).

Note that several elements of ARTT are being demonstrated via this exercise. A degree of increased tenderness is also likely in areas where drag is noted, where there is reduced ability to slide and to roll. Sometimes rolling the tissue will be more uncomfortable, adding the final element of ARTT (tenderness).

Exercise 4

Apply tests 1,2 3 to somebody else's sacrum and/or lower back and, as you do so, try evaluate directions of relative restriction in the ability of superficial tissues to slide. You are now on your way towards palpatory literacy.

Clinical summary

- Global evaluation via observation: static and during movement offers indications of areas that are restricted or dysfunctional
- Functional assessments allow you to identify specific structures that deserve further investigation
- Direct palpation isolates local areas of tissue change

Your only remaining concern is what to do about what you have identified. This book offers solutions to those concerns.

References

Barker, P.J., Briggs, C.A. & Bogeski, G. (2004) Tensile transmission across the lumbar fasciae in unembalmed cadavers: effects of tension to various muscular attachments. *Spine* 29(2): 129–138.

Chaitow, L. (2010) *Palpation and assessment skills*. Edinburgh: Churchill Livingstone.

Fourie, W. & Robb, K. (2009) Physiotherapy management of axillary web syndrome following breast cancer treatment: Discussing the use of soft tissue techniques. *Physiotherapy* 95: 314–320.

Franklyn-Miller, A. et al. (2009) IN: *Fascial Research II: Basic Science and Implications for Conventional and Complementary Health Care Munich:* Elsevier GmbH.

Fryer, G., Morris, T., Gibbons, P. et al. (2007) The activity of thoracic paraspinal muscles identified as abnormal with palpation. *JMPT,* 29(6): 437–447.

Fryer, G., Morris, T. & Gibbons, P. (2004) The relationship between palpation of thoracic paraspinal tissues and pressure sensitivity measured by a digital algometer. *J Ost Med*. 7: 64–69.

Fryer, G., Morris, T. & Gibbons, P. (2005) The relationship between palpation of thoracic tissues and deep paraspinal muscle thickness. *Int J Ost Med*. 8: 22–28.

Greenman, P.E. (1996) *Principles of manual medicine*. 2nd Edition. Maryland: Williams and Wilkins.

Grinnel, F. (2009) *Fibroblast mechanics in three-dimensional collagen Matrices. Fascia Research II: Basic Science Implications for Conventional and Complementary Health Care*. Munich: Elsevier GmbH.

Hammer, W. (1999) Thoracolumbar Fascia and Back Pain. *Dynamic Chiro Canada*. 31(10): 1.

Huijing, P. (1999) Muscular force transmission: a unified, dual or multiple system. *Arch Physiol Biochem*. 107: 292–311.

Janda, V. (1983) *Muscle function testing*. London: Butterworths.

Janda, V. (1996) Evaluation of muscular balance. In Liebenson Ceditor: *Rehabilitation of the Spine*. Baltimore: Williams and Wilkins.

Key, J. (2010) *Back Pain - A Movement Problem: A clinical approach incorporating relevant research and practice*. Edinburgh: Churchill Livingstone.

Langevin, H. et al. (2009) Ultrasound evidence of altered lumbar connective tissue structure in human subjects with chronic low back pain. Presentation 2nd Fascia Research Congress.

Myers, T. (2009) *Anatomy Trains*. 2nd edition. Edinburgh: Churchill Livingstone.

Stecco, L. & Stecco, C. (2009) *Fascial Manipulation*: *Practical Part*. Italy: Piccini.

Willard, F.H., Vleeming, A., Schuenke, M.D. et al. (2012) The thoracolumbar fascia: anatomy, function and clinical considerations. *J Anat*. 221(6): 507–536.

INDEX

A

abduction, hip, assessment 260–1
accelerometers 248–9
acid–base balance in tissues 25–6
active modalities of preparation for football training or competition 200–1
active stretching, martial arts training 157–8
acute programme variables in functional fascial training 174
adaptations (incl. remodeling) in musculoskeletal system 9, 253
  collagen 5–6, 7
  evidence for 15–16
  footballers 195–200
  to loading 5–6, 39–43
  range of motion 83–4
  specificity in 85–6
  speed of 8
administrative concerns in functional fascial training 174
agonist muscles and antagonist muscles, coupling/connections 186, 257
aikido 157, 158
algometer 242–3
  myometry with 245
alternate leg box jumps 180
amortization phase 219
Anatomy Trains (myofascial meridians) 45–58
  Pilates training 124, 125, 126, 127, 128, 129
animals, stretching 115–17
ankle hops, single leg 178–9
ankle joint of kicking leg, changes 196
ankle jumps, double leg 178
antagonist muscles
  agonist and, coupling/connections 186, 257
  force transmission to 4
anterior chain, diagonal 61, 65, 66
apparatus exercises, Pilates 124, 126, 127, 128
appendicular skeleton
  fascia 59
  muscles 60
arch/curl exercise in Gyrotonic® 139, 140–1
arm(s)/upper limb(s)
  bar deviation with 226
  bar jump with 226
  bar swing with 225
  extended overhead with resistance 175, 176
  swing, in walking 169

Arm Lines 49
  Pilates training 124, 125, 128
arthrogryposis 76
ARTT palpation 265–7
asanas (poses/postures)
  Corpse 111
  Dog see Dog Pose
  Triangle 52
assessment 241–66
  fascia-related dysfunction 253–66
  technologies 241–51
asymmetry (A) in ARTT palpation 263, 264
athletes 205–16
  coaching 205–16
  indentometry 243–4
  see also running
auto-release of myofascial after football training or competition 203
awareness (incl. sensory awareness) in fascial training 106–8
  dancers 149
  martial arts 159
  see also mindfulness
axial fascia 59

B

back (lower)
  elastic walking and 168
  walking and pain in 161
Back Line
  Double Prayer for 210
  Superficial see Superficial Back Line
balance
  dance training 151
  and injury risk in joint hypermobility
    general 73
    strength 73
  structural, Pilates and fascial release for 129
bar deviation 226
bar jump 226
bar swing 225
bears 117
Beighton tests (range of motion) 69
biochemistry 21–9
bioimpedance, electrical 244–8
biomechanics see mechanics
biotensegrity see tensegrity
Blakelee, Sandra and Matthew 156
body
  compartments, analysis 244–6, 247
  health, healthy fascia for 159

mass
  cell mass (BCM) 247
  fat free (FFM) 244, 245, 246, 247
  lean (LBM) 246, 247
  sequential delay of more distal body parts in fascial training 105–6
  stimulation in Gyrotonic® 136
  upper see trunk
  see also whole-body movements
body-mindfulness 153, 154–5, 158
bone injuries 191–2
bounces 95, 104, 108, 171
  mini-bounces 108, 213
  Pilates 123
  squat bouncing 222
  in stepping 104
  see also springiness
box jumps, alternate leg 180
boxing 155–6, 157
brain (incl. cerebrum)
  hormones 22
  insular cortex 25–6
  motor cortex 21
  see also central nervous system
breathing and respiration
  elasticity in 114, 117
    walking and 166
  in Gyrotonic® 140
  myofascial chains and 64
Busquet's muscle chains 64–5
  compared with Tittel's muscle slings 66, 67

C

C-fibres 22, 33
  tactile 37
cat, stretching 115–17
cell(s)
  body cell mass (BCM) 247
  response to loading/force/strain see mechanotransduction
  water in (ICW) 244, 246, 247
central nervous system 16–17, 21
  myofascial tone and disorders of 23–4
  see also brain; spine
cerebrum see brain
chair, Pilates 126
cheetah, stretching 115–17
chi (qi) 153, 154, 155, 157, 158
Chia, M. 154
children
  joint hypermobility 71
  playground activity 224